Accession no

D0414584

618.927 SUG

Children with Developmental
Coordination Disorder

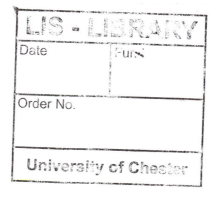

LIS - LIBRARY

Date	Fur..
Order No.	
University of Chester	

Children with Developmental Coordination Disorder

Edited by

DAVID SUGDEN PhD

and

MARY CHAMBERS EdD

both of the University of Leeds

Consulting Editor

PROFESSOR MARGARET SNOWLING

University of York

W

WHURR PUBLISHERS
LONDON AND PHILADELPHIA

© 2005 Whurr Publishers Ltd
First published 2005
by Whurr Publishers Ltd
19b Compton Terrace
London N1 2UN, England and
325 Chestnut Street, Philadelphia PA 19106, USA

All rights reserved. No part of this publication may be
reproduced, stored in a retrieval system, or transmitted
in any form or by any means, electronic, mechanical,
photocopying, recording or otherwise, without the prior
permission of Whurr Publishers Limited.

This publication is sold subject to the conditions that it shall not, by
way of trade or otherwise, be lent, resold, hired out, or otherwise
circulated without the publisher's prior consent in any form of
binding or cover other than that in which it is published and
without a similar condition including this condition being imposed
upon any subsequent purchaser.

British Library Cataloguing in Publication Data
A catalogue record for this book
is available from the British Library.

ISBN 1 86156 458 9

Typeset by Adrian McLaughlin, a@microguides.net
Printed and bound in the UK by Athenæum Press Ltd, Gateshead,
Tyne & Wear.

Contents

Contributors   vii
Preface   ix
Acknowledgements   xii

Chapter 1   The nature of children with Developmental
Coordination Disorder   **1**

Mary E. Chambers, David A. Sugden and Charikleia Sinani

Chapter 2   Motor impairment in DCD and activities of daily living   **19**

Reint H. Geuze

Chapter 3   Cognitive explanations of the planning and
organization of movement   **47**

Elisabeth L. Hill

Chapter 4   A dynamical systems perspective of Developmental
Coordination Disorder   **72**

Michael G. Wade, Dan Johnson and Kristi Mally

Chapter 5   DCD and overlapping conditions   **93**

Dido Green and Gillian Baird

Chapter 6   Progression and development in Developmental
Coordination Disorder   **119**

Margaret Cousins and Mary M. Smyth

Chapter 7   Assessment of Developmental Coordination Disorder   **135**

Dawne Larkin and Elizabeth Rose

Chapter 8   Early identification of children with
Developmental Coordination Disorder   **155**

Marian J. Jongmans

Chapter 9   Assessment of handwriting in children with
Developmental Coordination Disorder   **168**

Anna L. Barnett and Sheila E. Henderson

Chapter 10   Models of intervention: towards an
eco-developmental approach   **189**

David A. Sugden and Mary E. Chambers

Chapter 11   Neuromotor task training: a new approach
to treat children with DCD   **212**

Marina M. Schoemaker and Bouwien C.M. Smits-Engelsman

Chapter 12   A cognitive perspective on intervention for
children with Developmental Coordination Disorder:
the CO-OP experience   **228**

Angie D. Mandich and Helene J. Polatajko

Chapter 13   Overlapping conditions – overlapping management:
services for individuals with Developmental
Coordination Disorder   **242**

Amanda Kirby

References   267
Index   307

Contributors

Gillian Baird Newcomen Centre, Guy's Hospital, London, UK

Anna L. Barnett School of Psychology and Human Development, Institute of Education, University of London, UK, and Department of Psychology, Oxford Brookes University, UK

Mary E. Chambers School of Education, University of Leeds, UK

Margaret Cousins Department of Psychology, University of Central Lancashire, Preston, UK

Reint H. Geuze Developmental & Clinical Neuropsychology, University of Groningen, The Netherlands

Dido Green Newcomen Centre, Guy's Hospital, London, UK

Sheila E. Henderson School of Psychology and Human Development, Institute of Education, University of London, UK

Elisabeth L. Hill Department of Psychology, Goldsmiths College, University of London, UK

Dan Johnson University of Minnesota, Minneapolis, Minnesota, USA

Marian J. Jongmans Faculty of Social Studies, University of Utrecht, The Netherlands

Amanda Kirby The Dyscovery Centre, Cardiff, Wales, UK

Dawne Larkin School of Human Movement and Exercise Science, University of Western Australia, Crawley, Australia

Kristi Mally University of Wisconsin, La Crosse, Wisconsin, USA

Angie D. Mandich School of Occupational Therapy, Faculty of Health Sciences, University of Western Ontario, London, Ontario, Canada

Helene J. Polatajko Department of Occupational Therapy, Department of Public Health Sciences, and Graduate Department of Rehabilitation Sciences, Faculty of Medicine, University of Toronto, Ontario, Canada

Elizabeth Rose School of Biomedical and Sports Science, Edith Cowan University, Perth, Australia

Marina M. Schoemaker Institute of Human Movement Sciences, University of Groningen, The Netherlands

Charikleia Sinani Leeds Metropolitan University, UK

Bouwien C.M. Smits-Engelsman Nijmegen Institute for Cognition and Information, Nijmegen University, The Netherlands

Mary M. Smyth Department of Psychology, University of Lancaster, UK

David A. Sugden School of Education, University of Leeds, UK

Michael G. Wade University of Minnesota, Minneapolis, Minnesota, USA

Preface

Developmental Coordination Disorder is a developmental disability drawing upon disciplines associated with education, psychology and health and involves children with motor coordination disorders and associated difficulties. The motor difficulties lead to problems in everyday living and often have an effect on academic progress in schools. Although the condition has long been recognized, there has been a large upsurge of interest in the academic literature and clinical practice over the last 15 years. Despite this interest and attention, there are huge issues of a theoretical, clinical and educational nature that remain to be resolved and these include definitional and conceptual difficulties; issues related to co-morbidity and overlapping conditions; the dearth of a variety of assessment instruments leading to variability of diagnosis; and a lack of a cohort of intervention studies appropriately controlled. These issues, in turn, lead to confusion in the academic and educational/clinical field with parents of children with DCD having few definitive evidence-based sources from which they can obtain objective information and advice. There is also much debate about co-morbidity across the spectrum of developmental disabilities with DCD being one of a number including attention deficit disorder, dyslexia and autistic spectrum disorder.

This text brings together the strong research evidence base, marrying it with professional guidance such that researchers will be able to use it to direct and guide their investigations, and professionals will have the evidence to inform their practice. To accomplish this, a range of academics, clinicians and other professionals from around the world have contributed chapters in areas of their expertise. The essence of the book is for strong research evidence that will inform practice in both the clinical and research setting in the educational system, the health service and at home.

The text after the first chapter is divided into three sections: first, the characteristics and nature of the condition followed by assessment and diagnosis and finally, intervention. The first chapter by Mary Chambers,

David Sugden and Charikleia Sinani looks at the condition, examining formal definitions and descriptions together with some speculations and controversies. This chapter sets the scene for many of the issues raised in detail in subsequent chapters.

Five chapters make up the first section on *nature and characteristics* with Reint Geuze taking us through the core characteristics of the syndrome by describing and analysing the nature of the motor impairment. Elisabeth Hill focuses on planning and the organization of action using cognitive explanations looking at activities in daily living which are often a central focus of some clinical and professional groups. Mike Wade, Dan Johnson and Kristi Mally give us a highly original chapter on a dynamical perspective and DCD. Traditionally, concepts from cognitive models have been used to explain movements and actions but more recently, using information from complex systems and ecological psychology, dynamical systems offer new and exciting ways of analysing the condition. Dido Green and Gillian Baird take the currently hot topic of co-morbidity with in-depth analysis of overlap with such conditions as ADHD, dyslexia and autistic spectrum disorder. In addition, the often seen associated difficulties such as behaviour problems or poor self-concept, are examined. Finally in this section, Margaret Cousins and Mary Smyth examine the development and progression of the condition: Do children grow out of it? Do they compensate? Does it stay with them without intervention?

Three chapters comprise the second section on *identification and assessment*, beginning with a chapter on general assessment by Dawne Larkin and Elizabeth Rose who not only describe how assessment is multifaceted using different sources of information, but also note that it is inextricably linked to the intervention process. Marian Jongmans considers the assessment of young children with DCD, describing the adaptations of instruments for this purpose plus multiple sources of information together with some of the issues involved in early identification. Finally in this section, Anna Barnett and Sheila Henderson examine the assessment of handwriting. Those with clinical experience of DCD will recognize that handwriting is a distinct skill often separate from the global abilities of fine motor coordination and this chapter concentrates on this important topic.

In the final section on *intervention and management*, the lead-off chapter by David Sugden and Mary Chambers emphasizes that intervention should take place in the context of the child's lifestyle set in a family environment, being guided by principles gleaned from the motor development and motor learning literature. This theme is continued by Marina Schoemaker and Bouwien Smits-Engelsman in their chapter on neuromotor task training which notes that the heterogeneity of the population of children with DCD requires intervention to be flexible enough to draw upon different sources of information for guidance, including the developmental and learning fields. Using similar sources, Angie Mandich and Helene Polatajko present their CO-OP approach to intervention, which is a cognitively based approach involving the child in much of the decision-making process. Finally, Amanda Kirby, using her clinical experience and knowledge, brings many of the above chapters together by noting how much overlap there is between DCD and other developmental disorders and how this translates into clinical practice.

All of the authors have both research and clinical experience and the essence of the text is that research drives the practice which in turn informs the research questions to ask. The text aims to guide professionals through the most recent research on DCD, illustrating how this research provides the strong evidence for work with the children.

Acknowledgements

David Sugden would like to acknowledge his debt and gratitude to his mentor Jack Keogh, his guiding professor at the University of California. Mary Chambers's sincere thanks go to her long-suffering family for their continual support and encouragement, without whom the process would have been far more difficult. Last, to her Mum and late Dad go her thanks and gratitude for their love and support and for always standing by her; she dedicates her efforts to both of them.

CHAPTER 1

The nature of children with Developmental Coordination Disorder

MARY E. CHAMBERS, DAVID A. SUGDEN
AND CHARIKLEIA SINANI

Fundamental questions

Who are the children?

John, aged 8, is in Year 4 of primary school and his teacher describes him as having difficulties with tasks that involve motor coordination, noting that these difficulties are adversely affecting his schoolwork. He appears to be of average intelligence although he is a little behind in his reading (RA 7.4) but within the normal range. His manual skills are very poor, in that he finds it hard to manipulate small objects such as beads, blocks, puzzles and has great difficulty in writing, being slow, with the end product being barely legible. In the classroom he drops objects, bumps into people and furniture, and in the gym looks unsteady when running, jumping and climbing. His attempts at ball games usually end in failure and consequently he is now starting to be excluded from playground games with other children. At home, his parents report that he is disorganized and has difficulty in dressing if put under a time pressure such as rushing for the school bus. John has a very pleasant disposition, wants to succeed and is willing to work at the difficulties he encounters. On a standardized assessment instrument of motor impairment, the Movement ABC Battery (Henderson and Sugden, 1992) he scored 65 on the Checklist and 22 on the Test placing him in the bottom 5 per cent of the population for his age in the area of motor skills. He pays attention in class, is quite sociable with a number of friends but his poor motor coordination is noticed by friends and teachers and he is beginning to be embarrassed by it.

Peter, aged 9, is also in Year 4 at primary school and appears to be a very bright boy but it is difficult to assess his true potential because of his poor behaviour. He can hardly write, is extremely awkward in all motor activities and has a range of inappropriate behaviours. He has a reading age of 13, with an estimated IQ of around 130 placing him in the top 2.5 per cent of the population. However, his movements are so poor that it is very difficult for him to realize any of this potential. He studiously avoids all forms of movement activities and has a number of distracting attention-seeking behaviours which range from being the class joker to distracting his less able classmates. He engages in no playground games preferring to disrupt those who are involved, while his parents report that at home he spends much of his time in his room watching television, listening to CDs and using the computer. On the Movement ABC Battery he scored 80 on the Checklist and 26 on the Test, both in the bottom 5 per cent of his age group. His parents have had consultations with a paediatrician who has confirmed that Peter does not have cerebral palsy or any pervasive developmental disorder.

Caroline is 10 years of age and is in Year 5 of primary school and behind her age peers in all subjects, having a reading age of 7.5 and an estimated IQ of around 80. Her schoolwork is untidy and disorganized not only with poor handwriting but also with a history of forgetting books, homework, what work to do, writing implements and other items necessary for schoolwork. Her motor skills are very poor; she has difficulty forming letters, forgetting where to start and finish each letter; her manipulation skills are also very poor and she does not engage in any playground skills. On the Movement ABC Battery she scored 110 on the Checklist and 35 on the Test placing her in lowest 1 per cent of children in her age group.

Finally, Mark who is aged 10 has severe coordination disorders, particularly in total body movements. His gait is awkward and his teachers describe his running as 'arms and legs not in time with each other'. He often loses balance and falls over and his attempts to throw accurately or catch a ball nearly always result in failure. His handwriting is just legible but very slow, as are all of his manual skills. Crucially, Mark has other problems: although he is of normal intelligence, he is reading at the 7-year-old level and he has been diagnosed as dyslexic. In addition, he has low levels of concentration, is highly distractible and, although he has had no formal diagnosis, his teacher uses the term attention deficit disorder to describe him. He is currently attending a developmental clinic where assessment and diagnosis across a range of abilities are taking place.

These four children have different profiles, yet the first three, and possibly the fourth, could have a diagnosis of Developmental Coordination Disorder, recognizing that none of them would completely fulfil DSM-IV

(APA, 1994) criteria. DSM-IV (APA, 1994) is the Diagnostic Statistical Manual fourth revision, published by the American Psychiatric Association and is a widely quoted reference book for a range of psychological and developmental disorders.

Throughout the course of this book, children such as these will be described and analysed to examine characteristics, diagnosis and intervention. These four children epitomize some of the issues that are likely to be raised in the forthcoming chapters. Issues such as heterogeneity – we know that children with DCD are a varied group, but how varied are they and when do they stop being DCD and being part of another syndrome? Peter, for example, is bright with poor motor skills but also has behaviour difficulties; are these behavioural difficulties a consequence of his poor motor skills or are they co-concurring symptoms of another syndrome? John appears to be a classic case of DCD with poor motor skills that are affecting his everyday life and his academic progress despite being of average intelligence, whereas Caroline appears to be low functioning in all aspects of her school life with motor skills just being one of many. However, her motor skills do seem to be at a lower standard than her other school activities and one could ask whether this would be a sufficient condition to give a DCD diagnosis. Fundamentally, with Caroline, questions would be asked about a discrepancy notion in developmental disabilities and, indeed, whether a general learning difficulty would exclude a DCD diagnosis. For the former, analysis would focus on whether there was a significant discrepancy between her motor skills and the rest of her abilities; and, for the latter, the question would be whether a DCD diagnosis could or could not be explained by her overall learning difficulties. Both of these variables are part of the criteria laid down by DSM-IV (APA, 1994). Finally, with Mark the issue of associated difficulties or co-morbidity would be examined; a topic that will be raised in forthcoming chapters. Is Mark's problem one of movement coordination or is this simply part of a larger syndrome, one that the Scandinavians call deficits in attention, motor control and perception (DAMP) or Kaplan et al. (2001) would refer to as 'atypical brain disorder'.

Who is interested in the children?

Since the turn of the century there have been case histories of children who have coordination difficulties to such an extent that they interfere with the activities of daily living, with pioneering studies and literature starting to make their mark in the 1960s (Brenner and Gillman, 1966; Gordon, 1969; Gubbay et al., 1965; Illingworth, 1968; Walton, Ellis and Court, 1962). A paper in the *British Medical Journal* in 1962 probably marks the beginning of our scientific approach to the study of what today is called DCD; it noted a group of children with difficulties that could be mistaken for low intelligence or naughtiness but were more likely to be a consequence of their low motor skills. The disorder seen in primary school children involved a marked impairment in the ability to perform motor skills, resulting in poor functional performance at school. In the same year, Walton, Ellis and Court (1962) tried to describe this syndrome of motor difficulties which had severe clumsiness as the distinguishing feature. The authors could find no damage to pyramidal, extrapyramidal or cerebellar pathways and concluded that the disorder occurred not because of any lesion in a single area of the brain but because of a defect in cerebral organization. They observed that the cause of the disability was not simple and most importantly that the condition was not the result of abnormal maturation that could be corrected with the passing of time. They used the terms apraxic and agnosic to describe the children and noted that the difficulties were 'stubborn'. Since that time the research and literature have exponentially increased with a worldwide interest incorporating the children into the global category of developmental disability. However, the early work still raises fundamental issues and debating points that now have more data to help provide evidence-based practice.

The children provoke interest from a variety of professionals and academic researchers which, in itself, helps to broaden the scope of investigation and nature of the condition. Individuals who work with the children on a day-to-day basis are looking for answers to ongoing problems; thus, teachers and parents who constantly see the nature and the consequences of the condition are searching for guidelines and advice on how to work to best effect. Medical clinicians do not see the child as often yet are constantly asked for advice and help and other professionals, such as educational psychologists, occupational and physiotherapists, are required to offer guidelines for management of the condition. Academic researchers have investigated the condition using a variety of approaches and objectives ranging from those who have studied the underlying mechanisms in the disorder through those analysing assessment procedures to those examining the intervention process. From these, there are now claims that practices are being based on better evidence. Researchers are based in schools of psychology, education, paediatrics, physiotherapy, occupational therapy and, more recently, sport and exercise science and, together with charitable and private organizations, they are beginning to bring a range of research approaches that are being translated into clinical and educational practice.

The interest in motor activities has not just been one that has concentrated solely on motor competence for its own sake. For the past half a century researchers and clinicians have chronicled the links between motor and academic performances, with a host of studies in the 1960s, 1970s and 1980s, all examining the efficacy of utilizing motor activities for the promotion and improvement of academic performance (Kavale and Forness, 1995; Nicolson and Fawcett, 1994; 1999). This linkage has always attracted a following from the clinical and academic communities and currently there is much debate and interest on using motor activities to stimulate various parts of the brain such as the cerebellum and examining the concomitant improvements or otherwise in academic performance (Anderson and Emmons, 1996; Dennison and Dennison, 2001; Heiberger and Heiniger-White, 2000; Ornstein, 1998). Although overlapping with the core of researchers noted above, they are fundamentally regarding movement in a different manner. They are viewing movement as a means to an end; they are using movement in order to learn, whereas a group concentrating more on motor performance are viewing movement difficulties as the fundamental problem and any intervention is aimed at learning movement skills in a contextual situation. This 'moving to learn–learning to move' distinction is often not so much a dichotomy as a continuum with the balance being determined in each individual case. However, as will be seen in later chapters, there will be bias from particular researchers and clinicians which has theoretical underpinnings as well as practical outcomes.

What terms are used?

Many terms have been used to describe the condition and the descriptors used often reflect the emphases of the researchers' interests and also shed light on the difficulties experienced by children with movement problems.

Some of the terms used include *clumsy children* (Dare and Gordon, 1970; Geuze and Kalverboer, 1994; Henderson, 1994; Keogh et al., 1979; Lord and Hulme, 1987a; Losse et al., 1991), *clumsy child syndrome* (Gubbay, 1975a); *coordination problems* or *difficulties* (O'Beirne, Larkin and Cable, 1994; Sugden and Henderson, 1994); *motor coordination problems* or *difficulties* (Maeland, 1992; Roussounis, Gaussen and Stratton, 1987); *movement skill problems* (Sugden and Sugden, 1991); *movement problems* or *difficulties* (Henderson, May and Umney, 1989; Sugden and Keogh, 1990; Wright et al., 1994); *perceptuo-motor dysfunction* (Laszlo et al., 1988); *dyspraxia* (Iloeje, 1987; McGovern, 1991; Walton, Ellis and Court, 1962).

The most recent and formal term used to describe these children is *Developmental Coordination Disorder* (DCD). It appears in both the American Psychiatric Association (APA) *Diagnostic and Statistical Manual for Mental Disorders* (DSM-III-R (APA, 1987); DSM-IV (APA, 1994);

DSM-IV-TR (APA, 2000)) and the World Health Organisation (WHO) *International Classification of Diseases and Related Health Problems* (ICD-10: WHO, 1992a; 1992b; 1993) and was first classified as such in DSM-III-R (1987). The term DCD is currently used by most researchers including Henderson (1992); Hoare (1994); Missiuna (1994); Mon-Williams, Pascal and Wann (1994); Sugden and Wright (1995; 1996; 1998); Polatajko, Fox and Missiuna (1995); Polatajko et al. (1995) plus many others.

In the UK, the term DCD is now becoming more common but dyspraxia is the most widely used term with varying definitions encompassing a wide range of behaviours. It is also used by many professional organizations. In the UK there is a charity, the Dyspraxia Foundation, which exists to help people to understand and cope with dyspraxia; it is a resource for parents and children, teenagers and adults who have the condition and for professionals who help them.

How are children classified?

The classification in these manuals represents a very positive step forward, not only in terms of recognition of the disorder but also because of the credibility these manuals offer. Henderson (1994) notes that the fact that DCD now has a specific entry and is regarded as a separable developmental disorder of movement skills means that it requires diagnostic, aetiological and remedial attention in its own right.

As noted above, DCD has been given a number of titles, but establishing a common ground through the acceptance of a name for a disorder has positive, practical implications.

The American Psychiatric Association (2000) describes DCD as

> a marked impairment in the development of motor coordination (Criterion A) ... The manifestations of this disorder vary with age and development. For example, younger children may display clumsiness and delays in achieving developmental motor milestones (e.g. walking, crawling, sitting, tying shoe laces, buttoning shirts, zipping pants). Older children may display difficulties with the motor aspects of assembling puzzles, building models, playing ball and printing or handwriting. (pp. 56-7)

In addition, it has four diagnostic criteria: two inclusive and two exclusive.

A. Performance in daily activities that require motor coordination is substantially below that expected given the person's chronological age and measured intelligence. This may be manifested by marked delays in achieving motor milestones (e.g. walking, crawling, sitting), dropping motor and academic performances, with a host of studies in the 1960s, 1970s and 1980s, all examining the efficacy of utilizing motor activities for the promotion and improvement of academic performance (Kavale and Forness, 1995; Nicolson and Fawcett, 1994; 1999). This linkage has always attracted a following from the clinical and academic communities and currently there is much debate and interest on using motor activities to stimulate various parts of the brain such as the cerebellum and examining the concomitant improvements or otherwise in academic performance (Anderson and Emmons, 1996; Dennison and Dennison, 2001; Heiberger and Heiniger-White, 2000; Ornstein, 1998). Although overlapping with the core of researchers noted above, they are fundamentally regarding movement in a different manner. They are viewing movement as a means to an end; they are using movement in order to learn, whereas a group concentrating more on motor performance are viewing movement difficulties as the fundamental problem and any intervention is aimed at learning movement skills in a contextual situation. This 'moving to learn–learning to move' distinction is often not so much a dichotomy as a continuum with the balance being determined in each individual case. However, as will be seen in later chapters, there will be bias from particular researchers and clinicians which has theoretical underpinnings as well as practical outcomes.

What terms are used?

Many terms have been used to describe the condition and the descriptors used often reflect the emphases of the researchers' interests and also shed light on the difficulties experienced by children with movement problems.

Some of the terms used include *clumsy children* (Dare and Gordon, 1970; Geuze and Kalverboer, 1994; Henderson, 1994; Keogh et al., 1979; Lord and Hulme, 1987a; Losse et al., 1991), *clumsy child syndrome* (Gubbay, 1975a); *coordination problems* or *difficulties* (O'Beirne, Larkin and Cable, 1994; Sugden and Henderson, 1994); *motor coordination problems* or *difficulties* (Maeland, 1992; Roussounis, Gaussen and Stratton, 1987); *movement skill problems* (Sugden and Sugden, 1991); *movement problems* or *difficulties* (Henderson, May and Umney, 1989; Sugden and Keogh, 1990; Wright et al., 1994); *perceptuo-motor dysfunction* (Laszlo et al., 1988); *dyspraxia* (Iloeje, 1987; McGovern, 1991; Walton, Ellis and Court, 1962).

The most recent and formal term used to describe these children is *Developmental Coordination Disorder* (DCD). It appears in both the American Psychiatric Association (APA) *Diagnostic and Statistical Manual for Mental Disorders* (DSM-III-R (APA, 1987); DSM-IV (APA, 1994);

5

2000)) and the World Health Organisation (WHO) *ssification of Diseases and Related Health Problems* 992a; 1992b; 1993) and was first classified as such in ~~(1987)~~. The term DCD is currently used by most researchers including Henderson (1992); Hoare (1994); Missiuna (1994); Mon-Williams, Pascal and Wann (1994); Sugden and Wright (1995; 1996; 1998); Polatajko, Fox and Missiuna (1995); Polatajko et al. (1995) plus many others.

In the UK, the term DCD is now becoming more common but dyspraxia is the most widely used term with varying definitions encompassing a wide range of behaviours. It is also used by many professional organizations. In the UK there is a charity, the Dyspraxia Foundation, which exists to help people to understand and cope with dyspraxia; it is a resource for parents and children, teenagers and adults who have the condition and for professionals who help them.

How are children classified?

The classification in these manuals represents a very positive step forward, not only in terms of recognition of the disorder but also because of the credibility these manuals offer. Henderson (1994) notes that the fact that DCD now has a specific entry and is regarded as a separable developmental disorder of movement skills means that it requires diagnostic, aetiological and remedial attention in its own right.

As noted above, DCD has been given a number of titles, but establishing a common ground through the acceptance of a name for a disorder has positive, practical implications.

The American Psychiatric Association (2000) describes DCD as

> a marked impairment in the development of motor coordination (Criterion A) ... The manifestations of this disorder vary with age and development. For example, younger children may display clumsiness and delays in achieving developmental motor milestones (e.g. walking, crawling, sitting, tying shoe laces, buttoning shirts, zipping pants). Older children may display difficulties with the motor aspects of assembling puzzles, building models, playing ball and printing or handwriting. (pp. 56-7)

In addition, it has four diagnostic criteria: two inclusive and two exclusive.

A. Performance in daily activities that require motor coordination is substantially below that expected given the person's chronological age and measured intelligence. This may be manifested by marked delays in achieving motor milestones (e.g. walking, crawling, sitting), dropping things, 'clumsiness', poor performance in sports, or poor handwriting.

B. The disturbance in Criterion A significantly interferes with academic achievement or activities of daily living.

C. The disturbance is not due to a general medical condition (e.g. cerebral palsy, hemiplegia, or muscular dystrophy) and does not meet the criteria for a Pervasive Developmental Disorder.

D. If mental retardation is present, the motor difficulties are in excess of those usually associated with it (p. 58).

The World Health Organisation (ICD-10, 1992a) uses the term Specific Developmental Disorder of Motor Dysfunction as

A disorder in which the main feature is a serious impairment in the development of motor coordination that is not solely explicable in terms of general intellectual retardation or any specific congenital or acquired neurological disorder. Nevertheless, in most cases a careful clinical examination shows marked neurodevelopmental immaturities such as choreiform movements of unsupported limbs or mirror movements and other associated motor features, as well as signs of impaired fine and gross motor coordination. (WHO, 1992a, F82)

Other terms which ICD-10 notes are used include Clumsy child syndrome, Developmental Coordination Disorder as in DSM-IV and Developmental Dyspraxia (WHO, 1992a, F82).

This is elaborated by ICD-10 (1993) with the following criteria:

A. The score on a standardized test of fine or gross motor coordination is at least two standard deviations below the level expected for the child's chronological age.

B. The disturbance described in Criterion A significantly interferes with academic achievement or with activities of daily living.

C. There is no diagnosable neurological disorder.

D. The most commonly used exclusionary clause is that IQ is below 70 on an individually administered standardized test (F82).

Examining the classifications as set out by APA and WHO, certain aspects of DCD are highlighted in both manuals, but there are points that are absent in one or other citations and also explanations that are different. The first noted difference is in the title attributed to the disorder. The DSM-IV (APA, 1994) and DSM-IV-TR (APA, 2000) name the disorder 'Developmental Coordination Disorder' while ICD-10 (WHO, 1992a; 1992b; 1993), titles its classification 'specific developmental disorder of motor function' with DCD as one of three related terms used to describe the disorder. Despite this, there is considerable agreement between the two classifications regarding diagnostic features and differential diagnoses. Both state that there should be a marked (DSM-IV-TR) or serious (ICD-10) impairment in the development of motor coordination and that this interferes significantly with academic achievement and/or activities of daily living. Both state that the condition is not due to a diagnosable medical condition such as cerebral palsy. If mental retardation is present, the coordination difficulty must be in excess of what would be expected and ICD-10 states that all persons with an IQ of less than 70 should be excluded from this diagnosis.

Both classifications clearly state what DCD is not by eliminating certain medical conditions. In addition, ICD-10 recognizes that perinatal complications such as low birth weight or premature births may be linked to DCD. Both classifications mention the existence of associated features with DCD such as delays in achieving nonmotor milestones, for example, language development. However, only ICD-10 (WHO, 1992b) states that these features may include 'associated socio-emotional behavioural problems' (p. 250). Although DSM-IV-TR (APA, 2000) is possibly less detailed in its description of DCD, it does remark on the course and prevalence rate of the disorder. Together, these two classifications inform us as to the nature of DCD, although more is known about the disorder than is included.

Nature of the disorder

The knowledge gained over the past 30 years or so has been extensive but the exact nature of DCD from the literature has not, as yet, reached the point where a totally clear picture is presented (Sugden and Wright, 1998). Individual aspects of the disorder have been researched, highlighting distinctive behaviours; however, most reports can be seen to reveal the perspective and interest of the author and it is generally believed that the assessment and testing procedures influence what is found. Not only can the assessment procedures bias the findings in a certain direction but the methods chosen to report the findings may also have an effect. Throughout this text the contributing authors provide detailed descriptions and analysis of the nature of the disorder and present a complex detailed picture. Reint Geuze examines in detail the motor components of the disorder, while Elisabeth Hill looks at the planning and organization of movement; Margaret Cousins and Mary Smyth describe the progression and development of the condition while Dido Green and Gillian Baird look at the associated features and overlapping conditions in DCD. An exciting theoretical perspective is proposed by Mike Wade, Dan Johnson and Kristi Mally, using a dynamical systems framework.

Two procedures have been used to investigate the nature of DCD. The first and most common is to compare the behaviours of children with DCD with those of children classified as not experiencing DCD. This method follows a long-established tradition of inter-group analysis and distinctive aspects of DCD investigated in this way are well documented. However, an underlying question when performing inter-group analysis involves the concept of a syndrome: are differences found between DCD and non-DCD children clear, consistent and reliable enough to constitute a recognizable syndrome? This involves the issue of homogeneity and whether children with DCD form a homogeneous group. The second approach involves an examination of intra-group differences where difficulties seen within the DCD group are examined with a search for consistent subtypes.

Inter-group differences

Studies that describe diffeences between children with and without DCD range from general summaries to documentation of specific behaviours attributed to the disorder. The *British Medical Journal* (1962) lists many traits of children they refer to as clumsy; being in trouble at school, bad behaviour, experiencing difficulties with self-help skills and being awkward in their movements. A study by Walton, Ellis and Court (1962) followed children's development and observations are made about the delays of motor milestones in comparison with normally developing children. The authors found that the clumsy children displayed

> excessive clumsiness of movement, poor topographical orientation, inability to draw, to write easily and to copy. (p. 610)

Gubbay (1975a) found that the clumsy children differed significantly from the matched controls on nearly all the motor skills tasks and all the areas dealt with by the questionnaire, such as poor handwriting, low sporting ability, poor academic performance, bad conduct, clumsiness and unpopularity. These early studies focused on the tasks that children with DCD performed poorly in comparison with a control group.

A clear, consistent and reliable way of determining differences between DCD and non-DCD groups is precisely what any assessment instrument aims to give. However, in addition, many researchers have adopted the techniques of researchers from the motor control arena and examined some of the variables that have been shown to influence the control of movements and actions. For example, some researchers have looked at the differences between a sample of children with DCD and a matching control group on their abilities on variables involved in an *information-processing system*. The studies have involved a number of different protocols examining a range of variables from input through decision making through to output. Some have found children with DCD to be poorer at making visual and kinaesthetic judgements than control children and that poor judgements correlated with poor movement skill (Hulme, Biggerstaff, Moran et al., 1982; Hulme, Smart and Moran, 1982; Hulme et al., 1984; Lord and Hulme, 1987a; 1987b; 1988a; Wilson and McKenzie, 1998). In a slightly different vein, Mon-Williams, Pascal and Wann (1994) found no significant impairment of ophthalmic function in children with DCD, while recognizing that visual processing consists of much more than the provision of a clear retinal image and a deficit may lie elsewhere within the visual processing system. For example, Sigmundsson, Hansen and Talcott (2003) found that 'clumsy' children were significantly less sensitive than control children on a number of tasks of visual sensitivity, and Dwyer and McKenzie (1994) suggested that children with DCD are unable to employ efficient rehearsal strategies to maintain a visual image in a form that would enable them to act upon it. Schoemaker et al. (2001), when investigating whether children with DCD experience problems in the processing of visual, proprioceptive or tactile information, found that they performed slightly below the norm for tactile perception, while on the manual pointing task they made inconsistent responses towards the target in all three conditions (visual, visual-proprioceptive and evident). Estil, Ingvaldsen and Whiting (2002), examining ball catching, found a control group to be superior to children with DCD with respect to both spatial and temporal performance in intercepting a moving ball.

As kinaesthetic or proprioceptive functioning is an important variable in learning motor skills, an obvious question to ask is whether children with poor motor control have a deficiency in this area. Laszlo and colleagues (Laszlo and Bairstow, 1985a; Laszlo, Bairstow and Bartrip, 1988; Laszlo et al., 1988) found that after kinaesthetic training, the children with DCD made significant improvement in motor skill performance. Work evaluating the work of Laszlo and colleagues is reported by Sims and colleagues (Sims et al., 1996a; 1996b) who found kinaesthetic training to be effective but no different from a group receiving more conventional intervention. Other researchers have also found contrary evidence to that reported by Laszlo and colleagues (Laszlo, Bairstow and Bartrip, 1988; Laszlo et al., 1988). Sugden and Wann (1987) and Polatajko et al. (1995) both found that increased kinaesthetic acuity does not immediately translate into increased motor performance nor into generalizing new-found skills.

Many studies on visual and kinaesthetic processing have been incorporated into larger models of information processing and these not only include studies that explore the perceptual or input stage of the model but also concentrate on other aspects of information processing, such as the role of feedback and motor programming. Lord and Hulme (1988a) argued that children with DCD were not limited by an ability to develop a motor programme on a rotary pursuit task but they were restricted by impaired visual feedback control. They suggested that although children with DCD have a representation of what needs to be done, they are slow in processing information that affects other aspects of motor control, such as responding to errors. Smyth and Glencross (1986) suggested that children with DCD are deficient in speed of processing kinaesthetic information but not in speed of processing visual information, a finding supported by van der Meulen et al. (1991a) who proposed that the increased time delay the children with DCD showed when trying to track a target was a consequence of a strategy they employed to deal with their difficulties in motor performance and not due merely to impaired information processing. Wann (1987) suggested that children experiencing problems with handwriting employed movements that allowed greater visual control during movement execution. Again, this can be seen as a strategy used to compensate for difficulties in motor performance with a need to rely more heavily on visual feedback from the writing movements. Smyth and Mason (1997) found differences between children with DCD and a control group on their ability in proprioceptive matching and aiming but the same children displayed no differences in planning for end state comfort. Rösblad and von Hofsten (1994) suggest that the children with DCD were no more or less reliant on visual feedback to control their movements than control children with both groups slowing the movement to maintain their accuracy level. They suggest that the initial slower and more variable movements of the children with DCD are not attributable to visual information but to poor forward planning which interrupts the smoothness and efficiency of the movement, and anticipatory monitoring is replaced by feedback monitoring, which is both slower and more variable.

Other studies have found the *central decision-making capacity* of children with DCD to be slower to respond to stimuli but not inaccurate in their movements and concluded that the slowness was largely localized in the cognitive decision process response selection (van Dellen and Geuze, 1988; 1990; Vaessen and Kalverboer, 1990). Sugden and Wright (1998) suggest it is possible that children with DCD underestimate the requirements of the higher movement accuracy demands and, as a result, need more time to adjust their inappropriate movements. This could be due to inaccuracy in the perception of the accuracy demands or inaccuracy in the planning or programming of such movements. Henderson, Rose and Henderson (1992) found that children with DCD did not perform as well as control children in tasks with both cognitive and motor load, noting that it was not the motor loading that caused the decrement in performance but, rather, the cognitive loading in terms of the increased accuracy demands made by a reaction time task.

A number of comments can be made concerning the part played by information processing in the poor motor skills of children with DCD. First, information processing involves a range incorporating such abilities as sensory acuity, sensitivity, memory, decision-making, motor programming, feedback and strategies and differences in the studies often reflect what is being examined. Second, children in the studies differ by diagnosis with few identical criteria. Third, nearly all studies involve group data that are heavily influenced by heterogeneity in the group. The findings of the experiments concerning DCD and information processing suggest that there is evidence of visual and kinaesthetic deficits in children with DCD concerning the input aspect of the information-processing model, leading to difficulties in error detection and movement correction during execution. These perceptual difficulties result in less efficient motor programming in children with DCD, particularly when accuracy and anticipation are required. As the complexity and spatial uncertainty of tasks increase, children with DCD find more and more difficulties with motor control. Much of our knowledge of motor control differences between DCD and non-DCD groups comes from the information-processing tradition, and more detail of studies can be found in later chapters (Hill, Geuze) with an alternative perspective presented by Wade, Johnson and Mally.

Intra-group differences

There is the suggestion that the nature of DCD is such that the types of impairments seen in some children are not evident in others. This section examines how children with DCD differ sufficiently from within their own groupings to warrant *intra-group* analysis of this disorder. A number of studies exist which identify children with DCD as forming a heterogeneous group, in that the movement patterns they display are different in different children (Barnett and Henderson, 1992; Cantell, Smyth and Ahonen, 1994; Dare and Gordon, 1970; Dewey and Kaplan, 1994; Gubbay, 1975b; Henderson and Hall, 1982; Hoare, 1994; Sugden and Sugden, 1991; Wright, 1996; Wright and Sugden, 1996a; 1996b; 1996c). At a clinical level, one has only to look at the make up of the same total score on the Movement ABC from the individual three component parts to see how different profiles are evident.

The extent to which the children experience movement difficulties is the factor that is most commonly used to discriminate one subgroup of children from another. Sugden and Sugden (1991) use the notion of children *at risk* and children with *movement problems* when referring to the severity of the disorder. The cut-off points in norm-referenced tests, such as the Movement

Assessment Battery for Children (Movement ABC) (Henderson and Sugden, 1992), offer indications of the severity by reference to percentile charts. It is possible, however, to place children with DCD in subgroups from within the group on the basis of severity and on the nature of the disorder.

Hoare (1994) reported on subgroups of children with DCD by examining the results of the children's performance on kinaesthetic, visual, cross-modal (kinaesthetic and visual) and fine motor and gross motor tasks. Using cluster analysis she was able to define five subgroups of children with DCD and concluded that while all children with DCD experienced difficulties with their movements, there were examples where specific difficulties were far more evident within one subgroup than another. The work of Hoare (1994) has been supported by Wright and Sugden (1996a); they found four clusters of children who, while all experiencing difficulties generally, had specific problem areas. This study also revealed some patterns of associated behaviours, with one cluster considered to be the group with many difficulties, showing the clearest pattern of associated behaviours related to their movement difficulties; they are seen to be easily distracted, lacking in persistence, disorganized and confused about their school tasks. Dewey and Kaplan (1994) identified four groups including a control group showing no motor problems. Of particular interest in this study is the distinction between two groups, one displaying difficulties in the execution of motor skills with planning apparently remaining intact and one group showing difficulties in the planning. Miyahara (1994) also investigated the identification of subtypes of motor difficulties but, as this study concentrated on children with differing motor abilities who have a learning disability, it is difficult to translate to the DCD population (Macnab, Miller and Polatajko, 2001). Macnab and colleagues (2001) looked in detail at three cluster analysis studies, namely those by Dewey and Kaplan (1994), Hoare (1994) and Miyahara (1994). The authors conclude that cluster analysis is a useful tool in the identification of subtypes of DCD but stressed that it is imperative that the selection of variables should be guided by a clearly stated theoretical framework. What is clear from these studies on subtypes is that DCD children do have different profiles and these may have important implications for designing programmes of activities and strategies for intervention. However, it is also clear that not enough work has been conducted to enable us to determine stable subtypes of children with DCD.

A final thought on subtypes involves not simply looking at how children differ in their movement characteristics but how they differ in response to intervention, a proposition that has been examined in other developmental disorder literature such as ADHD and dyslexia. Sugden and Chambers (2003a) found that following a period of intervention, children with DCD not only differed in the final outcomes in their responses to intervention but also the manner in which they progressed throughout the period of the intervention. Four loosely defined groups emerged and, although they were not formally defined, this type of analysis would appear to be a fruitful ground for further study.

Associated behaviours

In both DSM-IV and ICD-10 there is mention of associated behaviours that accompany DCD with difficulties in academic achievement, behaviours, self-concept, poor motivation and attention being some of the most commonly noted. For example, Losse et al. (1991), when assessing children at 16 who had been diagnosed as clumsy at the age of 6, found that there was a higher incidence of low academic achievement, poor behaviour and self-concept problems in these children than in a control group. In other studies the higher incidence of associated behaviours is often quoted and it does raise some fundamental issues ranging from the pragmatic viewpoint of how one sets priorities for intervention to the more fundamental question surrounding the validity of separate syndromes in developmental disorders. This latter stance has been taken by Kaplan et al. (2001) who criticize the use of the term 'co-morbidity' when referring to developmental disorders because they say it makes an unsubstantiated presumption of independent aetiologies. The main thrust of their article is that independent discrete categories of developmental disorders do not exist and in addition, the term co-morbidity should not be used to describe overlapping symptoms. Instead, they propose use of the term 'atypical brain development' which does not refer to the condition itself but pulls together common aetiology which leads to varying symptoms. They claim this will lead to less time wasted in labelling and finding one specific syndrome that more or less fits the child and more on defining more specifically the strengths and weaknesses of the child, providing a behavioural profile which lends itself more easily to intervention. Parts of this have merit; clearly, there are overlapping symptoms and the concentration on a behavioural profile of the child does lead to more specific intervention and provides professionals and parents with definitive guidelines and targets. However, it is not convincing to use the term atypical brain development as a useful one and appears to be a throwback to the minimal brain dysfunction of the 1960s (MacKeith and Bax, 1963). This important topic area is taken in detail by Dido Green and Gillian Baird in a later chapter.

Development and progression

Most of the time motor behaviour is being assessed, it is done at one particular moment in time, providing a snapshot picture of the child's current capabilities reflecting complex interactions of biological, psychological and social processes. None of these processes are static: they are constantly evolving in a dynamic manner, which may result in a stable or changing condition in the child. The literature on stability or change in children with movement difficulties ranges from predictions between neurological examinations early in life to signs at school entry (Drillien and Drummond, 1983; Hall et al., 1995; Nichols and Chen, 1981) through school age predictions (Gillberg and Gillberg, 1983; Gillberg, Gillberg and Groth, 1989; Hellgren et al., 1993) to an examination of the condition later in life (Cantell, Smyth and Ahonen, 1994; 2003). A few children seem to recover from an early diagnosis but in many others the DCD condition remains and/or associated features such as behaviour, cognitive or self-esteem problems arise in its place. Margaret Cousins and Mary Smyth skilfully detail this complex area in a later chapter.

Issues and controversies

Definition and cut-off points

In a disorder as complex and varied as DCD it is not surprising that not only are there questions to be answered but also that firmly held different opinions are offered on all aspects of DCD. The heterogeneity of the condition makes it inevitable that different researchers and clinicians not only study different aspects of the condition but also see different samples and different characteristics from their sample. The definition as provided in APA DSM-IV or ICD-10 points to a number of questions. For example, in the motor core, which is Criterion A in DSM-IV, there is the whole question of assessment. Nowhere is there a 'gold standard' equivalent to the WISC in the cognitive domain (Henderson and Barnett, 1998) even though the Movement Assessment Battery for Children (Henderson and Sugden, 1992) is starting to build a more impressive database. But the problem remains as to what constitutes motor impairment; such issues as cut-off points are still not resolved and linking them to functional behaviour is a problem. Wright and Sugden (1996b) attempted to do this with their two-stage approach to identification, using both criterion referenced and normative measures, but one is still left with cut-off points that are identified more by clinical judgement and experience rather than by scientific methods. This problem becomes critical when increasingly administrators are asking professionals to make judgements such that financial support and resources can be allocated to the professionals in the field. Henderson and Barnett (1998) also identify the problem of what should go into a test of motor impairment. Various approaches have been used from standardized tests to functional checklists through to observational schedules. Should pure functional skills be examined or should there be a more detailed look at how the child interacts in context with his/her environment, examining the conditions under which this interaction takes place? Certainly, following a dynamic systems approach in our assessments procedures would lead to detailed observations of the movement in context with a study of the task to be learned, the conditions under which they are performed and the resources the child brings to the learning situation (see chapter by Wade, Johnson and Mally).

Earlier, it was noted that DCD appears to be a heterogeneous collection of disorders rather than a unitary condition. The evidence for this assertion comes from the very different profiles of children described as DCD with little commonality apart from the motor core, which can be made up of many different sub-units. A child can score in the lowest 5 per cent on the Movement ABC with a variety of profiles. Researchers have looked for subtypes among DCD children and although various clusters and factors have been proposed, there have been too few studies to make any definitive conclusions (Dewey and Kaplan, 1994; Hoare, 1991; 1994; Miyahara, 1994; Wright and Sugden, 1996a). This lack of definitive conclusions does not prevent us from keeping the concept of DCD, it merely notes that a group of children are having difficulty with motor skills and the overall profile of their difficulties will vary. What it does do is make it very difficult to ascribe some common underlying aetiology such as a visuospatial disorder or a planning disorder to the overall syndrome, as is common practice.

Activities of daily living and academic achievement

A number of issues surround Criterion B from DSM-IV which states that the condition interferes with activities of daily living or academic achievement. It is already noted that for over a half a century various professionals have used motor activities to ameliorate academic achievement, but Criterion B asks the question as to what the relationship is between motor performance and academic achievement. For example, is it indicating that there has to be a direct relationship between the two, suggesting that there is some underlying mechanism that is responsible for both? If so, the evidence for this is not good. Or is the relationship more of an indirect nature with variables such as motivation, self-concept and social emotional behaviour having an impact? Certainly, there is evidence that children's lack of confidence and competence in the motor domain has an effect in other arenas (Schoemaker and Kalverboer, 1994; Wall et al., 1985). The relationship between motor performance and academic achievement is a complex one and not at all straightforward. For example, if a child is given motor activities to improve reading through visual perception enhancement and the result is not encouraging that does not necessarily mean that a child's poor motor performance will not have an effect on academic achievement through indirect measures such as socio-emotional variables. Certainly, in the area of handwriting one could make the argument for a pretty direct effect if the child's perform-ance is so poor that it prevents them from accessing the curriculum.

There is also evidence that in a group of children with DCD there are long-term consequences for educational/academic achievement. Having movement difficulties in the early years does carry a risk of learning diffi-culties and, in many cases, these difficulties persist through adolescence (Drillien and Drummond, 1983; Gillberg et al., 1983; Gillberg and Gillberg, 1989; Gillberg, Gillberg and Groth, 1989; Hadders-Algra, Huisjes and Touwen, 1988a; Losse et al., 1991). However, as pointed out by these researchers, this coupling of academic achievement and motor perform-ance is not necessarily causal, with only the relationship being firmly established.

One would think that it would be relatively easy to judge the effect on activities of daily living. Certainly, there are many reports of children with DCD that stress poor self-help skills, poor recreation skills, not able to play with peers, but when one examines the detail there still remains the question as to what constitutes activities of daily living. Part of the Movement ABC is a Checklist with 48 items all purporting to measure daily activities. Other Checklists aim to achieve similar goals and some are age dependent (for example Bly, 2000; Chambers and Sugden, 2002; Doudlah, 1976; Wessel, 1976). However, the overwhelming majority of these are devised by professionals for other professionals and parents to fill in. More recently, work by Dunford, Street and Sibert (in preparation) took the unusual but logical step of examining functional skills from the viewpoint of parents, teachers and children with interesting results show-ing that the priorities in daily living had notable differences, with a recommendation that goals for therapy should be set collaboratively between the three groups as the same concerns are not always shared. This would fit with a more ecological and dynamic view of the child's dif-ficulties and approaches to intervention.

Exclusions and samples

Both Criteria C and D (DSM-IV) use exclusionary clauses for the defini-tion. The exclusion of children with an identifiable neurological disorder is mentioned in both DSM-IV and ICD-10 but with the more recent advances in brain imaging techniques it is more difficult to draw a distinct line between those with a known disorder and those without. As

Henderson and Barnett (1998) note, as it is now possible to detect small brain lesions in children with DCD, it is now more difficult to distinguish between DCD and conditions such as mild cerebral palsy and should such small brain lesions constitute a known neurological disorder, thus excluding the child from being diagnosed as DCD?

In the earlier description of the four children there is a debatable point as to whether a child has to have a discrepancy between his/her motor ability and intellectual competence such that the poor motor ability is unexpected. Again, this raises a number of issues and the two classifications take a different line on this question. DSM-IV takes a discrepancy line, noting that the condition can lie anywhere on the intellectual spectrum as long as the poor motor performance is in excess of any mental retardation that is present. ICD-10 takes a different approach using the term 'normal IQ' as the criterion. This issue is not unimportant as it could lead to different samples of children being involved in research studies, thus potentially biasing the results. It is also the case that in performing some parts of an IQ test children will be involved in visuospatial tasks and these may be repeated in some tests of motor impairment, again adding the possibility of bias.

Another form of possible variability in samples is the difference one may find in a group chosen through tests at a school and a group which is a clinical sample identified in a different manner. Many of the same tests are used but the latter is a referral group either by the parent or GP whereas the former is usually a research group chosen from a sample in a regular mainstream school. Sinani (in preparation) is using these different samples and examining the differences between them on representational gestures.

In this chapter little issue has been made about the naming of the condition; we specifically and strongly prefer the term DCD to all rivals including the popular UK term, dyspraxia. Henderson and Henderson (2002) outline the major reasons for this, noting that DCD is the internationally recognized term, that 'coordination' is the appropriate term for environmentally based actions and an opposition to bringing adult literature themes from acquired disorders such as apraxia into the developmental field.

In the subsequent chapters, many of the above issues will be addressed and elaborated. In addition, other controversies are raised from both theoretical and educational/clinical perspectives highlighting the dynamic and exciting nature of the debates that surround this condition, offering food for thought and avenues of exploration for research and practical consideration.

CHAPTER 2

Motor impairment in DCD and activities of daily living

REINT H. GEUZE

Introduction

The acquisition of complex motor skills is a striking phenomenon during human development. These skills allow us to interact with the environment, which is necessary for survival. Moreover, we are able to act on purpose and this opens the world of social interaction, play, sports, craftmanship and so on. Human development is a poorly understood process driven by changes of genetical and maturational origin and by input from the environment, in modern theories conceived as an emerging property of the interaction between these factors and their constraints (through self-organization). The result is well-known: the development of a newborn with a limited set of general and reflexive movements into an able-bodied and skilful youth and adult. Although developmental milestones may suggest a unitary pathway of development, there is ample evidence that at a more detailed level individuals differ as to when, how, and how well they acquire new perceptual-motor functionality and skills. It is against this background of developmental change and individual differences that developmental disorders should be evaluated.

In this chapter the sensory-motor impairment in Developmental Coordination Disorder is discussed. The first part includes a theoretical background, an analysis of what parts of the sensory-motor system may be affected, and a review of the evidence against the background of normal development. The second part of the chapter will discuss the relations between the motor impairments in DCD, academic performance and activities of daily living.

Case study

Jonne is a girl of 11 who participated in a research project by van Dellen and Geuze (1988). She is the oldest child in a family with three children. She performs at an average academic level in primary school. Following the Edinburgh Handedness Inventory she is right-handed, except for cutting with scissors. The Groningen Motor Observation questionnaire (GMO, van Dellen, Vaessen and Schoemaker, 1990), filled out by her teacher, indicates a lack of fluency in her movements, difficulty with rhythmical movements, inappropriate timing of movement and loss of control in stressful situations. She lacks dexterity, for example in ball games. Her GMO-score is under the 10th centile. The Test of Motor Impairment (Stott, Moyes and Henderson, 1984) shows a low to deviant score on nearly all of the items. She lacks speed and accuracy in the manual dexterity items and shows poor coordination between the hands. Ball skills are poor, especially with the left hand, and static balance is poor, too. During testing she is well motivated and cooperative. With a score under the fifth centile she is classified as displaying a motor difficulty. Parents and teachers are aware of her difficulties but have not taken action for intervention.

She is offered enrolment in a treatment programme (Schoemaker, Hijlkema and Kalverboer, 1994). Physiotherapy during three months twice a week results in improved speed in manual dexterity and coordination between the hands, but not in accuracy. Ball skills have improved. Static balance, however, remains a problem (more details are provided in case study 1 in Schoemaker, Geuze and Kalverboer, 1987).

In a follow-up study (Geuze and Börger, 1993) Jonne is tested again at the age of 16 years, and her mother is interviewed. Jonne attends a school for lower occupational education. She is a big, plump girl with an introverted nature, who does not interact with others easily. She likes to read and listen to music, apparently avoiding activities that require motor skills. She does not play a musical instrument because she knows she can't. She failed to learn to knit and type. She seems to compensate her problems partially with a sort of joyfulness, which makes her accepted by her peers. The Test of Motor Impairment shows little improvement. Accuracy and bimanual coordination are still poor, and so is static balance. Ball skills have improved but are still below average. The total score is still below the fifth centile using the 11–12 year norms.

From the case description above a number of important points come forward:

- the origin of her problems is in the sensory-motor domain, not in the cognitive domain or due to lack of motivation, attentional deficits or behavioural problems;

- Jonne's deficits are not restricted to one specific skill or domain of motor function;
- her condition of DCD is persistent, most likely extending into adult life;
- her condition seems to have consequences for daily life as it affected her participation in play and the learning of specific skills such as typing.

The essential questions of parents, teachers and researchers alike are 'What is the cause of this lack in sensory-motor skill?' and 'What can be done about it?' The latter question will be addressed by others later in this volume.

The main DSM criteria for DCD

The two main criteria for the DSM-IV classification of DCD (APA, 1994) are:

A. Performance in daily activities that require motor coordination is substantially below that expected given the person's chronological age and measured intelligence. This may be manifested by marked delays in achieving motor milestones (e.g. walking, crawling, sitting), dropping things, 'clumsiness', poor performance in sports, or poor handwriting.

B. The disturbance in Criterion A significantly interferes with academic achievement or activities of daily living.

Jonne clearly fulfils these criteria to be classified as DCD. Her motor performance in daily activities is substantially below that expected given her chronological age, as apparent from the Test of Motor Impairment. There needs to be no doubt that her intelligence is in the normal range because she shows normal progress in school (Criterion A). Her motor difficulties clearly interfered with activities of daily living, as she did not learn to knit and type, and avoided sports and skilled physical activities (Criterion B). Academic achievement was within the normal range, as she did not double a class or need special education or remedial teaching support.

The case study neatly illustrates an operationalization of the key-words in the criteria. These key-words are daily activities that require motor coordination, motor coordination, measured intelligence in Criterion A, and academic achievement, activities of daily living in Criterion B. It should be noted that DSM-IV does not provide a definition or operationalization of these concepts (for a discussion see Geuze et al., 2001). The operationalization as used in the case study is given in Table 2.1.

It will be clear there are several ways to operationalize each of the key concepts in the criteria and the assessment may be qualitative or quantitative. The criteria for the classification of DCD have recently been discussed extensively by Henderson and Barnett (1998) and Geuze et al.

Table 2.1 Operationalization of DCD Criteria A and B from DSM-IV in the case of Jonne

Criterion	Operationalization
Activities that require motor coordination A	Test of Motor Impairment, norms per age and sex, test items closely related to activities and skills required in daily life for a child of that age Teacher Questionnaire GMO (Groningen Motor Observation scale)
Measured intelligence A	Not measured, assumed to be in normal range because of normal school progress
Academic achievement B	Derived from school progress (no need for remedial teaching support or doubling a class)
Activities of daily living B	Interview with the mother at follow-up (age 16) about things she cannot do or do poorly that would be appropriate for a girl of that age

(2001). This chapter will concentrate on motor aspects and address the following questions:

- what is coordination?
- what are representative activities that require motor coordination?
- what are relevant activities of daily living?

Theoretical aspects of sensory-motor coordination, development and impairment

An analysis of sensory-motor impairment in DCD requires understanding of the components of the system and the functional processes that make them work. Different levels of analysis may be chosen.

As DCD includes the term coordination as the central aspect of the disorder, the term coordination will first be discussed and how it leads to functional behaviour. Then the main underlying system components and the functional processes that make them work will be addressed.

Coordination

Movement seems effortless for children with a normal development but it requires the concerted action of many components in the system with many degrees of freedom. The large number of muscles, over 700, with numerous motor units, and the rotational degrees of freedom of the joints pose serious problems for the control of movement. Separate cortical control of each of these units seems impossible, as it would require a huge information processing capacity of the brain. How then to accomplish complex actions such as catching a ball while running, which requires locomotion, postural control, visual perception of the moving ball and precise timing of arms and hand? The Russian physiologist Bernstein (1984) proposed that the control problem might be solved by constraining the number of degrees of freedom in the system. One way to do this is simply freezing joints so that they don't need to be controlled anymore. Another way is to assemble coordinative structures or synergies (Southard, 1991), in which parts of the sensory-motor system are coupled in a fixed relation at the level of motor units and muscles such that they act as a functional unit that is controlled by a simple set of parameters. Bernstein (1984) characterized the essentials of coordination as follows:

> The coordination of movement is the process of mastering redundant degrees of freedom of the moving organ, in other words its conversion into a controllable system. (p. 355)

Newell (1986) distinguished three aspects of movement:

- *coordination* which constrains the possibilities (degrees of freedom) of the perceptual motor system such that functional behaviour emerges;
- *control* which determines how the chosen coordination pattern is used, for example how fast the movement is going to be;
- *skill* emerges when the optimal set of control parameters is found, given the sensory-motor system, the task and the environment.

These aspects emerge as result of the interaction between the resources of the organism, the environment and the task (see Figure 2.1).

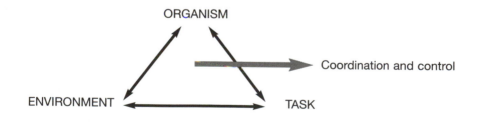

Figure 2.1 Coordination and control as a function of the interaction between organism, environment and task (after Newell, 1986).

Constraints

The concept of constraints is important for the understanding of development and related deficits because it connects the functional organization at the neural level with the functional capacities and limitations at the behavioural level. Among the biomechanical constraints of the system are maximum force of the muscles and limited range of motion of the joints. Additionally, constraints emerge from specific synergies or functional neural coupling between muscles or muscle groups. Other constraints are imposed on the system by task and environment (Figure 2.2). Newell (1986) proposed three categories of constraints that interact and determine the resulting coordination and control at the behavioural level:

1. *Organismic constraints*, which refer to limitations within the system (e.g. limited muscle force or information processing capacities). They may be divided in two types:
   - *structural constraints* which are relatively time independent; they refer to 'hard-wired' constraints in the perceptual-motor system and may act at different levels in the system (i.e. limited muscle force, perceptional constraints, limited speed of neural signal transduction due to incomplete myelination);
   - *functional constraints*, which may change on a much shorter time-scale. They depend on current weights of connections in the neural networks and are relatively easily adapted through experience and learning (i.e. when children learn new complex skills by imitation, training or instruction).

These concepts can be related to motor development and learning (Netelenbos and Koops, 1988). *Development* may be defined as the result of a self-organizing process of interaction between biological growth (or maturation) and spontaneous learning (exploration), generally in the direction of increasing functionality. It is characterized by a relatively slow rate of change. *Learning* can be distinguished from development as the process of change that is independent of biological growth. It is based on relatively fast changes of neural connections. In case of structural or functional deficits, functional reorganization is assumed to be subject to the same principles of self-organization and functional directiveness.

2. *Environmental constraints*, operating through external influences on the system. Examples are reduced vision due to fog, gravity, but also include rearing patterns, or the cultural conditions during development. Environmental constraints reflect the more permanent ambient conditions for the task and for motor development.

3. *Task constraints*, which are due to the specific demands of the task requiring specific sorts of coordination, e.g. handling a pair of scissors, picking up a glass of water. The task constraints may relate to the goal of the task, the way the task is to be executed (e.g. fast or slow), and the properties of the objects and the implements used in the task. Many tasks only require endpoint accuracy, such as picking up a pencil or pointing out a direction. How this is accomplished does not matter. In this case the constraints are mainly related to the endpoint. Other tasks require precise production of a movement trajectory such as in dance or handwriting, and there may be only one pattern of coordination that may accomplish the task at hand.

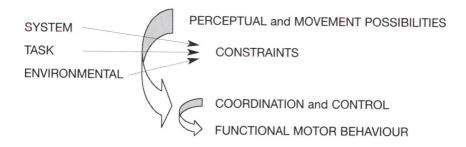

SYSTEM ——— PERCEPTUAL and MOVEMENT POSSIBILITIES

TASK ——— CONSTRAINTS

ENVIRONMENTAL ———

COORDINATION and CONTROL

FUNCTIONAL MOTOR BEHAVIOUR

Figure 2.2 Scheme of the emergence of functional motor behaviour through the influence of constraints.

During development the organismic constraints change as a result of biological change and because of their continuous interaction with the environment. The functional constraints may change due to learning and experience. Because of their plasticity, they enable the system to acquire functional skills and to adapt to changing structural constraints and changing task demands. Both structural and functional constraints may be involved in movement disorder. This implies that the present state of the child with a disorder will be one that is the result of both the underlying impairments and the adaptations the child's developing system has found to deal with its limitations (see Latash and Nicholas, 1996). The question of whether these adaptations have been beneficial or not is generally difficult to answer.

Motor impairment, a system analysis approach

From the previous sections it follows that perception, action and environment are inextricably bound and continuously interacting. Perceptual information is used for action, while action generates perceptual information that may be used to guide our actions and evaluate the result. Also, perceptual-motor development depends largely on interaction between the two. In a system analysis of the perceptual-motor system, three main subsystems may be distinguished; the perceptual system, the cognitive and memory system and the effector system. Functional processes in the nervous system acting upon and with information provided by these subsystems lead to purposeful and skilled action. In Figure 2.3 this has been schematically ordered. This scheme is justified by its close connection to general knowledge of the perceptual-motor system in a wide range of professions. Please note that this is just one of several system-analytical schemes that may be drawn.

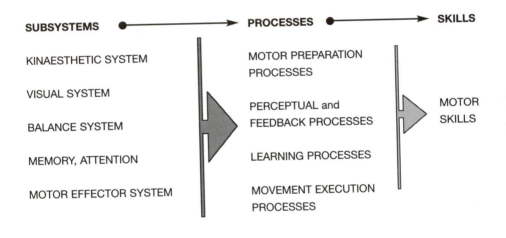

Figure 2.3 Schematic ordering of the main subsystems of the perceptual-motor system and the main processes that underlie motor skills.

Any defect in one of the subsystems or processes might lead to poor motor skills. Is there any evidence for a specific pattern of underlying impairment in the case of DCD? In an attempt to analyse perceptual-motor factors that contribute to the motor impairment in DCD, the literature on the development of these subsystems and processes will be reviewed, including how they relate to skills, and what is currently known about their relation with DCD.

Review of perceptual-motor development and impairment

Kinaesthesia

Position, velocity and force sensation (kinaesthesia) originates from sensors in the muscles and tendons. They provide information about posture, location and velocity of the limbs in space, and the forces exerted by the muscles. The information is used for the evaluation, planning and control of the movements and posture. Kinaesthesia may be partially redundant to other sensory information. It may be evaluated from tasks that rely mainly on kinaesthetic information.

Patients with complete loss of proprioception below the neck usually can perform planned movements with vision. Without vision, adaptation to perturbations of limb position or to a change of visual motor coupling is absent (Forget and Lamarre, 1995; Gentilucci et al., 1994; Guedon et al., 1998; Simoneau et al., 1999). Mirror drawing also nicely illustrates the influence of proprioception. Lajoie et al. (1992) report a deafferented patient who perfectly copied figures in a mirror, whereas control subjects needed many corrections due to conflict between visual and proprioceptive information.

There are two well-known tests that measure the sensitivity of position sense of the limbs. One is the Kinaesthetic Acuity Test (KAT – Laszlo and Bairstow, 1985b), the other a kinaesthetic pointing task (von Hofsten and Rösblad, 1988). The KAT evaluates the threshold angle between the arms after slow passive movement over a slope without vision of the arms. In the kinaesthetic pointing task, the index finger of one arm is passively moved to a target position on a table without vision and the subject matches this position with the index finger of the other arm underneath the table. Comparable tests related to velocity and force sensitivity, the two other main components of kinaesthesia, have not been found. The tests are limited to evaluation of end position after passive or active arm movement. One may doubt if this is sufficiently representative for the evaluation of kinaesthesia as it contributes to general motor performance.

Poor kinaesthetic sensitivity has been reported for 50 per cent children aged 5–6 years (Laszlo and Sainsbury, 1993). Developmental data show a gradual improvement of kinaesthetic sensitivity from 5 years of age to about 16 years of age (Laszlo and Bairstow, 1985b; Elliot, Connolly and Doyle, 1988; Visser and Geuze, 2000). A short training session with the KAT proved to be effective in improving kinaesthetic position sense and general motor skills, such as ball catching and posture, in 5- to 6-year-old children (Laszlo and Sainsbury, 1993). Von Hofsten and Rösblad (1988) found improvement of kinaesthetic pointing accuracy and reduced variability from 5 years onwards, with the largest change between 5 and 6 years, and further improvement up to 10 years of age. Elliot, Connolly and Doyle (1988) concluded that there is no association between kinaesthetic and motor performance measures independently of age.

A majority of children (aged 7–12 years) with perceptual-motor dysfunction (Laszlo et al., 1988) or moderate learning difficulties (Sugden and Wann, 1987) was found to suffer from dyskinaesthesia. Based on a number of KAT training studies, Laszlo concluded that kinaesthetic perceptual ability is a prerequisite for acquisition and performance of motor skills. These results seem to point at kinaesthesis as a main causal factor in the development of DCD. However, in other studies this conclusion could not be substantiated (Sugden and Wann, 1987; Elliot, Connolly and Doyle, 1988; Sims et al., 1996a;1996b; Sims and Morton, 1998). Sims and colleagues replicated and extended the training studies of Laszlo and her colleagues with a group of clumsy children aged 7–9 years, but found a short cognitive-affective training as effective in improving general motor skills (except for handwriting). Therefore, they concluded that

> nothing in the results of our studies offers any support for the opinion that kinaesthetic 'blindness' plays the unique causal role. (Sims et al., 1996b, p. 996)

A study of Harris and Livesey (1992) reported a positive effect of kinaesthetic training of young children on handwriting, whereas specific training of handwriting did not have an effect. Smyth and Mason (1998) did not even find a correlation between the KAT and the kinaesthetic pointing task, and the KAT did not predict differences in motor skills, although specific relations were found between other kinaesthetic tasks and the subscales of the Movement ABC test (Henderson and Sugden, 1992).

The kinaesthetic pointing task showed larger variable error, not constant and systematic error, associated with DCD in children aged 6–12 years (Schoemaker et al., 2001), but no differences in the age range of 11–16 years (Visser, 1998).

In summary, a majority of studies suggests that poor kinaesthetic sensitivity may contribute to the poor motor skills that are associated with DCD. In a meta-study of information-processing deficits associated with DCD deficient kinaesthetic processing was also found to be (weakly) associated with DCD (Wilson and McKenzie, 1998). The role of kinaesthetic sensitivity in the development of DCD is still veiled. The association between kinaesthetic sensitivity and poor motor skills seems to disappear in adolescence (Visser, 1998). Short training of kinaesthetic acuity at an age of 5–9 years may help to improve general motor skills of children with DCD.

Visual perception

Visual information is important in the control of our movements and posture in interacting with the environment. With eyes closed, the planning
and control of movement depends on proprioceptive feedback from cutaneous, kinaesthetic and vestibular sensors, and a spatial representation of
the environment. In many cases, the task cannot be performed without
vision, as in ball catching, or the quality of performance deteriorates, like
in walking. Visual deprivation in case of congenital blindness leads to a
delay of months in reaching the major developmental milestones
(Adelson and Fraiberg, 1974), but in the end blind persons reach most of
the perceptual-motor functionality of adults with sight. Most of the ophthalmic characteristics of the visual system, such as size of the visual field
and accommodation have matured before the age of 6 years, but depth
perception and acuity further improve up to about 12 years (Gallahue and
Ozmun, 1989).

In a developmental study of spatial perception Hulme et al. (1983)
report an increase in line matching ability in the visual and the kinaesthetic modality between the age of 5–6 years and 9–10 years. Substantial
relationships were found between the visual and kinaesthetic abilities and
a number of perceptual-motor skills. No such relationship was found for
cross-modal measures.

What is the role of visual perception in DCD? A study of 29 children
with DCD aged 5–7 years showed that ophthalmic difficulty and strabismus do not explain the motor problems in DCD (Mon-Williams, Pascal
and Wann, 1994). A series of studies by Hulme and Lord showed that children with DCD performed more poorly on size constancy judgements
and discrimination of area, slope, spatial position and line length. The
results could not be explained by variations in visual acuity (Lord and
Hulme, 1987a). Form discrimination ability related to drawing accuracy in
the DCD group but not in the control group (Lord and Hulme, 1988b).
However, the data did not show a consistent pattern of correlations with
general motor abilities. Henderson, Barnett and Henderson (1994) replicated and extended the latter study. They found perceptual deficits for the
clumsy children, but the correlations with drawing and TOMI scores were
virtually zero, both in the clumsy group and the control group. In a meta-
study of information-processing deficits associated with DCD, Wilson and
McKenzie (1998) found that the greatest deficiency was in visual-spatial
processing. This was evident regardless of whether or not the tasks
involved a motor component. Schoemaker et al. (2001) used the
Developmental Test of Visual Perception (DTVP-2, Hamill, Pearson and
Voress, 1993, revision of Frostig's milestone test battery) to study motor-
related and motor-reduced visual-perceptual factors in DCD. Less than 50

per cent of children with DCD had deviant scores in visual-motor skills, specifically in eye–hand coordination and visual-motor speed, or in the motor-reduced items, specifically visual closure and figure–ground perception. No correlations were found within the groups between visual-perceptual ability and motor skills as measured with the Movement ABC test. No consistent relations were present between visual, kinaesthetic and haptic perception within the group of children with DCD.

Conclusion: There is a clear association between visual-perceptual deficits and the poor perceptual-motor skills in Developmental Coordination Disorder. In the meta-analysis of Wilson and McKenzie (1998) this was the most dominant association. How these visual perceptual deficits affect the perceptual-motor skills in DCD is at present unclear.

Balance, postural control

Postural control and balance are usually considered prerequisites for most of our motor skills. They are implicated in skills such as walking and riding a bicycle, in stabilization of the body for handwriting and in anticipatory responses when reaching out to pick up an object. Control of the postural perceptual-motor system involves visual, vestibular, kinaesthetic and somato-sensory (e.g. skin pressure) perceptual information that is integrated in an adaptive way to maintain posture and balance. A simple measure of static balance used in most tests of motor performance is time to loss of balance. More refined stabilometry measures using a force platform are sensitive to age differences (Riach and Hayes, 1987) and vestibular dysfunction (Woolley et al., 1993).

During development the control of static balance is known to improve in several ways. First, the stability of static balance improves between 2 and 14 years of age (Odenrick and Sandstedt, 1984; Riach and Hayes, 1987; Usui, Maekawa and Hirasawa, 1995). Second, at the level of muscle activation efficacy increases with age, as evident from decreasing mean EMG-activation levels (Williams, Fisher and Tritschler, 1983), the emergence of more specific muscular synergies and decreasing visual dependence (Shumway-Cook and Woollacott, 1985). Third, responses to external mechanical perturbations (Berger et al., 1992; Roncevalles, Jensen and Woollacott, 2001) and adaptations to sensory conditions improve (Forssberg and Nashner, 1982; Foudriat, Di Fabio and Anderson, 1993). Static balance was found to depend strongly on visual information up to about 5 years of age (Shumway-Cook and Woollacott, 1985), and was still associated with the ability to perceive and process visual information in 11–13-year-old children (Hatzitaki et al., 2002). Typically developing children improve their reactive responses to light perturbations up to the age of 12 years (Foudriat, Di Fabio and Anderson, 1993).

Balance skills were found to be poor in quite a proportion of children with DCD (e.g. Visser, Geuze and Kalverboer, 1998; Wann, Mon-Williams and Rushton, 1998). Static and dynamic balance performance on TOMI items was reduced in adolescent children who were clumsy from the age of 5 years (Cantell, Smyth and Ahonen, 1994). Analyses of subtypes (Hoare, 1994; Macnab, Miller and Polatajko, 2001) show that there are subgroups of children with DCD and poor static balance. Average EMG activation level in static postural control has been found to be poor in children with motor problems (Williams, Fisher and Tritschler, 1983). Postural responses in reaching tasks indicated different timing of activation of shoulder and trunk muscles (Johnston et al., 2002).

In a detailed study of static balance carried out by the author, 24 children with or at risk for DCD with balance problems (DCD-BP) were selected and matched with 24 control children in the age range of 6–12 years, to explore the nature of their problems of balance control (Geuze, 2003). Additional groups of children (6–7 years, N = 25; 10–11 years, N = 16; with Movement ABC scores > 15th centile) were selected randomly to study developmental changes. Three experiments addressed the developmental and clinical differences in the control of static balance. In the first, the excursion of the centre of pressure (forceplate) was measured in conditions with/without vision while standing still on one or two legs. In the second experiment, EMGs were measured while standing on one leg. In the third experiment, a short unexpected force in the back lightly perturbed normal standing, and EMG and forceplate responses were measured. The results showed improvement of static balance with age, but only subtle differences between the DCD and control groups. DCD-BP children had more difficulty standing on one leg with eyes closed, showed slightly more co-activation and longer duration of recovery to the first perturbation. There was no correlation with the duration of static balance on the Movement ABC static balance item.

In summary, these studies indicate balance problems in a substantial proportion of children with DCD. When they are in balance, control seems rather normal but when larger fluctuations or unexpected perturbations occur these are more difficult for them to control. One explanation might be that they are slower to detect or respond to the spontaneous or unexpected external perturbations of balance. The relation between balance control and general motor skill is all but clear.

Memory and attention

Planning and control of movement depend on attentional and memory processes. These processes are also important for learning and improving movement skills. When a child learns to write he/she starts with copying letters, and information on form and size is stored in short-term memory (STM). After reproduction, the result is evaluated and during practice a movement trace is formed and stored in long-term motor memory. Later reproduction uses retrieval of the movement trace. Two sorts of memory seem particularly relevant. The perceptual-spatial memory stores information about the physical environment. The motor memory stores information related to the efferent activation pattern of the muscles and its afferent consequences of movement. Tests of memory usually measure the amount or quality of information that can be stored and retrieved correctly. The few studies that relate to DCD only concern STM or working memory. The Kinaesthetic Perception and Memory Test (Laszlo and Bairstow, 1985b) requires visual reorientation of a closed figure that has been scanned passively with the finger without vision. Another technique to study memory is delayed retrieval. Developmental studies generally show limited memory performance in children up to 6 years with increasingly better performance up to the age of 10 years (Ashby, 1983; Zaichkowsky, 1974); 4- to 5-year-old children were capable of maintaining and using precued information only with a response delay of 1 second, not 3 seconds or longer (Clark and Moore, 1981).

Attention may be conceived as the process of selecting information from the environment and the perceptual-motor system, including the selection of information from memory and proprioceptive information. A study on the development of exogenous orienting found that disengaging attention was only partly developed in 6-year-old children and nearly fully developed at 10 years of age, regardless of whether attention alone (covert attention) or attention and associated sensory and motor systems (overt attention) were involved (Wainwright and Bryson, 2002). Disengagement and visual orienting as measured by accuracy and reaction time were found to increase gradually from the age of 7 years up to adulthood (Schul, Townsend and Stiles, 2003). Apart from these fundamental attentional abilities daily perceptual motor tasks require selective and sustained attention. Sustained visual attention was found to increase up to about 8 years of age and level off between 9 and 12 years (Korkman, Kemp and Kirk, 2001).

The kinaesthetic perception and memory test differentiated between control children and children with DCD (Piek and Coleman-Carman, 1995). This might indicate that besides kinaesthesis, memory is also involved, but it has been argued that the cross-modal processing required by the task may be impaired. Dwyer and McKenzie (1994) found that after 15 seconds delay, clumsy children were markedly less accurate than control children in reproducing visual graphical geometric patterns. Skorji and McKenzie (1997) studied the reproduction of limb, head and whole body movement sequences after zero or 15 seconds delay. They conclude that compared to control children the memory of these children for modelled movements is more dependent on visual-spatial rehearsal. Together, these data suggest a higher rate of loss of information from working memory in perceptual-motor tasks in DCD.

Attentional deficits may also cause limitations of performance. During a tracking task van der Meulen et al. (1991b) observed attentional flaws in about half of the children with DCD of 6–7 years. Children with or suspected for DCD obtained significantly poorer scores on Child Behavior Checklist measures of attention (Dewey et al., 2002). The co-morbidity of DCD and ADHD suggests that attentional problems may play a role in the movement problems of children with DCD. In a cohort study (N = 409) of 7-year-old Swedish children Kadesjö and Gillberg (1999a) found 2.7 per cent with severe DCD, 4.6 per cent with moderate DCD, 1.7 per cent with severe ADHD and moderate or severe DCD, and 4.9 per cent with moderate ADHD and moderate DCD. In the Nordic countries there is consensus for a common diagnostic category named DAMP (deficits in attention, motor control and perception).

With respect to the fundamental attentional skills, children with DCD show deficits in specific conditions – with central (endogenous cue) as opposed to peripheral cues (exogenous cue) – that were not related to general motor performance measures (Wilson, Maruff and McKenzie, 1997). Further research with endogenous cues points at the possibility that difficulty of disengagement in children with DCD might be a difficulty to inhibit the initiation of incorrect stimulus-provoked responses (Mandich, Buckolz and Polatajko, 2003).

These studies show that poor attentional skills may be expected in quite a proportion of children with DCD. It is still unclear how the fundamental problems of orienting and disengagement of attention relate to their motor problems.

Motor effector system

Development of the effector system is characterized by a gradual decrease in central motor conduction time (afferent up to 5–7 years, efferent up to 10 years, Müller, Ebner and Hömberg, 1994) and an increase in force (between 6 and 10 years, Raynor, 2001; 5–12 years + adults, Smits-Engelsman, Westenberg and Duysens, 2003). During the growth spurt in puberty, force increases at an enhanced rate, especially in males (Beunen et al., 1988). The patellar tendon reflex, force production and EMG were studied in children with DCD and controls aged 6 and 9 years (Raynor, 1998, 2001). Raynor found slower building up of force once the muscle was activated in the younger group only. Decreased strength and power and higher levels of co-activation between antagonist muscle pairs of the knee were found in the DCD group and in the younger group compared to the older group. Slightly raised co-activation was also reported by Geuze (2003) for the ankle muscles during one-leg stance. Limited movement experience and co-activation of antagonist muscles may contribute to limited strength and power in children with DCD. These factors are likely to contribute to the slow movement performance that is characteristic for children with DCD (Geuze and Kalverboer, 1987; Henderson, Rose and Henderson, 1992).

A gradual development of force control is apparent from the studies by Forssberg et al. (1995) on the control of lifting objects, which gradually improves up to an adult level between the age of 5 and 10 years. Poor grip force control in the early phase of object lifting was documented in children with DCD by longer latencies and higher grip force, with larger variability between trials (Pereira et al., 2001). In isometric control of force with visual feedback the coefficient of variation of force decreased up to the age of 9–10 years (Smits-Engelsman, Westenberg and Duysens, 2003). Poor control of force and timing of simple motor actions have been reported in children with DCD (Geuze and Kalverboer, 1987; Lundy-Ekman et al., 1991; Williams, Woollacott and Ivry, 1992). These functions are assumed to be associated with basal ganglia and cerebellar function respectively. The enhanced variability that is usually found in timing, endpoint accuracy and force control has been attributed to noise in the nervous system.

Having reviewed the basic systems, the processes that act upon them will be considered (see Figure 2.3).

Movement preparation processes

Before a goal-directed movement is made, visual information has to be processed, relevant information extracted, which movement is appropriate has to be decided, a motor programme selected or assembled, parameters of force and timing set, followed by efferent activation of muscles, which need about another 50 ms to generate force. These processes are involved in movement preparation. In simple RT tasks the motor programme may be set beforehand. Thus, cognitive, attentional and memory processes are hardly of importance. Simple RT shortens with age and matures around 10–14 years of age, which is task-specific and subject-specific (see review Goodgold-Edwards, 1984). This can be largely explained by a decrease of conduction times between the motor cortex and the muscles (Müller and Hömberg, 1992). For the afferent pathways, adult values are reached by the age of 5–7 years and for efferent pathways around the age of 10 years (Müller, Ebner and Hömberg, 1994). Other authors report a longer period of decline of SRT, e.g. up to 15 years for acoustic SRT (Andersen et al., 1984) and visual SRT (Wickens, 1974). As central maturation is not completed until puberty and memory capacity and processing efficacy increase, this implies that the speed of information processing in more complex tasks may increase until at least the age of 15 years (for an excellent review of development of information processing see Wickens, 1974).

The ballistic phase of fast goal-directed movement is assumed to reflect the quality of the motor programme without influence of feedback processes (open-loop control) which typically have a delay of about 150 ms for limb movements. Poor selection and processing may lead to a non-optimal motor programme. Developmental data show that 6-year-old children are slower and less accurate than children aged 10 years and above. It has been reported that the development of accuracy lags behind between the age of 7 and 9 years, depending on the specific task. This is generally interpreted as a developmental transition from open-loop control followed by error evaluation to an integrated use of visual and kinaesthetic feedback in movement control (see the next section).

The simple RT of children with DCD aged 8–11 years is about 375 ms, 40 ms more than the RT of control children (Henderson, Rose and Henderson, 1992). This points at a slower central–peripheral conduction time or a less efficient (central) perceptual-motor coupling. In a two-choice RT task with choice of movement direction, children with DCD were about 150 ms slower in RT than control children and they made more errors. In more complex task conditions such as four-choice and incompatibility of direction between stimulus and response, the difference in RT between the groups increased dramatically up to 1 s. Evidence points to problems with the central process of response selection (van Dellen and Geuze, 1988).

With respect to the ballistic phase of fast goal-directed movement, it was found that children with DCD are slower, more variable and cover less distance than age-matched control children do (van Dellen and Geuze, 1990; van der Meulen et al., 1991a). This is an indication that the initial pre-programmed motor plan of children with DCD is less accurate. It may be concluded that children with DCD need more time for movement preparation and the result is less accurate.

Movement execution processes

Skilled movement is characterized by fluency and accuracy, and in sequential movements there is a smooth transition from one movement to the next. Development of movement execution has the following main movement characteristics:

- increasingly distal control of limbs;
- speed and accuracy increase (Sugden, 1980);
- fluency increases (van der Meulen et al., 1991b);
- decrease of attentional control.

Children with DCD have more variable and less fluent movement trajectories. Increased tension can be observed during manual tasks, which was interpreted as 'freezing' of degrees of freedom to decrease the complexity of movement control (Missiuna, 1994). Speed and accuracy of movements are reduced and variability is enhanced compared to controls (Geuze and Kalverboer, 1987; Henderson, Rose and Henderson, 1992; van Dellen and Geuze, 1990). With DCD, tracking quality (fluency) was found to be reduced, which could not be attributed to poor use of visual feedback (van der Meulen et al., 1991b).

Perceptual feedback processes

Visual and proprioceptive feedback may be used for correction of ongoing movement and for endpoint accuracy and offer the possibility to correct perturbation of ongoing movements. Slower movements are under cortical perceptual control called 'closed-loop control'. An example is precise tracking of a shape with a pencil, such as in the flower trail task of the Movement ABC test (Smits-Engelsman, Niemeijer and Van Galen, 2001). The first part of any goal-directed movement is under open-loop control (see movement preparation processes, above). This implies that for fast movements the second part, when close to the target, is influenced by feedback.

Studies by Hay and colleagues (see Ferrel-Chapus et al., 2002) show that on a number of task measures the motor performance of 7- to 9-year-old children is worse than that of children of 6 and 10 years. This temporal regression in movement control is interpreted as evidence for a change from dependence on visual information to an integrated use of different sources of perceptual information for movement control. Without vision, execution of movements is less accurate. Studies with deafferented subjects show that without kinaesthetic feedback movement control is nearly completely dependent on open-loop control or visual feedback and adaptation to perturbation and learning is absent without vision (see section on visual perception). Feedback is also used for the evaluation of the movement. For that reason, it plays a role in learning (see section on learning and autonomous control).

A good task to investigate the role of visual feedback is a visual-manual tracking task with and without visual feedback of the hand position. Quality of tracking improved and the delay between the target position and the hand position decreased from 6 years and did not reach adult levels at 11 years of age (van der Meulen et al., 1990).

Kinematic analyses of goal-directed movements showed that compared to age-matched controls children with DCD spent more time and needed larger corrections in the end phase of goal-directed movement (Geuze and Kalverboer, 1987; van Dellen and Geuze, 1990). These authors

suggested that inefficient feedback mechanisms contributed to the poor performance of the clumsy children. However, the studies by van der Meulen
and colleagues of goal-directed movement and visual-manual tracking conclude with another interpretation. The characteristic slowness and enhanced
variability of the ballistic phase and longer delay time and poor tracking quality were interpreted as indicating problems with open-loop control (van der
Meulen et al., 1991a, b). These studies agree on slow performance and poor
endpoint accuracy of goal-directed movement in the clumsy group, but not
on the interpretation. The author suggests that a poor feedback control system may well be responsible for the lack of movement control. First, the
longer delay time between the target position and the hand position makes
correction of the ongoing movement slow and more difficult. Second, such
slow processing of the perceptual feedback information and its transformation into corrective responses resembles the response selection deficit
reported by van Dellen and Geuze (1988). Third, taking the data on kinaesthetic sensitivity into account (see section on visual perception) it seems
likely that poor proprioceptive feedback contributes to poor movement control, too. This suggests a central processing deficit, which depends equally
on the processing of visual and proprioceptive information. For that reason,
in visual-manual tracking withdrawal of visual information of hand position
in the study of van der Meulen et al. (1991b) affects both groups equally, as
they now rely on proprioceptive feedback which is processed centrally much
in the same way as visual feedback is.

Learning and autonomous control

Before learning to write, distal control of wrist, hand and finger muscles
and their synergies should have developed to a certain extent. Instruction
and imitation teach the child how to hold the pencil. Endless practice
leads to optimization of performance (legible writing). Autonomous control, finally, reduces the demands for attentional capacity and frees the
brain of cognitive control in favour of other tasks. This example illustrates
the three main stages of learning (Fitts, 1964):

- in the cognitive phase one explores possible strategies and selects a
  solution of the movement problem;
- in the associative phase the chosen movement strategy is optimized;
- in the autonomous phase the component processes become
  autonomous: less subject to cognitive control, and less subject to interference from other ongoing activities.

There is a clear cognitive component in learning, both conscious and
unconscious, when solving the initial movement problem and in the
selection of relevant sources of information – visual or proprioceptive.

Development of skill is the outcome of interaction between maturation, experience and active learning. The rate and level of motor skill acquisition depend on characteristics of both the learner and the task. During development and learning motor skill is constrained by factors such as the complexity of the task, the performer's state of anticipation, the level of knowledge of results, the type of feedback, the extent and degree of variation of practice, the level of motivation or incentive, and the strategy employed (for a review see Goodgold-Edwards, 1984). Other constraints are found in cultural factors, e.g. some cultures don't use script; experience, e.g. in some countries children start learning to write at 5 years, whereas in other countries they start at 7 years; and competition between skills, e.g. children cannot learn all the different skills at once.

Motor problems have been associated with learning disabilities (e.g. Cermak et al., 1990; Dewey et al., 2002; Sugden and Wann, 1987). This might suggest that children with DCD might have a general learning disability that also affects perceptual-motor learning, either as a basic difficulty in the rate of learning or as a difficulty in applying what is learned to other similar skills (transfer). Few studies have addressed these questions. No difference in short-term learning was found in a rotary pursuit task with three 2-minute trials between control and clumsy children of 8–11 years of age. Their rates of regression of within and between trial improvement were equal (Lord and Hulme, 1988a). In a study of learning a new motor task and generalization children with DCD and their controls aged 6.5–8.5 years did not differ in rate of learning or in the extent to which they were able to generalize the learned movement (Missiuna, 1994). There is no evidence of a deficit in the rate of short-term learning or transfer in rather simple perceptual-motor tasks in DCD. What remains to be studied are learning and transfer and the development of autonomous control over extended time-scales and in more complex tasks.

Conclusion

In this review of motor perceptual-development and impairment, an arbitrary scheme of subsystems that underlie perceptual-motor performance and the processes that act upon them have been used. Against a background of theory and developmental data, the current state of evidence for specific impairment of the functioning of these subsystems and processes in children with DCD have been presented. The deficits that were associated with DCD were:

- poor kinaesthetic acuity, i.e. position sense of the upper limbs;
- poor visual perception;
- poor static balance and postural control;

- loss of information from visual-spatial short-term or working memory;
- poor attentional control;
- reduced strength and enhanced co-activation of muscles;
- slow movement preparation;
- enhanced spatial and temporal variability;
- slow feedback processing.

No evidence was found, however, for a short-term learning deficit.

The data come from studies that compared groups of children with DCD and age-matched control children. Developmental studies of children with DCD that explored developmental change with respect to these specific deficits are rare or not available. The limited set of longitudinal studies that have been published (for an overview see Geuze et al., 2001, Table 2) report developmental changes in DCD at the level of general motor performance. Only for kinaesthetic acuity the data showed that many children with DCD in the age range of 5–10 years have poor sensitivity, whereas for children aged 11–16 years kinaesthetic acuity was not found to differ from controls (Visser, 1998). Thus, the strength of association between the specific deficit and the perceptual-motor problems in DCD changes with age.

Although the impressive list of deficits above suggests that these functions all contribute to the poor motor performance of children with DCD, it should be noted that group studies can only indicate which deficits might contribute to the problems of the individual child. How far these deficits co-occur in the individual child is largely unknown. The few studies that report individual data show that as a rule of thumb only about half of the children with DCD contribute to the specific group differences (see Geuze et al., 2001). Studies on subtypes of DCD indeed show that subgroups of children with DCD exist with relative strength of performance in some perceptual-motor domains, and relative weakness in others (e.g. Hoare, 1994).

The analysis above reveals the limitations that children with DCD may have in specific aspects of perceptual-motor coordination (Criterion A of the DCD classification). It may be concluded that there is no single factor or clear pattern of factors that underlies DCD.

Consequences for activities of daily living

Turning to the activities of daily living as specified in the Criteria A and B in the DSM-IV classification of DCD. What are they? Organismic and environmental constraints determine the range of daily activities of the developing child. Among the global influential environmental factors are family habits and rearing style, cultural aspects, and school curriculum. The resulting set of daily activities will change with age.

The influence of organismic constraints is closely associated with the main developmental milestones such as head control, independent sitting, crawling and walking. Other motor milestones, like swimming, depend largely on experience and opportunity, independent of age. It is likely that these are culturally determined. In The Netherlands, for example, nearly all children learn to swim around the age of 5 years. But is swimming an activity of daily living? The DSM manual does not specify *daily activities that require motor coordination* (Criterion A) or *activities of daily living* (ADL) (Criterion B). The first may refer to the spontaneous and task-related motor behaviour of the child in its natural environment. For a child of school age this includes activities such as washing, dressing, eating, brushing teeth, transport to school, play, handling a schoolbag, writing, speaking, physical education activities, leisure activities and play at home, etc. ADL should not be considered as synonym for *daily activities that require motor coordination*. It would lead to circular reasoning between Criteria A and B. The term ADL is commonly used in the medical and paramedical professions to assess the level of functional independence in daily life and consequently the assistance a patient needs. The concept of ADL has been developed for adults, and agrees with the ICD-10 notion of handicap:

> a disability causes or may cause a disadvantage for a given individual that limits or prevents the fulfilment of a role that is normal for that individual (that is, a handicap). (WHO, 1980, pp. 25–30)

For a discussion see Vreede (1988). More recently it is also applied in populations of children with specific disabilities (see for instance Ottenbacher et al., 1999), for which instruments have been developed such as the Functional Independence Measure for Children (WeeFIM) and the Pediatric Evaluation of Disability Inventory (PEDI). The concept of ADL is difficult to apply to children with DCD. First, because for children with DCD compared to patients with severe medical conditions the level of interference with activities of daily living will be rather mild. Second, most of their activities require motor coordination, and for their development, play and leisure activities are as important as the activities related to independent living.

Criterion A is the single criterion that specifies the motor problem of DCD. The other criteria are supplementary to Criterion A. Criterion B simply states that some of these problems should have an impact on normal development. This suggests a causal relationship from A to B, which we may at most make plausible. Criterion B also implies that there may be coordination problems in the child that do not affect ADL, or that affect behaviour, for example as a result of social isolation.

Daily activities requiring motor control

The *daily activities that require motor coordination* should refer to motor performance that is representative for the child's age. One might argue that a single daily activity which is affected, for example poor handwriting, would suffice to fulfil both Criteria A and B. Thus, a child with poor handwriting skill without other motor problems would be classified as DCD (see case #11 of Table 2 of Smits-Engelsman, Niemeijer and van Galen, 2001). Most researchers prefer to rely on an evaluation of a wider representative set of human motor activities to classify a child as DCD. For this purpose questionnaires and motor performance tests have been developed. Age-related norms for total score are used to classify a child. Questionnaires ask for a subjective evaluation by parents or teachers of the quality of performance of the child in specific tasks derived from daily activities. An example is the Movement ABC checklist with 48 motor items. Motor tests provide a quantitative evaluation of the child's performance on a limited number of specific tasks that are assumed to be representative for the domain of motor activities in childhood. The Movement ABC test, for example, has only 8 items and the child should fail at least three items to be classified as DCD, and at least two for a borderline classification. Although there seems to be increasing consensus about the use of quantitative and normative motor tests for classification of DCD, the fundamental problem is which of the daily tasks that require motor coordination should be evaluated (Henderson and Barnett, 1998) and should this set change with development?

Activities of daily living

A full taxonomy of the daily activities of school children does not exist. Parents, teachers and therapists however, do have a notion of what a child should be able to do at a certain age. An important feature of motor tests is the extent to which the items reflect a child's activity in daily life. For the Movement ABC test this was an explicit goal. Items were chosen that bore as much resemblance as possible to the activities a child performs in the classroom and at play (manual of the Movement ABC, p. 10, Henderson and Sugden, 1992). However, the Movement ABC is a test of motor skill rather than an evaluation of activities of daily living. The Vineland Adaptive Behavior Scales (VABS) were designed to assess personal and social sufficiency of individuals with and without disabilities from birth to adulthood. It has subscales for daily living skills and motor skills but has not often been used in research on DCD. An exception is a study by Miller et al. (2001b) on the effect of cognitive treatment for children with DCD. Unfortunately, they only report effect size of treatment at subscales level, without details of daily living skills. They do report the three skills that Canadian children with DCD aged 7–12 years wanted to improve most: writing, printing and bicycling.

Table 2.2 lists five categories of activities that the author considers representative and age independent. Each category can be divided into specific activities that may be age dependent. The main activities that are considered to be representative for school children are included.

Table 2.2 Categories of daily activities that require motor coordination, and main specific activities within each category assumed representative for schoolchildren

Category of ADL activities	Specific activities that require motor coordination
General	Locomotion, gesturing, speech etc.
Regular activities at home	Dressing, personal care, eating/drinking, activities in household or gardening etc.
School-related activities	Physical education activities, schoolground play, handwriting, activity related to transport to school
Organized training	Music lessons, sports training, hobby club course
Voluntary leisure activities, hobbies	Swimming, climbing trees, drawing, building from wood, constructional play, children's games, ball play etc.

Activities of daily living and DCD

Although it is clear that most children with DCD, selected or referred, have been observed to be hampered by their clumsiness in everyday motor behaviour, the specific ADL that is affected has been rarely described. Even with a thorough knowledge of the literature on DCD, it is striking how few articles report concrete activities that were affected. Most of them describe the skills at a more abstract level of coordination, test score or movement difficulty. An exception is a study by Watkinson et al. (2001) who defined culturally subaverage engagement in physical play as a relevant type of ADL for DCD, and developed a validated self-report protocol for its assessment. Table 2.3 lists a review of reported difficulties related to ADL from 23 case studies (for references see Geuze et al., 2001, Table 2 case studies) of children referred to as clumsy, awkward, apraxic, dyspraxic, having motor coordination problem, motor learning difficulty, perceptual-motor dysfunction, poorly coordinated – descriptions considered equivalent to DCD (Missiuna and Polatajko, 1995). It is clear that these activities relate to 'independent living skills' and play, and they fit into the categories of Table 2.2.

Table 2.3 ADL-related difficulties reported in 23 case studies of clumsy children. Entries have been ordered with respect to frequency of report. Difficulties that were only reported once were not included

Reported ADL-related difficulty	Frequency (% of children)*
Writing/printing	83
Constructional play	35
Ball skill	35
Drawing/copying	30
Speech	30
Dressing	30
Hop, jump, skipping rope	30
Locomotion/fall/running	22
Use of knife and/or fork	22
Buttoning	17
Tying shoe laces	17
Balance	17
Walk stairs	13
Ride tricycle or bicycle	9
Typing	9

* not prevalence

A pilot study of ADL and DCD

In a pilot study of children's ADL an adaptive questionnaire (Geuze, in press) was used in a telephone interview with parents of 15 children with DCD and 18 control children in the age range of 6–11 years. The categories as listed in Table 2.2 were used and parents were asked to rate their child on the specific activities within each category. The questionnaire was adaptive in the sense that parents could spontaneously add information related to the question that was more than a straight answer and the interviewer could ask for more specific information. Additional questions related to the child's motor milestones, medical history and current status, and behavioural problems. It took 10–30 minutes to complete the interview. Table 2.4 lists items that were found to be sensitive to differences between the groups.

The main ADL items associated with DCD problems in the age range of 6–11 years were:

- home: eating, dressing, individual limitations (using a hammer, putting in earrings);
- school: handwriting, sports, independent transport to school, academic progress;
- other: dropped out of organized sport or learning a musical instrument because s/he could not do it;
- milestones.

Table 2.4 Differences between children with DCD (n = 15) and control children (n = 18) with respect to motor milestones, ADL and academic performance. Pilot data of an adaptive questionnaire telephone interview with parents. Data refer to the percentage of children in each group reported to have (had) problems.

Milestones

% of children late and/or slow	Control child parents' answer	DCD child parents' answer
Independent walking	5%	33%
Learning to ride a bike	11%	54%
Learning to swim	0%	54%

ADL problems

Type of question	Control child parents' answer	DCD child parents' answer
ADL problems at home		
• dressing	0%	47% (mostly shoelaces)
• eating	35%	60% (spilling, cutting with knife)
• other	0%	27% (stairs, earrings, hammer)
ADL problems at school		
• handwriting	30% poor	57% poor, 20% bad
• gym	5% poor	20% poor, 7% bad
• other	5% (cutting with scissors)	7% (handicrafts)
ADL problem transport	5%	20%
• safely riding a bicycle		
ADL sports	33% not active	27% not active, 20% failed
ADL musical instruments	63% not active	73% not active, 7% failed
ADL leisure; involvement in:		
• non-motor (read, computer, tv)	57%	73%
• fine motor	57%	60%
• gross motor activities	79%	47%
School – academic (present)	passing 100%	just passing 33%
• ever doubled a class	16%	33%

Additionally, co-morbid signs of ADHD and anger due to frustration were reported in the DCD group.

Two cases may illustrate individual variation. The first is an 11-year-old boy with a Movement ABC test score of 14, specifically in manual dexterity. He was slow in learning to ride a bike. His main current motor problems that his mother reported were poor coordination abilities, messing with food, tying shoelaces, cutting with scissors, poor handwriting, and instability in riding a bike such that he could not safely go to school by bike. School progress was normal. The second case is a girl of 11 years with a Movement ABC test score of 13, mainly due to poor posture and balance skills and to a lesser extent to poor manual skills. Her father reported sufficient ADL competencies but really poor handwriting. School progress was normal. Remarkable here is the incongruence between the Movement ABC balance subscore and the parent's report of sufficient quality of ADL. Apparently, in this case insufficient control of balance and posture had been compensated for and had not resulted in affecting ADL except for handwriting, perhaps. The outcome of the pilot study confirms earlier reports of ADL (see Table 2.3), underactivity in pastime activities and hobbies with motor involvement (Cantell, Smyth and Ahonen, 1994) and enhanced prevalence of reduced school progress (Henderson et al., 1991; van Dellen, Vaessen and Schoemaker, 1990).

The adaptive questionnaire seems suitable to get a quick overview of limitations in ADL of the individual child. For a full account of ADL other sources of information may prove to be valuable: the child itself (see the CO-OP approach of Polatajko and co-workers, e.g. Martini and Polatajko, 1998; Miller et al., 2001b), and the teacher.

In a second pilot study, a similar questionnaire was applied to 468 Dutch students (mean age 19 years, range 19–23 years) in their first year of Psychology. They answered the questions of their current status of motor competence and retrospectively for their primary school period. In 4.3 per cent of cases (n = 20) the question 'Do you find yourself clumsy?' was answered positively. However in 45 per cent of these cases a medical condition was likely to cause or contribute to the lack of proficiency. An incidence of 2.8 per cent of cases with DCD (cases with medical condition excluded) was estimated from a set of retrospective and current specific questions on motor skills. Remarkably, these cases did not report problems in ADL, probably because they avoided activities that would bring limitations. In contrast, nearly all students with chronic or temporary medical problems reported problems in ADL. Although this sample is far from representative, these data provide a first view of the persistence of DCD into adulthood.

LIBRARY, UNIVERSITY OF CHESTER

Conclusions on ADL and DCD

Conclusions that may be drawn from the review of case studies (Table 2.3) and the pilot study (Table 2.4) are:

- all children with DCD were affected in ADL, but some very marginally;
- a number of control children were also reported to meet problems in ADL!;
- DCD children's ADL differs from the adult clinical type of ADL;
- ADL is relevant information for any study on DCD;
- ADL changes with age (e.g. legible writing is not relevant for a 6-year-old).

Conclusion

This chapter reviewed and discussed the motor problems of children with DCD in relation to the Criteria A and B of the DSM-IV classification. It is shown that there is evidence for a large number of possible deficits in sub-systems and processes that are associated with DCD. How they contribute to the perceptual-motor problems of the children is largely unknown. Between the individual children they are variedly present, making samples of children with DCD non-homogeneous. The review and pilot studies provide information on the ADL for children that is relevant in cases of DCD. Here too, the relation between limitations in perceptual-motor competence and impact on ADL is largely unknown. We presently lack knowledge of the consequence of DCD for the child's development and the emergence and prevention of impact on ADL.

CHAPTER 3

Cognitive explanations of the planning and organization of movement

ELISABETH L. HILL

By the time typical children reach infant school they have in place key movement skills such as running, hopping, jumping, throwing, kicking and writing (Gallahue and Ozmun, 1995; Haywood and Getchell, 2001). While these skills will continue to be refined throughout childhood, they reveal that children possess sophisticated movement planning, organization and execution skills even at this young age. In this chapter the potential cognitive explanations for Developmental Coordination Disorder, a disorder in which movement skill does not develop in the typical way, will be reviewed, and, where possible, studies will be considered in terms of their parallels to activities of daily living.

Typical development of skilled action

Movement is an essential ability which allows us to respond and interact adaptively with the environment. While tending to take movement for granted, it is involved in everything we do. Many movements, such as postural adjustments and blinking occur automatically, while others are more obvious in everyday life (e.g. eating, dressing, writing). Furthermore, many human skills involve sequencing movements in new and unusual ways, playing the piano or doing gymnastics, for example.

Broadly speaking the development of movement skill has been shown to occur with age (e.g. Hay, 1979) and to show some degree of consistency over time. The fact that skilled action develops implies that the central nervous system stores information previously experienced and that this information expedites future behaviour. This is taken by many to imply that movements can be preprogrammed (by a feedforward, or open-loop mechanism) on the basis of prior experience. Schmidt (Schmidt, 1988a for example) has proposed the concept of a 'motor program', a set of preprogrammed muscle commands reducing the need for feedback control. Individual motor programs could be described as stored responses for specific movements which include information on the necessary conditions, speed and force for a movement as well as information concerning the sensory consequences of an intended movement. This general motor programme will be adapted appropriately for each situation in parallel to the execution of the movement itself. In this way, developed movement skills can show variation, implying that on-line changes can be made to existing motor programmes, adjustments which suggest that there is a role for feedback (or closed-loop) control in skilled action. Thus, evidence points to the use of open-loop (preprogrammed) as well as closed-loop (feedback) control in skilled movement (for an up-to-date model see for example Wolpert, Miall and Kawato, 1998). Imagine walking. It is easy to see how the initial, core response is preprogrammed in the healthy adult. But, constantly receiving changing sensory information while walking alters the exact nature of gait. Vision of objects in our path as well as visual and tactile information concerning the slope and stability of the ground (e.g. ice, heathland) are examples of environmental constraints which may cause alteration of gait in order to maintain stability. Incoming, changing information such as that just described is under closed-loop control, with on-line feedback being used to adjust the preprogrammed response so that it becomes efficient in a given situation.

As alluded to above, the development of skilled action is influenced by all sensory systems (Sugden, 1990). Vision and proprioception are key senses that interact to elicit skilled actions. Vision provides information both about the environment and the individual's place in it while proprioception contributes internal information concerning the movements of the body (Gibson, 1966). In the absence of vision, and consequent reliance upon proprioception, task performance has been reported to decrease (Sugden, 1990), thereby highlighting greater efficiency when the two systems interact.

Theoretical approaches to the question of how skilled action develops can be categorized broadly in terms of maturational theory (where development of skilled action is a consequence of unfolding structures in the nervous system; e.g. Gesell, 1946), information-processing theory (where action is viewed as taking place in discrete hierarchical stages, see Figure 3.1; e.g. Connolly, 1970) and the dynamic systems approach. In this latter account behaviour is described as arising from the interaction of multiple systems including the central and peripheral nervous systems, muscle, joint and limb systems, as well as external forces such as gravity and perceptual information, e.g. optic flow. According to this framework, motor skill development is an *emergent* process, where motor behaviour is *self-organized* rather than prescribed (see Smith and Thelen, 2003 for a review).

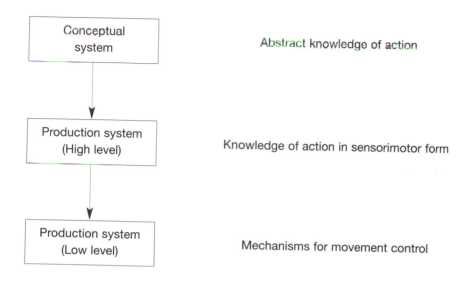

Figure 3.1 Basic diagram of Roy's (1983) model of the action system (adapted from Roy and Square, 1985, p. 113). In this model, the developed action system plans and controls actions through two interacting functional systems, the conceptual and production systems. The conceptual system integrates incoming sensory information about task context with a stored knowledge base for action which may include knowledge about the properties of an object as well as of task-specific actions. The conceptual system provides an abstract representation of action. The production system uses information from the conceptual system to develop or access a set of production rules that will help to guide limbs in time and space. Generalized action programmes are integrated with the necessary perceptual-motor processes for organizing and executing actions, actions which are acted out through muscular activity. According to this model, action production is dependent upon first having a conceptual representation of an action.

Developmental Coordination Disorder

The development of motor coordination occurs gradually from birth but what happens in cases where this development does not occur in the typical manner? One example is seen in the condition 'Developmental Coordination Disorder' (DCD). This condition has been recognized officially as a clinical entity only since the publication of the 3rd edition of the Diagnostic and Statistical Manual of the American Psychiatric Association in 1987. DCD is a neurodevelopmental disorder defined in terms of a child experiencing movement difficulties out of proportion with general development and in the absence of any medical condition (e.g. cerebral palsy) or identifiable neurological disease. For a diagnosis to be given,

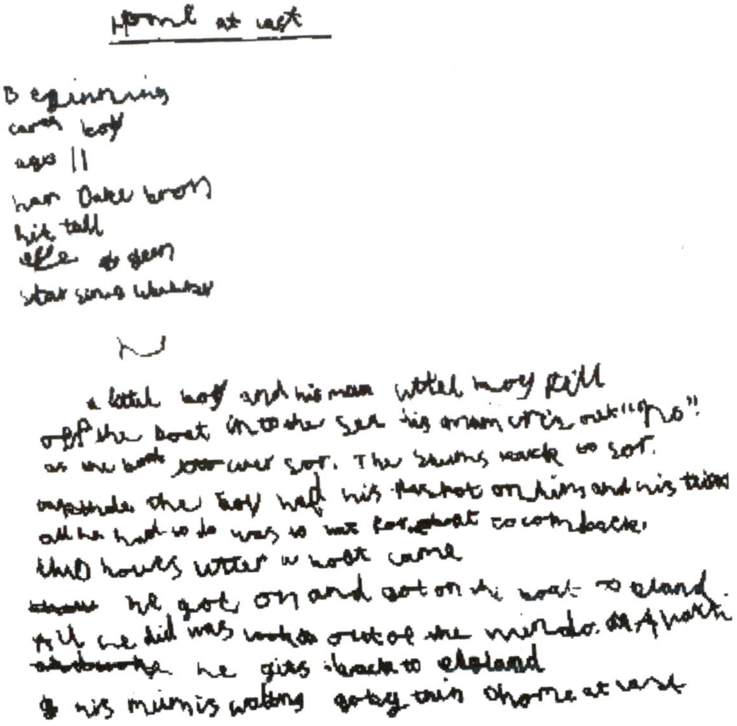

Figure 3.2 Example of the free handwriting of a 10-year-old child with DCD.

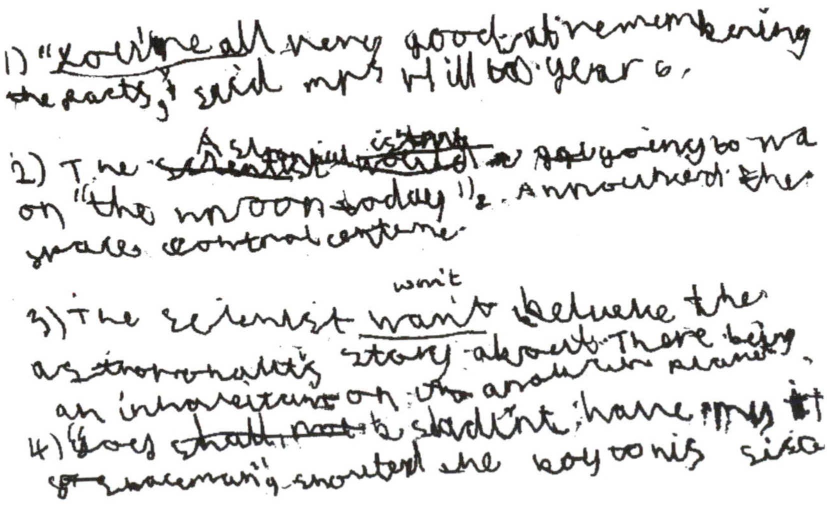

Figure 3.3 Example of a passage copied by a 10-year-old child with DCD.

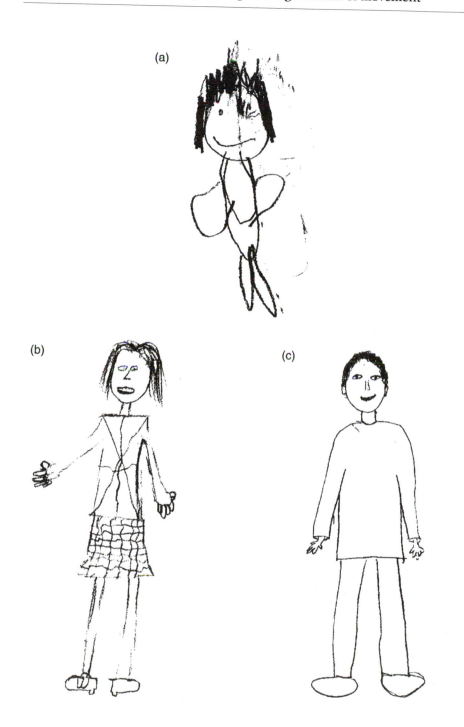

Figure 3.4 Example of the drawing of a 10-year-old child with DCD (Fig. 3.4a) vs. other typically developing 10-year-old children (Figs 3.4b and 3.4c).

movement difficulties must interfere significantly with activities of daily living such as dressing, eating and walking or with academic achievement. An illustration of the level of difficulties experienced by children with DCD is shown in Figures 3.2–3.4 which give examples of the handwriting, copying and drawing abilities of children with DCD.

Over the past three decades, a variety of labels have been coined to describe DCD. Descriptive terms such as clumsy child syndrome (Gubbay, 1975a) have been used, in addition to terms such as developmental dyspraxia (Denckla, 1984) and specific developmental disorder of motor function (World Health Organisation, 1992a). The term dyspraxia is now reasonably well-known by the general public, at least in the United Kingdom, with the national parent support group being known as the Dyspraxia Foundation. However strictly speaking dyspraxia relates to a specific type of motor difficulty. Thus in this chapter the term DCD will be used to refer to the general condition and the term dyspraxia to a specific type of deficit.

Developmental dyspraxia

The use of the term 'developmental dyspraxia' has its roots in the adult neuropsychological literature and is used developmentally by some as an all-embracing term for movement difficulty. In contrast, others adhere to a strict definition of the term developmental dyspraxia, as it is used to define adult apraxia. Namely a very specific movement difficulty relating to the production of purposeful skilled movements in individuals whose motor effector and somatosensory systems are intact. Following this definition, it is clear that developmental dyspraxia could be one symptom of a DCD syndrome. Much of the literature has focused on whether specific Developmental Coordination Disorders are synonymous with, or separate from dyspraxia (e.g. Dewey, 1995; Missiuna and Polatajko, 1995; Miyahara and Möbs, 1995), with no definite consensus emerging.

One particular problem has been the lack of an official operational definition of developmental dyspraxia in the literature. Dewey (1995) has attempted to provide such a definition that would distinguish developmental dyspraxia clearly from developmental disorders of motor function and control. She proposed that developmental dyspraxia should be defined as a disorder of gestural performance affecting both familiar and unfamiliar action sequences in children whose basic motor effector and somatosensory systems are intact. Dewey's definition of developmental dyspraxia allows both for subtypes of gestural disorders to be identified and for different underlying mechanisms to cause these subtypes of the disorder. Experimental studies of dyspraxia have provided some understanding of a subset of the motor coordination difficulties of those with DCD.

Experimental studies of dyspraxia

Traditional tests of apraxia, and thus of dyspraxia, look at the production of meaningful (or representational) vs. meaningless gestures. A representational gestures task requires that the participant demonstrate *familiar* actions. These can be either transitive (requiring the use of an object, such as combing the hair with a comb, cutting paper with scissors) or intransitive (movements that do not require an object, such as salute, hitchhike, make a fist). Actions can be elicited in different response conditions, the predominant ones being to verbal command, imitation and using the object itself. In the verbal command condition, the participant is asked to demonstrate an action, which in the case of the transitive condition is done in the absence of the actual object. In the imitation condition, the experimenter mimes the action (again, in the absence of the object in the transitive condition), and the participant is required to copy this exactly. A typical performance profile sees transitive gestures performed more poorly than intransitive gestures, and all gestures performed more poorly to verbal command than to imitation. Most superior performance is seen, predictably, when demonstrating an action using the required object.

One argument is that poor performance on a representational gestures test in patients could arise from a comprehension deficit. To assess gesture production independently of this, participants can be asked to imitate meaningless (unfamiliar) single hand postures and sequences of these postures. Such a task has the advantage of using gestures that cannot be ascribed a verbal label, thereby removing an explanation of poor performance in terms of a comprehension deficit rather than a movement difficulty. Thus, a comprehensive apraxic battery allows a number of effects to be considered, including the effect of input modality (verbal command vs. imitation), movement complexity (single posture vs. sequence), type of limb gesture (transitive vs. intransitive), representational nature of gestures (meaningful vs. meaningless), and gesture performance vs. actual object use. Examples of these are shown in Table 3.1.

A small number of studies have investigated praxis errors in tests of meaningful gestures in typically developing children. The quantitative pattern of performance on tests of representational gestures seen in adults, with transitive gestures performed more poorly than intransitive gestures and gestures to verbal command more poorly than to imitation, is also observed in healthy children (Kools and Tweedie, 1975; Overton and Jackson, 1973). Age-related changes have been reported in the qualitative nature of the responses produced by children when completing a task of representational gestures (Kaplan, 1968). Thus accurate performance on a task of representational gestures has been shown to increase with age in typically developing children.

Table 3.1 Examples of tests used to assess apraxia, showing a breakdown of task components including movement complexity (single posture vs. sequences), type of limb gestures (transitive vs. intransitive) and the representational nature of gestures (meaningful vs. meaningless). The transitive and intransitive pantomimed gestures can be performed both to verbal command and imitation

Type of apraxia test	Example
MEANINGFUL MOVEMENTS:	
Transitive gestures:	
Action with single object	Comb hair, stir coffee with spoon, saw wood.
Action with multiple objects	Make tea or toast, bake cake, look up a number in phone book and dial it.
Simple pantomimes	Mime brushing teeth with toothbrush, or cutting paper with scissors.
Complex, narrative pantomimes	Mime act of making a cup of tea, or writing letter and posting it.
Intransitive gestures:	
Symbolic gestures	Blow a kiss, hitchhike, cross fingers for good luck.
Natural, expressive gestures	Wave goodbye, indicate anger towards somebody.
MEANINGLESS MOVEMENTS:	
Single movements	For examples see Figure 3.5
Sequences	Close fist, thump sideways on table; fingers and thumb extended, but closed on table-top. Back of hand slaps the table across other arm, rotates, palm slaps back at the start position

Children with DCD and developmental motor deficits perform significantly more poorly than their typically developing peers on tasks of representational gestures but show the same hierarchy of performance difficulty; namely, transitive gestures are performed more poorly than intransitive actions, and gestures to verbal command more poorly than to imitation (Dewey, 1993; Dewey and Kaplan, 1992; Hill, 1998). This pattern of performance has also been reported in those with sensorimotor dysfunction (Dewey, 1991), specific language impairment (Hill, 1998) and learning disabilities (Cermak, Coster and Drake, 1980), and is true in both quantitative and qualitative analysis of task performance (Hill, Bishop and Nimmo-Smith, 1998).

To complete the assessment of dyspraxia in DCD, Hill (1998) assessed the production of single and multiple meaningless postures in children with DCD. These children had no difficulty copying single hand postures such as those shown in Figure 3.5 in relation to their typically developing peers, although in some instances they were significantly slower to produce an accurate posture. Furthermore, these same children showed no difficulty in the copying of short, meaningless hand sequences, although Dewey and Kaplan (1992) reported that their sample of children with DCD did have difficulty copying meaningless hand sequences, in comparison to their typically developing peers. Zoia and colleagues (2002) assessed limb gesture performance using a variety of input modalities (imitation, visual + tactile, visual, verbal) in a group of children with DCD in relation to typically developing children aged 5–6, 7–8 and 9–10 years. The performance of the children with DCD in relation to typically developing children throughout the four input modalities was suggestive of a maturational delay, with the difference increasing with age. This finding is supported by Hill's (1998) study in which a younger control group – who acted as a motor match for the DCD group – was included as well as an age matched control group. Taken together, these studies indicate that developmental dyspraxia – a difficulty in the production of gestures – is a component of the symptomatology seen in DCD.

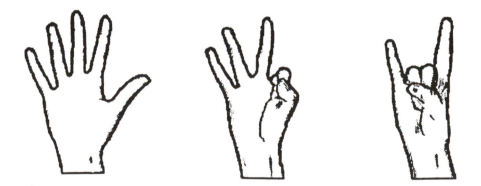

Figure 3.5 Examples of the meaningless single hand postures used by Hill (1998). Hand postures were taken from Kimura and Archibald (1974).

Cognitive explanations of DCD

Various hypotheses have been suggested in an attempt to identify the underlying mechanism(s) whose impairment contributes to DCD. A brief overview of the main approaches is presented below. This covers

descriptive approaches, explanations of DCD in terms of motor programming ability and perceptual accounts of DCD. It should be noted that
most of the published research has investigated children, rather than
adults, with DCD, hence the use of the term 'children' to refer to research
participants. This does not by any means deny the longitudinal nature of
the disorder (Losse et al., 1991; Cantell, Smyth and Ahonen, 1994).
Furthermore, it stresses the need for adult studies investigating the cognitive causes of DCD.

Descriptive studies of DCD

In this area of research functional everyday tasks with which the child with
DCD has difficulty (e.g. buttoning; Barnett and Henderson, 1994) are
investigated systematically. Such work can highlight the precise output
problems that such children experience daily with a specified task.
Barnett and Henderson (1992), for example, investigated drawing ability
in children with DCD, finding that the more uncoordinated a child was,
the poorer their drawing ability. Whereas drawing skill tended to remain
stable or improve in well-coordinated children, it fell further behind
chronological age norms with time in those with DCD.

The findings of descriptive research can help to increase awareness of
the actual output difficulties of the child with DCD, as well as to help
teachers and other professionals to identify children with DCD who have
not yet been diagnosed officially. Thus, while the descriptive approach
cannot tell why DCD occurs or how it is mediated, it can point to the
problems encountered by the child with DCD and raise awareness of their
difficulties.

Motor programming explanations of DCD

A second research approach investigates the problems of children with
DCD using chronometric techniques such as aiming, interception and
tracking tasks. Much of this work focuses on: (1) the preparation and
organization of motor responses, and (2) timing control as studied
through tapping tasks.

Response selection

In a simple reaction time aiming task, children with DCD have been found
to have significantly prolonged movement latency and movement duration, as well as increased variability of these compared to age-matched
controls (Henderson, Rose and Henderson, 1992). Performance on the
Test of Motor Impairment (TOMI; Stott, Moyes and Henderson, 1984) was
a powerful indicator of movement duration, suggesting that the greater

the degree of impairment shown by a child with DCD, the longer the time taken to complete a movement.

By evaluating their reaction time data with reference to that of typical adults and patients with Parkinson's disease, Henderson, Rose and Henderson (1992) suggested that the prolonged response latencies seen in children with DCD reflect problems in the search for and retrieval of stimulus–response (S–R) mapping from working memory, but only when there is little S–R compatibility *along with* responses that are demanding to produce. This compatibility effect may therefore be an indicator of general resource depletion in the planning and control of action, rather than a direct reflection of a specific processing deficit underlying poor coordination.

Henderson, Rose and Henderson (1992) also presented the same children with a 'coincidence timing' task in which a series of auditory tones were presented at regular intervals and children were required to synchronize the arrival of their finger at a target with the presentation of the fifth tone. In this task, absolute timing error was found to be significantly greater in the children with DCD. Increasing the time between each tone presented in the countdown resulted in equally poor performance for children in both the DCD and control groups, suggesting that the problems of children with DCD arise from an inability to generate responses with reliable timing rather than from a poor cognitive process of time estimation. This finding lends support to the suggestion that a general deficit in planning and action control influences the behaviour of children with DCD.

In a number of studies, researchers in the Netherlands have investigated the perceptual anticipation of children with DCD and age-matched controls through the medium of choice reaction time tasks (e.g. Geuze and van Dellen, 1990; van Dellen and Geuze, 1988). Perceptual anticipation is measured as a decrease in reaction time when children have received a precue indicating to which target they will be expected to move. While children with DCD had significantly slower reaction and movement times, along with increased variability on these tasks, these children profited from precuing in the same way as their typically developing peers. This finding may indicate that children with DCD have more problems translating a stimulus code into a response code when this translation requires more transformations (van Dellen and Geuze, 1988). Following this account, response selection is a cognitive decision process that is likely to be involved in any adequate explanation of perceptual-motor deficits. It is suggested that an impairment in the cognitive decision process of response selection may, at least in part, contribute to the slow performance of children with DCD on these tasks. However, in a follow-up to the van Dellen and Geuze (1988) response selection study, Geuze and Börger (1994) found that although 50–70 per cent of the 12-year-olds with DCD studied 5 years previously (those reported in 1988) were still performing poorly on the TOMI, the differences of response selection between the children with DCD and their typically developing peers had disappeared. Thus the role of response selection in DCD remains unclear.

These simple and choice reaction time studies suggest that it is a central deficit in the planning and control of action, rather than a specific processing deficit, that contributes to the poor coordination of the child with DCD. Such findings are consistent with studies adopting the descriptive approach which have revealed that slowness is a major characteristic of the performance of children with DCD on everyday tasks such as drawing (Barnett and Henderson, 1992) and buttoning (Barnett and Henderson, 1994).

Timing control

Studies of timing control have investigated movement coordination by considering the stability of the intervals between taps when required to tap regularly. If a lack of ability to adapt to specific constraints is found in children with DCD when tapping, this may point to nonoptimal functioning of the central nervous system in these children. Williams, Woollacott and Ivry (1992) investigated timing control in children with DCD on a tapping continuation task (children were required to tap in time with a tone and to continue tapping once the tone had ceased). The Wing-Kristofferson model of repetitive movements (Wing and Kristofferson, 1973) was used to identify the locus of the timing control difficulties seen in the children with DCD.

The Wing-Kristofferson model is a linear model that looks at the nature of the representation of a movement sequence by focusing on order errors in the execution of sequences during regular tapping tasks. When tapping out regular sequences using one finger, the variability of interresponse intervals (the length of time between consecutive taps) can be measured. Two sources may be responsible for the variability of interresponse intervals, the first being a timekeeper process which triggers the response at the required interval, and the second a motor delay, the mechanism that intervenes between the trigger and the response. This two-component model predicts that successive interresponse intervals will be negatively correlated. If an interresponse interval is longer than the average, this will be followed by one shorter than the average more often than would be predicted purely by chance. Research has shown that the timekeeper process and motor delay are independent, suggesting that these two mechanisms have distinct physiological representations (Wing, Keele and Margolin, 1984).

Applying the Wing-Kristofferson model to their data, Williams, Woollacott and Ivry (1992) found that children with DCD had significant difficulty with timing control when compared to their well coordinated peers. Variability in the timed, rhythmic responses of those in the DCD group could, for the most part, be explained by the Wing-Kristofferson model in terms of a problem in the central timing mechanism (the time-keeper process) rather than in a peripheral mechanism involved in response implementation (the motor delay component). This finding ties in with that of the continuation tapping task reported by Henderson, Rose and Henderson (1992) as well as with other studies of continuous tapping in DCD (e.g. Geuze and Kalverboer, 1987; 1994; Hill and Wing 1999). Overall the findings of tapping studies point to evidence for a general timing difficulty in children with DCD. The consequences of this for everyday activities and learning are not difficult to imagine.

The evidence from timing control studies relates also to the reaction time literature. Both sets of findings suggest that some kind of central planning deficit is related to DCD, rather than a problem arising at the peripheral level of response implementation. If this is the case then the difficulties of a child with DCD could lie in organizing certain timing dimensions of central motor programmes. A likely source of such central timekeeping problems could be the cerebellum. Indeed, some evidence for at least a subgroup of DCD showing cerebellar-type difficulties has been postulated by Lundy-Ekman et al. (1991).

If it is the case that impairment in a central timing mechanism contributes to the problems of children with DCD, then this would have consequences for learning. If you are unable to map successfully the temporal aspects of a task onto its spatial component when catching a ball, for example, then inaccurate feedback will be incorporated into the existing schema for ball catching. Inevitably, this would impair the ability to make appropriate adaptations to the task and performance would never be improved adequately. Timing is an intrinsic component of any everyday task, thus an explanation of DCD in terms of a deficit in a central timekeeping component of the motor system may be a valid one. Future work needs to investigate further the underlying temporal components of functional everyday tasks in naturalistic settings (see Barnett and Henderson, 1994 for a study which does this). Such an approach can provide an indication of the extent of the temporal dysfunction that the child with DCD faces on a daily basis in activities of daily living and academic tasks.

Microscopic movement planning

A further approach to understanding the nature of difficulties in the planning and organization of movement in DCD comes from studies investigating the coordination of the timing of microscopic aspects of movement such as the coordination of the start or end of a movement with grip force (the amount of squeeze exerted by the fingers when holding and moving an object). When adults hold an object while making vertical movements there are differences in the coordination of grip force with movement onset (see Figure 3.6). Specifically, when making upward movements adults increase their grip force at the onset of movement (in the acceleration phase). In contrast, when making downard movements adults increase their grip force only towards the end of the movement (in the deceleration phase). These differing patterns of anticipatory grip force adjustments indicate acquired knowledge about environmental effects on movements (Flanagan and Wing, 1993; see Wing 1996 for a review). Arguably this task acts as an analogue for moving a cup to and from the mouth to drink. While there have been no studies charting the developmental course of coordination between grip force and movement phase when making vertical movements with objects, Forssberg and colleagues have documented developing coordination of the grip force and movement onset in infants, children and young adults when simply lifting an object to hold it steady above a table top (Forssberg et al., 1991; Forssberg et al., 1992). They have shown that anticipatory grip force adjustments in lifting an object develop until approximately 8 years of age, with some refinement continuing after this point.

In two case studies, Hill and Wing (1998; 1999) have investigated how the developmental curve in lifting and making vertical movements while holding an object might be altered in impaired development, and specifically in boys with DCD in comparison to their peers. In their first study,

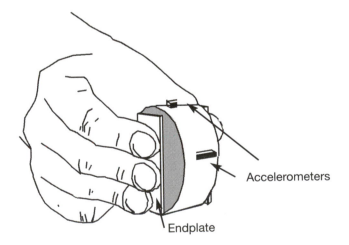

Figure 3.6a Moving an object: participants move the force transducer up or down using a precision grip, as shown. (redrawn from Wing, 1996)

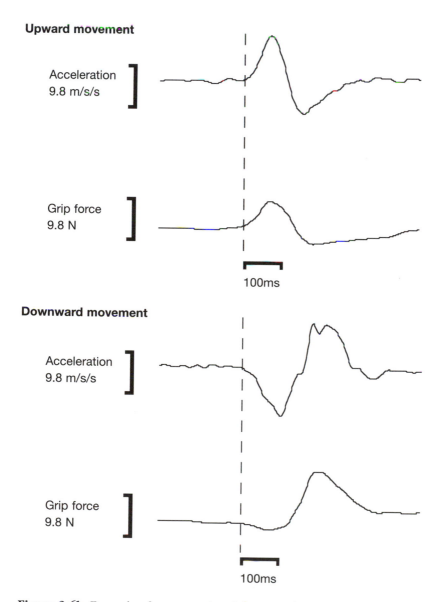

Figure 3.6b Example of an upward and downward movement trace showing the coordination between onset of grip force increase and movement onset/end.

vertical upward and downward movements were made while holding an object, while in the second study different children repeated this task, but also undertook a lifting task, a time production (tapping) task and holding an object subject to unpredictable perturbation (a test of reflexes). By combining performance on this series of tasks, it was possible to postulate the locus of motion planning difficulties seen in DCD. A number of differences were observed between the child with DCD and control child. In the first study, Hill and Wing (1998) showed that an 11-year-old child with DCD increased his grip force earlier when making downward, but not upward, movements in comparison to a typically developing control child.

In the second study, the child with DCD showed an earlier rise in grip force when making both upward and downward movements (Hill and Wing, 1999). This was seen in parallel to greater variability in the timing of voluntary actions in the child with DCD when undertaking the tapping task and longer grip reflexes in the child with DCD in comparison to his typically developing peer. However, no differences were seen between the two children in the coordination of grip force and movement onset when lifting an object to hold it a short distance above the table top. These findings suggest that the difficulty in this particular child with DCD relates to the timing of movement execution. The authors speculate that at least part of the observed deficits might be explained in terms of inaccurate prediction, fitting in with the model of Wolpert, Miall and Kawato (1998) that planning any particular movement involves selecting appropriate feedforward (and inverse) models from a larger set that spans all possible movements. These models will be selected according to context, something that may not be used to an individual's advantage in those with DCD. Wolpert, Miall and Kawato (1998) identify this function with the cerebellum, which ties in with the findings cited by Williams, Woollacott and Ivry (1992) above. Furthermore, Kooistra et al. (1997) have shown that the motor problems of children with congenital hypothyroidism, a condition believed to affect the cerebellum, are likely to be related to peripheral processes associated with motor execution rather than to central cerebellar processes associated with motor timing.

In their studies, Hill and Wing showed that two children with DCD experienced certain significant diffficulties in their planning and/or execution of movements at the microscopic level (at a time scale of half a second or less). In the future, clearer understanding of the planning, organization and execution of movements by children with DCD at the microscopic level of motion may have far-reaching implications for therapeutic training methods to help them maximize the efficiency of their movements and consequently minimize the difficulties that they experience with the manipulation of objects in daily living, such as when eating. This detailed approach offers a positive new methodology for investigating the planning and execution of movement in both typical and atypical development although clearly further larger and more detailed studies are essential before the total value of the methodology can be evaluated.

In sum, a number of classic as well as more novel techniques have been used to investigate the movement production problems of childen with

DCD. These studies suggest that a crucial deficit exists in the planning and control of action, and that this contributes to poor coordination. Furthermore, children with DCD have significant difficulty with the timing of both individual movements, and sequences of movements, when compared to their well coordinated peers. Taken together, such findings suggest that the difficulties of an individual with DCD could lie in the organization of certain timing dimensions of movement, with the cerebellum being a possible source of such problems.

Perceptual explanations

A third approach to the understanding of DCD has focused on the links between problems of perception and impairment of movement in an attempt to identify the specific information-processing deficits that might underlie the movement problems seen in the individual with DCD. In particular, specific deficits of visual and kinaesthetic perception have been suggested.

Visual perception

Adequate visual-perceptual input is crucial for accurate skilled movement. Visual perception is important so that distance and spatial relationships are perceived correctly and movements are guided accurately. Charles Hulme and his colleagues have considered the issue of a deficit of visual-perceptual processing in children with DCD in order to assess the role that perceptual impairments may play in the difficulties of those with DCD. If it is the case that children with DCD cannot perceive a situation accurately, then their movement plan and its execution will be based on 'misinformation'. Indeed, the work of Hulme and his colleagues has shown evidence of wide-ranging deficits in the perceptual processing of visuospatial information in children with DCD.

Hulme and his colleagues (Hulme et al., 1982; Hulme, Smart and Moran, 1982) based their research on the premise that there are three distinct perceptual systems which must each function appropriately before successful interaction can occur between the systems. Specifically, these three systems are: (1) a visual-perceptual system, (2) a kinaesthetic-perceptual system, and (3) an inter-sensory system linking vision and kinaesthesis (kinaesthesis provides information concerning body schema through internal information).

Hulme et al. (1982) showed that children with DCD had significantly poorer visual *and* kinaesthetic perception than their typically developing peers when children were required to match the length of lines presented successively both within and between the visual (V) and kinaesthetic

(K) modalities. Line matching occurred in four conditions: V-V, K-K, V-K, K-V. In the visual modality the child saw a line, while in the kinaesthetic modality the child felt the length of a rod. The initial stimulus was then removed from vision/touch prior to matching. Motor skill correlated significantly with accuracy of line length matching in the visual, but not in the kinaesthetic only or cross-modality matching conditions. This finding suggested that difficulties in the visual perception of distance and spatial relationships may be an important determinant of the poor motor coordination experienced by children with DCD. Alteratively visual-perceptual deficits and motor performance may be linked because they depend upon the same cause, rather than being linked directly themselves.

Before proceeding with further details of later studies conducted by Hulme and his colleagues, it is necessary to draw attention to two issues arising from the study described above. First, the experimental design fails to rule out the possibility of a memory impairment leading to the observed performance, though this explanation has been eliminated by a later study in which children were required to match lines presented simultaneously (Hulme, Smart and Moran, 1982). In addition, visual acuity difficulties were not investigated in the Hulme et al. (1982) study, though again these were ruled out in a later study (Lord and Hulme, 1987a), as well as by Mon-Williams, Pascal and Wann (1994) and Mon-Williams and colleagues (1996) using a different paradigm.

In a later study, Lord and Hulme (1987a) examined the range of the visual-spatial perception deficits that had been reported previously in children with DCD. In this study, size constancy judgements, visual discrimination of shape, area and slope were made by children with DCD and their typically developing controls to visually presented stimuli. Children with DCD performed significantly worse than controls on all but the shape discrimination measure. As a result, Lord and Hulme proposed that visuospatial deficits contribute to serious problems of motor control. They place this deficit within an information-processing framework of motor control suggesting that visual-perceptual ability is involved in most motor skills and that dysfunction at this level of the motor control hierarchy has a knock-on effect: If initial perceptual input is poor then accurate decision making about movement cannot occur. Furthermore a visuospatial deficit is likely to decrease the chances of error detection and correction during a motor activity, leading to inefficient or inaccurate output being executed.

In a study that focused on how children with abnormalities in motor development remember movements, Skorji and McKenzie (1997) reported that the memory of children with DCD when imitating movements modelled by the experimenter was more dependent upon visuospatial rehearsal than the memory of typically developing children, providing further evidence for the involvement of a visuospatial impairment in DCD. Inevitably the process between visual-perceptual input and motor output is a complex one, making it difficult to untangle the exact level at which the system breaks down.

The probable complexity of the route between visual-perceptual input and motor effector output is highlighted further in a study by Lord and Hulme (1988b). In this study, the role of visual-perceptual ability in drawing was assessed in relation to the issue of whether a visual-perceptual deficit is the cause of DCD. Children with DCD and controls completed tasks of visual discrimination (identifying two stimuli as 'same' or 'different'), tracing and drawing with and without vision. Visual-perceptual ability correlated with drawing ability *only* in the DCD group, a finding which the authors explained in terms of visual-perceptual function influencing motor performance *only* if the former skill is poor, hence the significant correlation between visual-perceptual and drawing abilities in the DCD, but not the control children.

To summarize the work on visual-perceptual ability and its relation to motor output in children with DCD, the findings are difficult to interpret convincingly, perhaps owing to the probable complexity of the processing stages occurring between the visual-perceptual modality and motor output assessed in these studies. In a recent meta-analysis to identify information processing factors that characterize DCD, Wilson and McKenzie (1998) analysed 50 studies, reporting that the greatest observed deficit was in visual-spatial processing, irrespective of whether or not tasks involved a motor component. It is also possible that the problems of children with DCD may arise from an abstract problem of understanding spatial coordinates, which is not tied to any one modality. This would lead to problems with visuospatial tasks, although the problem is not actually in the visual system, it is equally present in other sensory systems, e.g. tactile or vestibular. A valuable focus for future research will be to consider cross-sensory interactions in individuals with DCD.

Kinaesthetic perception

An alternative perceptual explanation of the difficulties experienced by children with DCD has focused on kinaesthetic sensitivity. Like vision, kinaesthetic perception (sense of position in space and movement of the body and limbs) is a crucial source of movement activity. (One point of difference between some researchers is the use of the words 'kinaesthesis' and 'proprioception'. Strictly speaking, proprioception is a broader term used to cover all sensory systems involved in providing information about position, location, orientation and movement of the body and its parts.

Certain authors use the two terms somewhat interchangeably. In the current chapter the term kinaesthesis is preferred, but where authors have used the term proprioception, their definition of the term will be described.) Imagine yourself catching a ball. An important aspect of this task is an appreciation of the fact that the environment is constantly changing as the ball moves closer to you. Movements of the eyes, head, arms and hands must be coordinated and synchronized with the movement of the ball, if it is to be caught. To be successful at this task it is critical that you have an intact and accurate sense of kinaesthesis. If this is inadequate or nonexistent then you will fail the task, the ball will be missed and, doubtless, you will experience a certain degree of embarrassment.

One does not tackle the task of catching a ball as a novice each time that we come back to it. In fact, preparation for catching is essential. We learn quickly that we can anticipate the stance and position that we must adopt in advance of the ball arriving into our hands. An experienced catcher will take up this position for both body and hands before the ball has been thrown, adapting these once the trajectory of the ball becomes evident. This latter task requires an understanding of time and space so that the eye can be coordinated with the trajectory of the ball. The catcher must be sensitive to time in order that the hands will be opened, not only in the right part of space, but also at the right moment in order to catch the ball accurately.

It can be seen that a task such as catching a ball seems fairly simple to a person with intact kinaesthetic perception (provided conditions such as the size or visibility of the ball are adequate), but that it may be a task of extreme difficulty for somebody who has a deficit of kinaesthetic perception. Such an individual would have great difficulty predicting where to place their hands in order to catch the ball successfully.

Kinaesthesis is an internal source of information, being compiled from information collated from the four classes of kinaesthetic receptors (joint receptors, tendon organs, muscle spindles and skin receptors). This process produces a global perception of movement and position by indicating the relative position of body parts and by providing sensory information about the extent, direction, speed and force of movements. Consequently kinaesthesis is involved in the efficient acquisition and performance of motor skills (Laszlo and Bairstow, 1983). DCD may, then, be related to a deficit in the kinaesthetic receptors or in the processing of information from these receptors. This could give rise to the motor difficulties of children with DCD since they may be basing their movements on inaccurate cues, leading to less accurate motor plans being formulated, muscles being activated inappropriately and inaccurate feedback being provided. Inevitably this becomes a circular problem with poor motor input leading to inaccurate feedback and vice versa.

Judith Laszlo and her colleagues have investigated their suggestion of a deficit of kinaesthetic perception through the development of their 'Kinaesthetic Sensitivity Test' (KST; Laszlo and Bairstow, 1985b). The KST is divided into two parts; the first a test of kinaesthetic acuity and the second a test of kinaesthetic perception and memory. The equipment for the *Kinaesthetic Acuity Test* is placed on a tabletop in front of the child and involves two ramps, which can be positioned at angles from the horizontal. On each ramp is a peg which can be slid up and down the ramp. A masking box is placed over the equipment. Each trial proceeds in the following way: the slope of each ramp is altered, with the slopes of the two ramps differing for each trial, ensuring that one slope is steeper (termed 'higher' in the test instructions) than the other. Children place a hand on each peg (under the masking box). The experimenter moves a child's hands simultaneously up the ramps and down again, after which the child indicates which hand was 'higher'. Thus the child is required to discriminate the heights of two inclined runways and the test is described as measuring the ability to discriminate limb position following passive movement, something which Laszlo and Bairstow claim to be dependent upon kinaesthetic sensitivity.

The test of *Kinaesthetic Perception and Memory* is a pattern representation task, in which a child must restore a displayed pattern to the orientation the pattern had when previously traced. Children's hands are guided (in the absence of vision) around an arbitrary shape, after which the experimenter alters the orientation of that shape. Vision is restored to the child who must then return the shape to its original configuration. Thus, the child must integrate kinaesthetic and visual information (a crossmodal task) in order to complete the task correctly, a requirement that makes the test of kinaesthetic perception and memory a test of higher kinaesthetic processes. For both the tests of Kinaesthetic Acuity and of Kinaesthetic Perception and Memory, Laszlo and Bairstow (1985b) provide normative data derived from the study of British and Australian children as well as of Australian and Canadian adults. Performance improves with age with children aged 12 years performing approximately similarly to adults on Kinaesthetic Acuity. On the Kinaesthetic Perception and Memory test the performance of children aged 12 years is superior to that of younger children but substantially poorer than that of the adult normative sample. Laszlo and colleagues (1988) reported that children with DCD perform worse than their typically developing peers on both tests.

Unfortunately, while the results of Laszlo's work with the KST have been replicated at least partially (see Piek and Coleman-Carman, 1995), many others have failed to find significant difficulties on either part of the KST (Hoare and Larkin, 1991; Lord and Hulme, 1987b). Using this particular kinaesthetic test, it is therefore difficult to ascertain whether a difficulty with kinaesthetic perception is related to DCD. As Wann (1991) has argued, there are certain flaws present in many tests claiming to measure kinaesthesis, for example, most are based around a series of static judgements and therefore measure proprioception rather than kinaesthesis, many impose a memory load, and those where the limbs are not placed in matched orientations measure the egocentric mapping of proprioceptive cues, rather than proprioceptive sensitivity per se. However, some form of kinaesthetic deficit may account for the uncomfortable and inefficient postures and actions generally adopted by children with DCD, who may not be able to 'feel' that a posture is awkward (because of some dysfunction in the kinaesthetic system; Cantell, Smyth and Ahonen, 1994; Hill, 1998; Smyth and Mason, 1997; 1998). It is a possibility of course that a posture which looks and would be uncomfortable for the motorically unimpaired person does not feel uncomfortable to an individual with DCD.

A number of researchers have attempted to investigate the issue of a kinaesthetic deficit in DCD in other ways. T.R. Smyth has conducted a series of studies using chronometric techniques in order to investigate the visual and kinaesthetic processing of children with DCD. In a reaction time study which investigated the processing of visual and kinaesthetic information, Smyth and Glencross (1986) found that abnormal coordination was associated with difficulty in processing kinaesthetic but not visual information, providing evidence for a specific deficit in DCD. Later studies in the same series have also identified a kinaesthetic deficit in DCD (Smyth, 1994; 1996). In addition, these two studies manipulated the experimental set-up further in order to investigate the nature of the kinaesthetic deficit. The results of these simple and choice reaction time tasks provided evidence to suggest that abnormal motor coordination was not the result of poor motor programming (Smyth, 1994). A possible explanation lies in a difficulty in the cross-modal translation of information (Smyth, 1996), a finding supported by Piek and Coleman-Carman (1995) who reported that Laszlo and Bairstow's test of Kinaesthetic Acuity discriminated between children with DCD and controls *only* when administered actively, and not when administered passively as stated in the test manual.

Further evidence of a kinaesthetic or proprioceptive deficit in DCD has come from studies adopting a target location and pointing task reported initially by von Hofsten and Rösblad (1988). These authors use the term proprioception to mean information about the body obtained from receptors located most noticeably in the joints, muscles and tendons. This test assesses the use of visual, proprioceptive and visual + proprioceptive information. The child sits at a table, on which is placed a circle made of a number of points marked with pins. The task is to place a pin under the table at the correct point which 'matches' the location of a specified pin on the tabletop. In this way, proprioception is measured as the ability to use information obtained through touch. The child either sees (intramodal), feels (intermodal) or sees and feels the pin on the tabletop before sticking a pin under the table in the corresponding location. Studies by Smyth and Mason (1998) and Sigmundsson and colleagues (e.g. Sigmundsson, 1999; Sigmundsson, Ingvaldsen and Whiting, 1997) have shown that children with DCD perform more poorly in terms of absolute error on both inter- and intramodal matching. In the case of the Sigmundsson studies this result was explained as arising from the particularly poor performance of the children with DCD when performing with the nonpreferred hand. Smyth and Mason focused more on a comparison between the matching conditions, reporting that when the conditions were analysed together, performance in the proprioceptive-only condition was significantly worse than that observed in the visual and visual-proprioceptive conditions, which themselves were not different from one another. This result, like those reported in the series of studies by T.R. Smyth suggest that it is when kinaesthetic (or proprioceptive) processing is required in isolation from visual processing that performance difficulties in this domain occur for children with DCD. Mon-Williams, Wann and Pascal (1999) conducted a series of cross-modal matching tasks, finding that the particular difficulty of those with DCD was in making cross-modal judgements that required the use of visual information to guide proprioceptive judgements of limb position, providing further evidence that proprioceptive skill may be a problem for those with DCD.

To summarize, although it does seem that there is at least some kind of kinaesthetic processing difficulty in DCD, no clear picture has transpired. Taking the studies together, the only clear point that emerges is summarized neatly by Hoare and Larkin (1991) who state that kinaesthesis is a

> global, multi-modal construct, and task specifics may dictate many of the relationships between this and motor ability in both clumsy and normal children. (Hoare and Larkin, 1991, p. 677)

It is clear that more detailed, theory-driven experimental manipulations are needed before reliable conclusions can be drawn.

Evaluation of perceptual explanations

Unfortunately neither the visual-perceptual nor the kinaesthetic explanations of DCD have withstood fully the test of time. Replication of both the work of Charles Hulme and particularly of Judith Laszlo has failed frequently to repeat their results (e.g. Barnett and Henderson, 1992; Henderson, Barnett and Henderson, 1994; Hoare and Larkin, 1991). Owing to the diverse methodologies adopted in the visual and kinaesthetic literatures, it would be useful in a future study to assess the effect of visual vs. kinaesthetic training in an intervention study, to investigate whether training in one modality has a beneficial effect compared to the other. Laszlo's kinaesthetic training could be given to one group, while another could be given visual-perceptual training, using a visual spot-the-difference task, for example.

It is unlikely that either a visual or a kinaesthetic deficit is the single contributing factor to DCD. An alternative explanation is that the sensory systems (e.g. visual, vestibular, kinaesthetic) may be interlinked in order to provide accurate spatial information, and that without each component of the system being intact, the system cannot operate accurately (Henderson, 1993).

Summary

Undoubtedly, children with DCD experience significant difficulties with fine and gross motor control, the planning and execution of movement and visuospatial skill. Unfortunately, the question of why children with movement difficulties have such problems remains unanswered. One drawback of the research to date is that it assumes that the functional architecture of the motor system is invariant across typically developing children and those with DCD. It would seem more likely that this is not the case, owing to the possible abnormality of processes such as visual-perceptual development from birth. This would have long-term consequences for motor development. Such a deficit would have implications for development from infancy onwards because acquisition of function must depend at least in part on the adequate development of skills which have developed earlier in the developmental process. In this case, poor perceptual-motor skills may be related to mild perceptual-motor dysfunction early in development which has interfered with the development of more complex motor skills. If this is the case, the relationship between perceptual-motor difficulty and DCD may arise not only from impaired perceptual-motor difficulty at the time of assessment, but also from the impaired acquisition of perceptual-motor skills during development. Furthermore, little research has been conducted investigating aspects of postural control in those with DCD (see Johnston et al., 2002, for an exception).

Considering the prevalence of motor difficulties in a range of developmental disorders, with estimates of DCD alone ranging from 6 to 10 per cent (American Psychiatric Association, 1994 and World Health Organisation, 1992a respectively), it is imperative that further understanding of the motor difficulties seen in these disorders must be obtained. The greatest challenge and avenue for progression in understanding DCD will be to identify and develop a theoretical and functional cognitive framework. Causal modelling of the links between behaviour, cognition and biology (see Morton, 2004) will be invaluable to this end (see Figure 3.7). Without such a framework, intervention studies and practical day-to-day management of DCD will continue to be variable in its success and the problems of self-esteem will continue to be felt more fully than is optimal. Despite the difficulties associated with the investigation of motor skill development, the development of such an understanding must not be ignored.

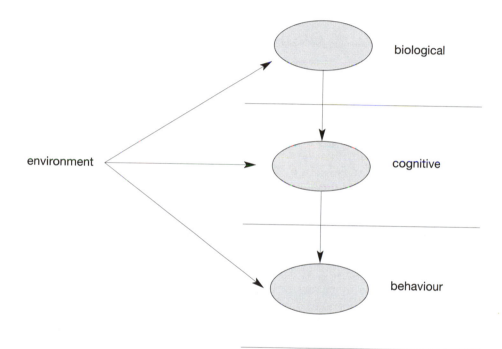

Figure 3.7 Illustration of the causal modelling approach.

CHAPTER 4

A dynamical systems perspective of Developmental Coordination Disorder

MICHAEL G. WADE, DAN JOHNSON AND KRISTI MALLY

Introduction

Developmental Coordination Disorder (DCD) is an established clinically diagnosed condition representing approximately 6 per cent of children. It is reliably identified by parents and teachers, and treated to some degree by occupational and physical therapists and other trained professionals. All of these individuals seem to 'know it when they see it', and standardized tests such as the Movement ABC (Henderson and Sugden, 1992) and the TGMD (Ulrich, 1985) confirm these clinical descriptions. Identification and opportunities for delivering appropriate therapeutic interventions for the treatment of DCD have met with considerable success despite the limited understanding of the root cause of DCD. The underlying processes that constrain the expression of a normal range of motor skill behaviour are less well understood. Research on DCD has produced limited insights as to a reliable account of the observed behaviour. Henderson and Henderson (2002) noted 'the gulf between experimental studies of normal performance and studies of individuals diagnosed with DCD seems wide and deep'. Scholars in Europe and less so in North America have addressed both the theoretical and empirical issues regarding the underlying processes which account for the observed clinical behaviours presented by individuals diagnosed with DCD. This can at times be both challenging and frustrating because children with DCD often exhibit unremarkable skill levels for tasks such as reaching, grasping, walking etc., but experience considerable difficulty with more complex activities such as using scissors to cut out patterns; using a knife and fork; catching a ball etc., in other words activities where the demand characteristics require either more complex coordination and control, or attentional effort, or both. Not surprisingly children with DCD often have co-morbidity issues, one of which is attention deficit disorder (ADD), which adds further to the challenges of seeking an explanation for the diagnosis.

The contributions made by information-processing (IP) theory are well represented in this volume in the chapters by Geuze and Hill. It is hoped that presenting a dynamical systems perspective will provide a contrast to the information-processing orientation. The contributions that the IP perspective has made to our broad understanding of skill acquisition across the lifespan are substantial. This chapter tries to provide a different theoretical approach which is commonly referred to as dynamical systems (DS) theory. In order to make appropriate contrasts between information-processing theory and dynamical systems theory the authors have, throughout this chapter, compared the different styles of enquiry and also critically reviewed and analysed some of the constraints of the IP theoretical orientation as well as the difficulties that *all* investigators are challenged with when conducting scientific enquiry on developmental coordination disorders. This chapter presents an overview of dynamical systems, provides a critical review of information-processing research related to DCD, tackles some of the inherent problems in measurement, and contrasts measurement styles in the information processing domain with the kinds of experiments and dependent variables used from an ecological dynamic systems perspective. Towards the end of the chapter a review of some of the current work employing dynamical systems theory is presented followed by some suggestions for future research. Where appropriate there is a comparison between both theoretical orientations in order to emphasize the essential differences of the two approaches.

Primer on dynamical systems

The extant published research encompasses broad theoretical approaches that include standard information-processing models; motor deficits seen as a neurological dysfunction focusing on comparisons between both cerebella and basal ganglia function. More recently, efforts to exploit the dynamical systems approach to better understand coordination and control deficits in individuals with DCD have appeared in the literature.

For those unfamiliar with the dynamical systems orientation, it incorporates ideas from the ecological psychology proposed by James J. Gibson (1979) and the notion of coordination dynamics proposed by the Russian physiologist Nikolai Bernstein (1967). Implicit in DS research is the assumption that objects and their potential for action are directly perceived via what Gibson (1979) refers to as affordances, which he defines as 'a specific combination of the properties of its substance and its services taken with reference to the animal.' (Gibson, 1977). This information is used to organize action within the context of the task demands and the environment in which the activity is to occur. The majority of fundamental motor skills we can all perform with relative ease, including individuals diagnosed with DCD. It seems that skills requiring more complex manipulations are a challenge for children with DCD. The DS perspective views these activities within the context of a possible difficulty in directly perceiving the affordance of the task and assembling the necessary coordination and control dynamics in order to harness the degrees of freedom demanded for successfully executing the task. The central departure here is that the mechanisms that enable skilful behaviour are not viewed so much as specific internal mechanisms or devices, but more the systems ability (or inability) first to perceive the affordance and then to self-organize action as a function of environment, task and the individual performing the activity. This assumes that any skilful activity is a direct result of the interaction between task, performer and environment (Newell, 1986, Keogh and Sugden, 1985). By way of introduction, a good starting point would be the philosophical basis of the information-processing approach which dominated cognitive science through much of the twentieth century and from which dynamical systems theory is a radical departure.

The seventeenth-century philosophers Descartes and Locke influenced much of twentieth-century behavioural and biological scientific enquiry. Descartes and Locke promoted the separation of body and mind (dualism) which argued for either an exogenous or an endogenous referent that controls or generates the periodic profile evident in living systems. This view influenced not only research on coordination and control, but also much of the sciences of modern psychology, biology and neuroscience. The notion of an internal referent or comparator, which either imposes order or controls action, has been the hallmark of much of the research on human and animal behaviour over the past 50 years.

The study of complex systems in physical biology and its application to research on the coordination and control of human movement offer a very different paradigmatic view of how action and motor skills might be organized and executed. The study of complex systems applies the mathematics of nonlinear dynamics and thermodynamics and proposes that the many and varied elements that make up the universe exhibit a capacity to self-organize in response to state changes. More importantly, the same ideas may apply equally well to patterns of behaviour and not only to molecules and cells. Kelso (1988), in referring to the term 'complexity', noted the following in regard to the emergence of complex behavioural patterns:

> From our point of view ... the mapping of complex patterns of behavior onto lower-dimensional laws may be even more crucial as we consider those 'typically biological' features of physical systems – their ability to

perceive, coordinate actions, memorize, learn, and anticipate – including intentional and linguistic aspects. (Kelso, 1988, p. 4)

The idea that coordination arises via the system self-organizing rather than being a slave to a central executive is appealing because it offers an opportunity to resolve what is now commonly referred to as 'Bernstein's Problem'. The Russian physiologist Nikolai Bernstein, whose work was first published in English in 1967, remarked that the richly varied coordination movements exhibited by people and animals possessed a simplicity of control despite the enormous complexity of the nervous system involved and the environment in which all of this activity took place. To Bernstein this simplicity was derivable from low-dimensional informative structures; and the paradox faced by scientists interested in explaining coordination is in the lawful restrictions on the behavioural degrees of freedom as a basis for the infinite number of qualitative distinctions among coordination patterns. Periodicity or rhythmicity has long been recognized as characteristic of both living systems and the living universe itself. Coordination (i.e. the bringing of parts into proper relations) is a complex problem of organization. The human body consists of approximately 10^2 joints, 10^3 muscles and 10^{14} cells. How all the degrees of freedom for any human action are coordinated is an insurmountable problem if viewed from a computational perspective. Over the past 25 years, considerable research effort has been directed towards explaining the coordination and control of movement. Generally, the IP approach has been to assume an intelligent executive (the 'ghost in the machine') that must unavoidably become more intelligent as the magnitude of the coordination problem grows! The alternative approach, influenced by the study of complex systems, argues that coordination is influenced by the properties of nonlinear systems. Thus, to provide a description of the principles that underlie coordination, research has focused on examining low-dimensional regularities that have lawful properties and low-dimensional informative structures (optic and haptic invariants) (Turvey, 1990).

Solving problems of coordination in intact normal systems is challenging, but seeking an account for the atypical motor behaviour of children diagnosed with DCD adds to the challenge. Descriptive information on atypical development in the standard terminology both of psychology and movement science is well known (e.g. slower rates of task acquisition, higher variability in performance, uneven strategic development, slower reaction time, etc.). Scientists have only recently begun investigating the capacity of an atypical individual to exhibit self-organizing behaviours relative to problems of control and coordination. Standard descriptive accounts usually point to neurological damage of one kind or another, and inferences are then made regarding an impaired capacity to 'compute' acceptable solutions to the problems posed by movement skills that require coordination and control (see Keele and Ivry, 1990; Williams, Woollacott and Ivry, 1992). As an alternative, the DS approach seeks to determine whether or not the low-dimensional regularities that might account for the capacity to self-organize in intact living systems are present in atypical populations. This approach (i.e. searching for dynamic patterns in complex systems) attempts to describe atypical motor behaviour by examining the action system's capacity (or inability?) to exhibit the charac-teristics of preferred rhythmic stabilities. Thus a dynamical systems view of DCD may be grounded in a child's capacity to exhibit self-organization. This hypothesis needs to be tested and, if found reliable could lead to the development of clinical tools for use both in early detection and in the development of appropriate intervention strategies to address the prob-lem of DCD.

Research overview and criticism

Deficits in timing mechanism

Over the past 16 years the literature has been saturated with research focusing on problems associated with the timing of rhythmic movements. Timing research from an information-processing (IP) framework typically involves either a unimanual or bimanual rhythmic tapping task. The bulk of this work has consistently demonstrated that children with DCD are more variable in several aspects of timing, including movement time, reaction time, on target time and cycle interval time (Geuze and Kalverboer, 1987; 1994; Lundy-Ekman et al., 1991; Henderson, Rose and Henderson, 1992). Deficits in the mechanisms that control the timing of action may indeed be responsible for some of the difficulties experienced by children with DCD, and while much of the reported research refers to these 'deficits in the mechanisms', few studies sought to directly measure or isolate the targeted mechanism! One must exercise caution when pag-ing through the DCD timing literature as the claims by investigators are rarely consistent with respect to the methodology, the theoretical model and the results.

Neurological basis of timing and force variables

Lundy-Ekman et al. (1991) took the timing model proposed by Wing and Kristofferson (1973) one step further, using it to divide children with DCD into two groups; those with timing difficulties and those with force difficulties. They proposed that both internal and peripheral timing parameters were mapped onto the cerebellum, and that force parameters were mapped onto the basal ganglia. They hypothesized that DCD could therefore be sub-typed into a cerebellum group and a basal ganglia group as a function of both soft neurological signs and observed motor problems.

This study has several methodological problems. First was participant selection, whereby children were assigned to one of two groups based on either a soft cerebellum sign or soft basal ganglia sign, and a score at or below the 40th percentile on the Bruininks-Oseretsky Test (BOT) (1978). Some children in the original group displayed soft neurological signs, but scored too high on the BOT to be considered for this study. This suggests that clumsiness was likely not a prevalent characteristic shared by those labelled with soft neurological signs, which contradicted a central hypothesis of the study. The authors devoted significant journal space to 'warning' against the use of soft neurological tests, while ironically making strong conclusive statements using the results of these very same tests! Much of their theorizing was based on an earlier study (Ivry and Keele, 1989) which reported an association between a 'hard' neurological connection between the cerebellum and basal ganglia and motor problems, involving timing and force respectively. The Ivry and Keele study reflects the current World Health Organisation (WHO) definition of DCD. The *Classification of Diseases and Related Health Problems* (ICD-10; WHO) states that motor coordination difficulties observed in these children are not explicable in terms of any specific congenital or acquired neurological disorder. There appears to be little support for the claim that DCD could be divided into two specific groups based on the specific neural substrates.

Our cursory review of DCD research literature is illustrative of both the general deficiencies and the inherent challenges in the research. The deficiencies arise either from the difficulties unique to the study of atypical populations or from the methodologies employed in the investigations. Two difficulties related to the study of unique populations are apparent in the reviewed research. First, small samples of subjects are used in comparing DCD and non-DCD groups (e.g. Wann, Mon-Williams and Rushton, 1998). Although this no doubt arises from problems of subject procurement and diagnosis of subjects with DCD, it limits the validity of the findings. Second, the recurring problem of co-morbidity in DCD research makes efforts to identify specific underlying processes that contribute to the disorder a source of frustration. The presence of attention deficit hyperactivity disorder (ADHD) along with DCD is especially common, with estimates of co-morbidity as high as 65 per cent (Sugden and Wright, 1998). From a DS perspective, both the properties of the perception-action system and the attentional capabilities of individuals are significant elements in the emergence of coordinated movement. In fact, the interaction between the various system components is a necessary and sufficient condition for the self-organization of behaviour propagated by DS adherents. As such, it is reasonable to suggest that (a) a dynamical systems approach predicts the occurrence of the observed co-morbidity and (b) a non-traditional experimental approach, one that recognizes the interactions between system components, will be required to uncover underlying processes.

A more general problem in much of the DCD literature is a lack of innovation in the methodologies employed. Many studies of the characteristics and underlying causes of DCD are replications of studies conducted with non-DCD populations. Although these studies have been useful in comparing the performance of DCD children with other groups of children, they reveal little about the underlying processes that might contribute to DCD. In general, these studies have not used the more complex tasks needed to reveal the presence of a coordination disorder. For a particular experimental condition, the lack of task complexity may be evident in either the actual movement skill required of subjects or in the perceptual information made available to subjects, especially since it is generally agreed that it is the more complex coordination tasks which are the hallmark of DCD! The perception of organism–environment relations, an important informational constraint in the emergence of coordinated movement, involves the detection of higher-order informational patterns. In tightly controlled experimental settings, these patterns may not be available to subjects. As such, the studies may be criticized for lacking ecological validity; that is, they constrain the full expression of the normal, complex interactions between individuals and their environment. The DS perspective emphasizes that this might prevent the experimental observation of effects that result from the imposition of normal environmental constraints on the movement system.

The research to date has largely examined the perceptual-motor component of DCD from an information-processing approach: sensory information viewed as input, followed by motor response as output. It is assumed that disruption occurs in the sequential processing of the information necessary to control movement, with the disruption targeted at either the processing stage or the execution of a motor response (Wilson and McKenzie, 1998). As a result, researchers have looked for the underlying causes of DCD in distinct perceptual or motor processes. The ecological view which is inherent in DS theory seeks a very different interpretation of the underlying mechanisms. In contrast to an information-processing approach, the ecological view holds that information from the senses is complete (direct) and does not require 'enhanced' association or representation (Gibson and Pick, 2000). If cognitive processing is not necessary for perception, the information available to the senses must be sufficient in itself to specify the facts of the environment (Turvey and Shaw, 1999).

Gibson (1966) described the detection of this information as 'recognizing subtleties of invariant stimulus information and the registering of concurrent co-variation from different sensory organs'.

The ecological approach emphasizes the reciprocity of perception and action, and thus it seems a mistake to view behaviour as separate components of perception, cognition and action and study them in isolation (Cisek, 1999). This is a radical departure from the distinct, sequential perception and action stages of the information-processing model. This coupling of perception and action is expressed by Gibson's (1966) statement that 'there is an output to perceptual systems and an input from motor systems'. Along with linking perception and action, an ecological perspective recognizes the interaction between the nervous system, the body and the environment, and that credit for adaptive behaviour cannot be assigned to any one part of this system (Chiel and Beer, 1997). Just as the perception and action systems are coupled within the organism, so is the organism coupled to the environment, and it is a mistake to separate the two (Cisek, 1999). If these levels of interaction exist, it is reasonable to question the value of measuring isolated perceptual skills in relation to coordination disorders. One may question therefore whether they are measurements at a meaningful level of organization.

Attempts to determine the role of perceptual ability in coordination disorders have often involved either the isolation of perception from motor action or the isolation of specific perceptual skills. The result, perhaps desirable in experimental settings, is a simplification of the perceptual demands on the participants. This may be misguided because such experimental designs may unintentionally eliminate the interactions that result in the problems associated with the disorder, i.e. patterns of information that occur across modalities or perception that may be dependent on motor output (Clark, 1999). To the extent that researchers eliminate these factors, they may be missing the significant expressions of the role of perception in DCD.

The study of visual perception in children with DCD provides an example of what may be a misguided approach. Deficits in visual perception have been considered a likely signature of DCD (Wilson and McKenzie, 1998). This is reasonable from an information-processing approach; a deficit in this ability would be expected to disrupt the processing chain that leads to coordinated motor action. As such, one would expect to find a strong relationship between visual perception deficits and DCD. This however is not the case, as studies have failed to clearly establish that a perceptual skill problem is an underlying cause of the disorder (Schoemaker et al., 2001). The failure to establish this connection may be a consequence of testing the effects of isolated skills without regard for more complex interactive effects. A DS approach neither assumes nor requires a direct causal relationship to be established because direct sequential processing of information is not a valid assumption. It may work for engineering models and computer machine language but perhaps not for complex coordination of natural biological motion.

The above criticisms apply in some degree to all theoretical persuasions. No approach is immune from the difficulties associated with a 'messy' disorder such as DCD. The authors do suggest, however, that the insights gained from dynamical systems and ecological interpretations of DCD will aid in the development of experimental approaches that might prove useful in the investigation of the 'tough' questions surrounding DCD.

Problems of measurement

The quality of a science is reflected in part by its capacity to measure and record particular phenomena reliably. It is also probably true to say that generating specific metrics for a particular set of phenomena is considered more 'sophisticated' than mere description. Unfortunately, in the study of movement patterns in children the measures used, particularly by those imbued with either of Cronbach's (1957) two psychologies, have relied more on product measures. This has constrained the development of explanations for the observable changes in the movement patterns of children.

Error scores per se record only the variability of the performer to complete an action accurately. This kind of measurement offers only limited inference about the process that underlies motor skill development. In fact, an error score may sometimes misrepresent the process by which it was achieved! While it is recognized that the product (outcome) is usually what is important in the real world, an understanding of the process is required for explanations of the regularity observed in the development of control and coordination in children. The traditional product (task) approach to the study of motor development is founded on some rather tenuous assumptions. First, there is the assumption that the investigator has selected a valid task that accurately represents a wide range of other skills, and second, that experimental results of performance on this task (measured by error scores) can be generalized to other skills. This approach tends to use tasks in which the measurement of movement through kinematic methods is not always practical, so that often limited information is gleaned about how the performer produced the movement (Schmidt, 1988b). This approach is less concerned with the process that generated the performance than with how the skill is learned. Thus the relationship between product and process is not readily apparent. Here, process is inferred by outcome, logical but often speculative. On the other hand, the process-oriented approach is interested only in the underlying structure of motor performance. A focus on internal processes that are not directly observable requires more exotic methodology that records limb movement or movement of the entire body, and/or electromyographic recordings of the electrical activity of muscle during a skilled response. Inference is still part of the theorizing but is supported by more than scores of a target outcome.

Measurement and the ecological approach to motor development

Traditional theories of motor development, be they neural-maturational (e.g. Gesell, 1946; McGraw, 1945) or cognitive perspectives (e.g. Piaget, 1952) are based on a class of concepts one could generally describe as prescriptive. These theories of the development of skill are anchored to the idea that representations (i.e. symbolic knowledge structures) existing within the central nervous system are fundamental to the control of action. Both views also assume that development of skill is due to the development of prescriptions for action at some level of representation. Skill is thought to emerge as a result of the maturation of the neuromuscular system. In other words, maturation leads to the unfolding of a predetermined pattern – that plans exist before the behaviour emerges. Such traditional theories would explain the onset of walking in children as a point at which the neuromuscular system had developed to a level where it could support such activity. Again, implicit in this view is that the potential for walking exists in the neural substrates in immature form until differentiation permits this prescriptive action to emerge.

These traditional ideas about the emergence of motor skills have been challenged from the DS perspectives of the development of control and coordination. A conceptual basis for these contemporary approaches is grounded in Gibson's (1966, 1979) ecological psychology, Kugler and Turvey's dynamical systems approach (Kugler and Turvey, 1987; Kugler, Kelso and Turvey, 1980; 1982) and Reed's (1982) theory of action. At the heart of these approaches is the idea that coordination and control emerge not from prescriptions for action, but as a consequence of the constraints imposed on action. Constraints reduce certain configurations of response dynamics with the resulting pattern of movement a reflection of the 'self-organizing optimality of the biological system', rather than specifications from prescriptive knowledge structures (Newell, 1986). The central dispute is about whether the order and regularity in motor development can be attributed to internal prescriptive representations of action (information processing) or to self-organizational characteristics of the biological system and its interaction with the environment. The differences between these two views of motor development lie not only in the interpretation of data, but also at the level of analysis (Schmidt, 1988b).

Measurement techniques nontraditional to the study of motor development are now being applied by those of the ecological persuasion in their examination of the processes of skill development. Investigators now realize the value in recording topological descriptions of behaviour, and are incorporating methodologies and techniques which permit such description. Kinematic measures employing motion analysis via digital video techniques are assisting investigators to expand the frontier of the ecological perspective of motor skill development. Thelen and Cooke (1987) used kinematic techniques in a study to investigate the relationship between the stereotyped movement pattern of infant stepping and the development of adult locomotion. Detailed video analysis and EMG data were employed to compare infant stepping with an adult gait pattern. They concluded that mature walking evolves from infant stepping, and that the gradual changes in the organization of the step during infancy may be evoked 'by the dynamic functional demands of up-right locomotion' (p. 392), in addition to the development of balance, postural control and strength. They also argued that the changes in the organization of gait during infancy must be explained as an emergent property of the dynamics of the system, with no need for recourse to centrally represented gait patterns to account for changes in locomotor behaviour. This approach to the study of motor development is the 'new kind of science' referred to by Turvey and Carello (1981) and it requires a new way to observe and record behaviour. With the advancement of this type of enquiry more sophisticated kinematic techniques and a greater reliance on topological description of movement are now the norm for the development of theoretical explanations for the processes that contribute to the emergence of skilled motor behaviour.

An important focus of the DS perspective is the individual's sensitivity to information in the environment relative to his or her actions, what constitutes information, and how the information is used to control movement. To describe the relationship between the animal and the environment in extrinsic metrics (e.g. recording diameter and height in metres or feet), and further to suggest that the child uses these extrinsic units to control behaviour, undermines the notion of ecological realism and is unacceptable (Turvey and Carello, 1981). Because, in this view, the actor and the environment are functionally inseparable units that are intrinsic to an organism–environment system and share common bases in both 'such that certain parts and processes of the system define the units in which other parts and processes are measured' (Turvey and Carello, 1981, p. 317). Extrinsic measures can be transformed into performer-scaled units by selecting the dimension of interest and transforming it into a body-scaled metric by dividing the dimension value by the performer value. This yields a body-scaled ratio in which the extrinsic values cancel, expressing an invariant person–environment relationship across persons of different body sizes (Davis and Burton, 1991). For example, Warren (1984) concluded that the stair-riser height requiring minimum energy expenditure should not be stated in terms of absolute (extrinsic) units; rather the optimal height is just about one quarter of the leg length for both tall and short climbers. By using this intrinsic measure, Warren concluded that the optimal riser height was constant over scale changes in the system. In a study of road-crossing behaviours in children and adults (Lee, Young and McLaughlin, 1984), the temporal gap between vehicles in a simulated (yet realistic) road-crossing task was scaled to the subjects by computing the ratio of this time gap and the actual time the subject needed to cross the street. This resulted in a performer-scaled metric in which a value of 1.0 afforded crossing the street. As a challenge one might ask if children with DCD can identify relevant environment dimensions scaled relative to the performer, such as those illustrated above. Answers to such questions would better help understand the interaction between actor and environment, and that this understanding is founded upon the realism of intrinsic measures. Individuals with DCD will have such 'body-scaled' or 'intrinsic' measures available but may not be sufficiently sensitive to them, or are not directly attentive to them! This will impact their ability to successfully acquire or express the complex skill activities which they currently find difficult to achieve.

Thus the DS perspective poses the following questions with respect to children diagnosed with DCD:

1. Can the DCD child demonstrate preferred rates of periodicity or rhythm?
2. Are these preferred rates stable across a relatively wide spectrum of vector fields?
3. If the boundaries of this field are exceeded, can the system reorganize at a new stable state?

The classic examples in quadrupeds are the four stages of coordination dynamics of the horse, namely walk, trot, canter and gallop. For humans walking and running are two different levels of biomechanical organization. The above might be important 'first steps' in determining the coordination and control states of children diagnosed with DCD.

How DS can assist in investigating DCD

As noted above, the use of error scores has limitations, and while the magnitude, direction and variability of errors provide insights regarding motor skill performance, error information as to how skill behaviour emerges from the developing organism is largely speculative. Rhythmicity, or periodicity, is a characteristic of most living systems and can be found at different levels of analysis: mechanical, physiological and biochemical, to name but three. There is a large body of evidence in the life sciences, in the study of human movement and in psychophysiology to demonstrate that such systems exhibit periodicity that responds to or reflects the essential interaction between the organism and its immediate environment. The study of biological clocks has a long history, as does the study of biochemical systems with their periodic characteristics of secretion. Within the contemporary field of kinesiology and the study of human movement, the dynamic systems approach has, as one of its key elements, the study of periodic activity. This can be demonstrated in several movement domains and while space does not permit an exhaustive review, a few instances will illustrate the point.

Earlier work from the authors' laboratory (Wade, 1973; Wade and Ellis, 1971; Wade, Ellis and Bohrer, 1973) examined the play and motor behaviour of groups of normal and mentally handicapped children in free play settings that manipulated both social group size and the complexity of the play environment. The research tested the hypothesis that a periodic relationship was predictable between a system that required chemical support for energy expenditure and renewal, and behavioural need to maintain a hypothesized optimal level of arousal. Periodicities were detected in the play behaviour of young children measured by continuously monitored heart rate, as well as corroborating observational data that reflected patterns that could be assigned to both cycles of energy expenditure (work/play) and habituation to a play environment that was modulated by levels of arousal. It is interesting to note that in a second study this characteristic periodicity found in the play of typical children was absent in a sample of mentally handicapped children (Wade, 1973). These early studies demonstrated that the interplay between the biochemical constraints of the system and the arousing properties of the environment couple in such a way as to emit measurable or detectable periodicities. Periodicity has also been detected in foetal motor activity. Robertson (1985) detected cyclic motor activity in the human foetus during the second half of pregnancy.

Investigating periodicity requires the collection of time series data and the use of Fourier transform and associated spectral analysis to reliably detect the existence of such periodic activity. While this is not a new technique, it is receiving increased empirical attention as equipment for recording continuous movement and the analytical capabilities of microcomputers improve. Periodicity is a particular characteristic of the temporal basis of activity that is relevant for studying developmental issues as well as general problems of control and coordination of motor skills. At one level, the absence of periodic behaviour in the organism over a range of movement behaviours may be an initial signature of dysfunction, to appear later as both cognitive and motor disabilities (Burton, 1990; Wade, 1973; 1990).

Central to Gibson's ecological approach to perception and action (Gibson, 1979) is the assumption that perceptual systems are coupled with action systems. David Lee and others (Bertenthal and Bai, 1989; Butterworth and Hicks, 1977; Lee, 1980; Lee and Aronson, 1974; Stoffregen, 1985) have all investigated the coupling between changes in perceptual information and the motor activity of the organism as reflected in the maintenance of upright posture and whole body sway. The results of these studies suggest that this coupling is a critical element of skilled activity. Thus, when recording levels of motor development in children, which are reflected in poor, average or enhanced levels of skilful behaviour (coordination and control), the periodicity exhibited may well reflect the sensitivity of the organism to this perception/action coupling.

Ecological psychology argues that periodicity of a different kind is demonstrated in the interplay between perception and action. Central to this ecological view is the notion that our perceptual systems rely on the activity of the organism in discovering and interacting with and within its environment, such that perception and action become equal partners in the life course of living systems. The coordination and control exhibited by the organism in interacting successfully with environmental demands are reflected in the periodic nature of living systems. Our earlier work demonstrated periodicities in the play activity of children; in a similar fashion, the dynamics of perception/action coupling, via ambient arrays from perceptual flow fields, may reflect our capacity to directly perceive information from the environment. A good example of this is the optical flow field generated by moving an enclosure backward or forward about a subject. Such movement specifies motion of self (ego-motion) to the subject. Just as periodicity emerges from the proposed epistemic system of the organism (Berlyne, 1960), which resonates on the physiological regulatory mechanisms to produce work/rest cycles in the organism, so might the dynamic properties of perception/action coupling of a living system demonstrate periodicity, as motion specified from the environment couples to the movement of the perceiving individual.

Stability

The dynamic properties of perception/action coupling demonstrated in children (Bertenthal and Bai, 1989; Lee and Aronson, 1974) and in adults (Stoffregen, 1985) represent another form of periodic behaviour. The correlation between the oscillation rate of the moving room and the sway motion of an individual in that room was high ($r = .7$; Stoffregen, 1985) and reliable. This oscillatory coupling is above postural threshold (0.1–0.3 Hz), and presumably the stability of this relation will be relatively constant across a range of values above threshold but below a breakdown point (chaos). A similar example might be a group of runners or joggers who couple to a preferred rate of stride cadence. This 'preferred' jogging rate may not be representative of any single person in the group, but represents a preferred rate or attractor about which fluctuations represented by each individual runner can be tolerated.

With respect to children diagnosed with DCD one might assume the general hypothesis that a periodicity principle operates as an attractor that is present in these individuals and would seek to determine if individuals with DCD would exhibit same or different periodic characteristics or levels of tolerance before breakdown.

Recent studies using dynamical systems

Volman and Geuze (1998) took the study of DCD in a different direction from that of the IP literature discussed thus far. Although they credited information-processing theorists with insightful attempts, they felt the IP approach failed to account for the spatiotemporal organization of patterns of movements. An alternative approach (dynamical systems) which refutes the notion that timing is regulated by a central timekeeper was to view the temporal pattern as an emergent property that was the result of the dynamic interaction between task, environment and performer (Newell, 1986). Volman and Geuze (1998) examined and compared the phase dynamics of rhythmical tapping tasks in children with DCD and matched controls. Results indicated that children with DCD had patterns of coordination that were less stable in anti-phase coordination compared to in-phase coordination. Further, DCD participants required more time to restore their initial pattern after a perturbation (Volman and Geuze, 1998). This latter finding might have ecological relevance because it suggests that children with DCD have more difficulty responding to small environmental perturbations. Volman and Geuze (1998) referred back to earlier findings of slower movements seen in children with DCD. This slower movement may be an intentional strategy (attractor state) in order to remain in a more stable state. Children with DCD may simply slow down in order to maintain control and coordination of a given task. Further it was suggested that DCD participants were having difficulty maintaining their posture and were unable to give the task their full attention. Such a hypothesis could direct research down an entirely different path; with an interest in not only the neuromotor difficulties, but also in the task demand and the context of the environment.

As noted above, caution must be exercised when reading the timing literature about DCD. Information-processing theory proposes problems with a 'central timekeeper'. The Volman and Geuze (1998) study suggests that children with DCD have less stable rhythmic coordination than their matched controls. A hierarchical timekeeper model cannot explain these stability differences, since these models fail to account for the inherent stability properties, such as the resistance to perturbations, or the loss of stability and phase transitions when frequency is increased (Volman and Geuze, 1998). A DS approach credits this reduced stability to a weaker coupling between rhythm units, and not to a specific locus of dysfunction at the neural level. The results of Volman and Geuze (1998) differed from those of Lundy-Ekman et al. (1991), because Volman and Geuze (1998) could not credit soft neurological signs related to cerebellum or basal ganglia as being associated with specific clumsy characteristics.

Although the DS approach is more holistic for studying the difficulties experienced by children with DCD, it has thus far been unable to unravel any specific information that could aid in the development of more effective assessment tools or treatment strategies. Certainly, deficits in the mechanisms that control the timing of action may be responsible for some of the difficulties experienced by children. However at present it remains simply a part of the larger interactive picture.

The role of vision

The role of vision in maintaining balance has been tested extensively using several paradigms including blurring participants' vision (Edwards, 1946), oscillating a cube around the participants' heads (Witkins and Wapner, 1950), and using a 'moving room' (Lee and Aronson, 1974). Wann, Mon-Williams and Rushton (1998) used Lee and Aronson's (1974) moving room paradigm to record the postural sway of children and adults. The 'Swinging Room' was a large box open at one end and at the bottom. The 'walls' facing the participants were covered with wallpaper. The room was suspended on a rope and swung freely (to a simple harmonic motion) to give the illusion that the participant was moving. The goal of their study was to examine the effect of optical flow on posture. Specifically, Wann, Mon-Williams and Rushton (1998) asked whether participants had the ability to maintain their equilibrium in the face of perturbations in optic flow information. They looked at two parts of the frequency response function: gain and phase. The term gain refers to the estimate of amplitude or energy transfer whereas phase refers to the estimation of transfer lag.

Six children with DCD from a neurodevelopmental therapy clinic participated. These children scored in the bottom fifth percentile when assessed with the Movement ABC (Henderson and Sugden, 1992). They had normal IQs and were at various stages of a therapeutic intervention programme. Three control groups were also used: typically developing children age-matched to the children with DCD, nursery-school children, and adults.

The room oscillated at three different amplitudes which were scaled differently for each group and corresponded to 40 per cent (a sway within their balance limits), 80 per cent (a sway at their balance limit), and 120 per cent (a sway beyond their balance limit) of the participants' foot size. Each participant stood in the room and was presented with eight trials. Of the eight trials, six consisted of two trials at each of the three amplitudes; one consisted of the room stationary, and one in which the participant was asked to close his/her eyes for the duration.

Measurements of posture were recorded as a function of head movement. When examined as a group, the children with DCD responded essentially the same as the age-matched controls. Wann, Mon-Williams and Rushton (1998) examined the individual responses of the children with DCD and found that the responses of two of the children in the DCD group were equivalent to their age-matched controls. When those two children were removed from the DCD group and the remaining four children were compared to the control, they found that children with DCD had higher gains across all conditions! Three of the children in the DCD group swayed with gains as high as the nursery school children. Two of the children swayed less when their eyes were closed than they did in the eyes-opened condition. This finding resembled the results found when using participants who had low vision (Wann, Mon-Williams and Rushton, 1998).

Since they were more influenced by the room oscillation than the other controls, nursery-school children appear to be more reliant on visual information to maintain balance. Vision appears more important to younger children than proprioceptive information. The variability in performance among children with DCD and the small sample size, make generalization of performance invalid, thus revealing little about the differences in both gain and sway amplitude between children with DCD and their age-matched controls.

New directions for DS research on DCD

So far, information that focuses on the nature of dependent variables used and the implications that they have for studying movement behaviour has been reviewed, as well as a discussion of two contrasting theoretical paradigms of movement behaviour. One adopts an ecological stance and studies movement development more from an emergent properties perspective (dynamical systems) and the other takes a more traditional view and seeks to understand the acquisition of motor skills via a more computational learning perspective (information processing). Both approaches have made contributions to our understanding of how movement develops in children. The rapid advance in technology made available in the past decade suggests that this progress will only accelerate in the future. What is certainly true is that each perspective requires a fundamentally different style of enquiry.

As noted above, DS theory relies on a crucial philosophical point of departure; namely, a commitment to realism, which eliminates the Lockean notion of ideas and promotes a direct relation between the organism and the environment. Thus, for the realists, the model construct for the development of coordination and control is that it is autonomous, self-organizing and possesses no 'between things'.

With respect to the perceptual abilities of children with DCD, information-processing research has focused on deficits in visuospatial, kinaesthetic, and cross-modal processing across a number of motor control operations (Wilson and McKenzie, 1998). No clear causal relationship has emerged from the research to date. Although several studies have described deficits in various perceptual skills, in each case the causal relationship has been questioned in subsequent research (Sugden and Wright, 1998). From a dynamical systems perspective, DCD may be described as an expression of deficits associated with the ability to detect relevant perceptual information – specifically in the ability to detect or differentiate higher-order patterns of information across modalities. This stands in contrast to the view that DCD may be explained in terms of deficits in the processing of specific modalities of sensory information.

In their meta-analysis of information-processing deficits associated with DCD, Wilson and McKenzie (1998) reported on 50 studies, which included 983 children with DCD and 987 control children. Meta-analysis was used to determine the relative importance of proposed perceptual deficits, compared to the magnitude of the deficits. The following findings were reported:

1. Motor impaired children were inferior on almost all measures of information processing.
2. Perceptual deficits existed independent of motor problems, and effects were significant even when a motor response was not involved.
3. Performance (time) pressure was not necessary for deficits to be displayed.
4. Visuospatial deficits showed the strongest effect, even without motor response.
5. Kinaesthetic and cross-modal effects involving motor responses were moderate.

The authors concluded that visuospatial processing is implicated in DCD, although a causal role cannot be established. Both kinaesthetic and cross-modal perceptions were found to be inferior in children with DCD, but the authors indicated the need to test their effects without contamination from a motor response.

Visual-proprioceptive matching ability was studied in a group of 29 children with DCD and a control group of 29 children selected from the same classes at school (Mon-Williams, Wann and Pascal, 1999). The children with DCD made more errors than the control group in tasks involving spatial matching (unseen hand to a seen location) and limb matching (one limb to the other unseen limb). The DCD group also seemed to lack the advantage that the control group gained from having vision of one limb. In contrast to the control group, the children with DCD made the most errors on a visual-proprioceptive spatial matching task, indicating difficulty in making cross-modal judgements. In one proprioceptive limb-matching task, the DCD children's performance became worse when visual information was added, while the control group's performance improved under the same conditions. The authors concluded that cross-modal judgements assisted skill acquisition, and that some DCD children were unable to make these judgements. They also recommend further research into the effect of redundant information on the performance of children with DCD.

The processing of visual, proprioceptive and tactile information was investigated in 19 children with DCD and 19 age- and sex-matched control children (Schoemaker et al., 2001). Visual perception was tested using the Developmental Test of Visual Perception, tactile perception was assessed with the Tactual Performance Test, and the ability to use proprioceptive information was tested using a manual pointing task developed by von Hofsten and Rösblad (1988). The children with DCD performed significantly worse than the control group on all tests of visual-motor integration. On tests of motor-induced perception, two out of four subtests did not reach significance – form constancy and figure-ground, while two subtests were found significant – position in space and visual closure. Children with DCD performed slightly below the norm for tactile perception. On the manual pointing tasks, the children with DCD were more inconsistent in their responses whether they could use visual, proprioceptive, or visual-proprioceptive information. It was concluded that no consistent pattern of deficits exists in the DCD children, which is consistent with the heterogeneous nature of the disorder, and that no causal relation exists between motor and perceptual impairments. Furthermore, the authors suggested that the motor component contributed more to poor performance than the perceptual component.

Henderson, Barnett and Henderson (1994) attempted to replicate and extend the findings of Lord and Hulme (1987a) who had identified visuospatial deficits as a likely cause of clumsiness. Sixteen children with motor difficulties and 16 matched controls were assessed on the Test of Motor Impairment, various graphic tasks, and a measure of visuospatial discrimination. The clumsy children performed significantly poorer than the control group on a test of visuospatial discrimination, but no relationship was found between the magnitudes of the perceptual and motor impairments. When visual feedback was withheld in graphic copying tasks, the superior performance of the control group did not diminish, indicating that superior performance was not specifically dependent on a difference in visuospatial skill. The authors suggested that the defective processes in clumsy children may not be modality-specific, and that previous experiments by Lord and Hulme (1987a) that claimed to establish visuospatial deficits as the likely cause of motor impairments were of fundamentally inappropriate design.

Newnham and McKenzie (1994) investigated the cross-modal transfer of shape information between modalities by clumsy children. Eighteen clumsy children and 18 non-clumsy children were compared in their ability to transfer sequential shape information between the haptic and visual modalities in a matching-to-sample task. In the cross-modal matching of a haptic standard to a visual shape, the clumsy children were not significantly different from the non-clumsy group. In the matching of a visual (V) standard to a haptic (H) shape, the clumsy children made consistently faster and less accurate responses. For intramodal performance (V-V or H-H), there was no significant difference between the groups. The authors suggested that deficits in a specific visual to haptic translation process involving poor visual memory might be present in the clumsy children.

The central issue from a dynamical systems perspective is the systems sensitivity to the available perceptual information. The two key systems here are vision and touch (haptics). There is a growing body of promising research particularly concerning haptics that suggests that in much the same way as the visual system detects motion via optical flow, so the haptic correlate of this is an individual's ability to make judgements about the length and use of objects wielded freely in spaces, e.g. Carello and Turvey (2000). Such information is derived from the moment of inertia about the fulcrum of the activity, namely the wrist, in such a way that individuals can accurately describe, via the 'tensor', both the length and size characteristics of implements that they wield without directly observing them. Further accurate judgements are possible about the potential use that these objects hold for action. Visual perception beyond sensitivity to optical flow (Lee, 1980) includes sensitivity to coordination dynamics expressed via such protocols as point-light displays.

The ecological-dynamical systems perspective recognizes that organisms exist as part of a larger, self-organizing system. While not denying that individual internal processes contribute to the functioning of the organism, it is suggested that the investigation of properties arising from interactions between the organism and its environment hold considerable promise for discovering the underlying dynamics of coordination disorders. This approach motivates two distinct but related directions for future research: one focuses on the role of ecologically relevant perceptual information in constraining action, the other on the underlying dynamics common to all complex biological systems.

Gibson's ecological psychology, with its emphasis on the detection of information that specifies relations between the organism and its environment (affordances), provides a conceptual framework for uncovering the perceptual processes relevant to the development of coordination. Indeed, the ecological approach suggests that the essence of coordination is the fit between an organism's actions and the environmental conditions. The ability to detect this action-relevant perceptual information (the perception/action cycle) might well differentiate DCD and non-DCD children, indicating a possible underlying factor in DCD. As noted above, sensitivity to optic flow (Lee, 1980), perception of object properties from haptic information (Carello and Turvey, 2000), and the perception of body-scaled animal–environment relations (e.g. Warren, 1984), are established lines of research that should be further explored with children diagnosed with DCD.

At an even more fundamental level, a dynamical systems approach motivates the investigation of coordination dynamics that underlie both perception and action (e.g. periodicity, phase relations, systems stability, non-linear phase changes). Experimental paradigms involving the systematic manipulation of these parameters, and subsequent comparisons between DCD and control groups, might reveal differences in sensitivity and adaptability to the underlying dynamics of coordinated movement.

Dynamical systems emphasise the interdependence of all the components and processes that comprise an animal–environment system. This suggests possible relationships between coordination disorders and other aspects of a child's development. If, as the dynamical systems approach maintains, different aspects of behaviour are organized according to the same dynamic properties, reduced sensitivity or adaptability to these properties is likely to influence a range of other behaviours. If this is true, we should not be surprised at the observed prevalence of co-morbidity in children with DCD, and we should recognize the potential influence of coordination difficulties on a child's social, emotional and cognitive development.

CHAPTER 5

DCD and overlapping conditions

DIDO GREEN AND GILLIAN BAIRD

Introduction

Questions regarding the presence or extent of associated and/or co-existing developmental disorders with DCD are not merely academic but also concern clinical issues directly linked to understanding the presentation and therapeutic needs of the children. It has been long understood that children with one developmental disorder are likely to have symptoms of another, and that impaired motor skill acquisition could be a marker for neurological dysfunction, injury and/or immaturity of the brain.

Follow-up studies of children who had experienced some neurological insult in the neonatal period in the 1970s showed them to have impairments in verbal ability, copying forms, concept formation, visuospatial ability and motor coordination which were linked with later learning difficulties in school affecting literacy and numeracy (Francis-Williams and Davies, 1974). A significant number of babies of very low birth weight were found to have learning difficulties especially perceptual-motor problems and lower performance than verbal abilities on intellectual testing (Francis-Williams and Davies, 1974). Conceptualized as 'the continuum of reproductive casualty' due to minimal brain damage (MBD, Pasamanick and Knobloch, 1966), similar terminology and thinking were applied to the child who had no adverse birth history but who appeared to have developmental problems with poor motor skills and difficulties in other aspects of learning in the absence of a generally low intellectual ability. In this paradigm, MBD was seen as a milder form of the damage done by anoxia or infection. However, the label of minimal brain damage fell out of favour as there was seldom any evidence of brain damage in most children with developmental or psychiatric problems and although children with brain damage had an increased risk of psychiatric disorder, there was little evidence for the existence of a meaningfully distinctive behavioural syndrome that differed from other psychiatric conditions (Rutter, 1982). Such arguments were also used against the concept of Minimal Brain Dysfunction as the diagnostic entity of a genetically determined disorder (Wender, 1971).

To aid research principally in childhood psychiatry, developmental disorder definition moved towards concepts of more specific impairments defined by discrepancy criteria – when impairment in the skill cannot be accounted for by a general learning difficulty or other disorder. Developmental disorders such as Speech and Language Impairment (SLI), specific reading, spelling and maths disorders, as well as individual and distinct psychiatric diagnoses such as Attention Deficit Hyperactivity Disorder (ADHD) and Pervasive Developmental Disorder (PDD) emerged in the *Diagnostic and Statistics Manuals* and *International Diagnostic Classification of Diseases* with several revisions (DSM-III, APA, 1987; DSM-IV, APA, 1994; ICD-10, WHO 1992b). Research studies concentrated on the 'pure' disorders believing them likely to give clues regarding specific features and thus increase understanding of these conditions.

The subsequent debate regarding the distinguishing characteristics that define discrete or specific developmental conditions is one that permeates many academic papers (Biederman, Newcorn and Sprich, 1991; Henderson and Barnett, 1998; Rispens and van Yperen, 1997; Whitmore and Bax, 1999). This continuing discourse notwithstanding, the concept of 'coordination impairments' as a distinct diagnostic condition was recognized within the DSM-III in 1987 under Developmental Coordination Disorder (DCD; APA, 1987) and in the ICD-10 in 1992 under Specific Developmental Disorder of Motor Function (SDDMF; WHO, 1992b, ICD-10). The *extent* to which the presence of other motor, learning and/or psychiatric symptoms would warrant additional labels or rule out DCD or SDDMF as a primary diagnosis has, however, remained poorly defined.

From the clinical perspective, the complexity of impairments has always been clear to parents and clinicians. Research studies, both cross-sectional and longitudinal, are again recognizing that symptoms of many developmental disorders overlap, albeit to varying degrees in different individuals, which may change over time. An increasing number of cross-sectional studies are being undertaken looking for the degree of contiguity between key developmental symptoms. The frequency of co-morbidity among children with coordination difficulties is attested by the work of Kadesjö and Gillberg (1999b), Kaplan et al. (1998; 2001), Kavale and Nye (1985–86), O'Hare and Khalid (2002), Silver and Hagin (1990) and Sugden and Wann (1987). Kaplan and colleagues (1998) investigated the overlap between reading (dyslexia), attention and motor deficits and found sufficient evidence to recommend that the common occurrence of at least two out of three of these problems should be considered the norm rather than the exception – potentially attributing a contributory status versus an associative one. (These authors opt for a more general descriptive term of atypical brain development to describe these children rather than multiple, yet more specific terminology, such as a combination of labels to include dyslexia, dyspraxia, dyscalculia and dysgraphia.) Longitudinal studies have highlighted other problems from which these children or young persons may suffer and which are often of greater impact in the longer term. For example, learning, behaviour, social and emotional outcomes are adversely affected in many adolescents and young adults who have had or continue to suffer from DCD (Geuze and Börger, 1993; Hellgren et al., 1994; Losse et al., 1991; Rassmussen and Gillberg, 2000; Schoemaker and Kalverboer, 1994; Sigurdsson, van Os and Fombonne, 2002).

This chapter will look at studies which have attempted to identify co-existing conditions with DCD, and also those which have looked for DCD in particular conditions including babies with normal birth histories and those of low birth weight. Discussion will follow as to whether the quality of DCD is the same in all conditions and finally consider some theoretical views and clinical/educational implications of the findings.

It is worth a brief diversion to consider terminology. The co-occurrence of symptoms of different disorders is often referred to as co-morbidity. Co-morbidity means two or more diseases, which brings an assumption of separate and different aetiologies and the term is therefore criticized by some (Kaplan et al., 2001). The present use of 'co-morbid, co-existing or overlapping' makes no such aetiological assumption nor does it infer primacy of one condition over another.

Distinguishing DCD through measurement of the impairment

There are several key questions for any review of DCD before looking systematically at overlapping conditions. Some are covered in different chapters of this book and will also be considered within the context of this chapter:

1. Is DCD one condition?
2. Is DCD a delay or disorder, the tail of normal distribution or different from the normal pattern?
3. How separable is DCD from a motor disorder such as mild cerebral palsy?
4. How separable is DCD from the problems of general learning?

Although most studies identify and measure DCD on the basis of contrasting motor attainments with those of age matched peers, the identification of DCD has taken various forms depending on the theoretical presumptions regarding aetiology. Measurement selection is frequently influenced by the importance given to aspects of motor development and performance such as: whether neurological signs are used to include or exclude children; whether the planning and learning of new skills is considered differently from the execution of learned skills; whether impairments in gross and fine motor competences are both necessary for a DCD diagnosis; what cognitive tests are used for inclusion or discrepancy criteria; whether tests should be sex specific etc. The range and choice of tests used in diagnostic procedures will affect the type of motor difficulty identified.

Measurement of motor skills or clumsiness in their execution has focused predominately on performance – speed and accuracy – in relation to chronological age (and sex and laterality) on particular tasks which have been standardized (for example: ball skills, balance, fine motor posting activities) rather than the functional achievement of complex skills involving motor activities in everyday life and circumstances. Although, recently O'Hare, Gorzkowska and Elton (1999) have developed such assessments to be used in conjunction with more traditional standardized motor tests. Within their more global battery are included activities such as stuffing an envelope, putting together a pen, tying a knot and opening a padlock.

Supplementary tests defining more qualitative aspects of motor development have varied from the incorporation of visual-spatial and perceptual testing to analysis of motor planning and 'soft' neurological signs. The use of gesture to evaluate motor planning has been frequently undertaken with adult onset apraxia and more recently with children with DCD (Agostoni et al., 1988; Dewey et al., 1988; Green et al., 2002; Hill, 1998; Hill, Bishop and Nimmo-Smith, 1998; Smyth and Mason, 1997). The ability to replicate a gesture reflects the frontal/prefrontal lobe's capacity to store the representation of the goal and also stimulate the image of the goal that is built from the observed gesture. Children with coordination difficulties have been found to have difficulty in generating and replicating both transitive (representational) and intransitive (non-representational) gestures.

Another aspect of movement quality that has been analysed in studies reverts back to the concept of neurological immaturity with the measurement of 'soft' signs – movement patterns and reflexes which are either present in the younger child or in a more severe presentation indicative of overt neurological damage (Hadders-Algra, 2002; Touwen, 1979). The analysis of these 'soft' signs was recommended by Bax and Whitmore in the school entry medical examination to support the identification of children who may require additional educational support (1987). Although the measurement of these 'soft' signs can be done with considerable precision, the reliability of these evaluations as used on a daily basis amongst health professionals to distinguish normal variance in movement quality from the atypical has however been challenged (Wilson et al., 2000a).

The questions regarding the separability of DCD from mild cerebral palsy and learning difficulties and developmental immaturity versus disorder are not necessarily answered by most tests used to diagnose DCD. Furthermore, Crawford, Wilson and Dewey (2001) illustrated the differential outcome which resulted from variations in test selection on groups of typical children, children with/without DCD and children with/without ADHD. These points must be borne in mind when considering the prevalence of co-existing conditions in DCD.

Singularity or heterogeneity of DCD – are there agreed subgroups?

One of the key questions surrounding the specificity of DCD is whether there are distinguishable subgroups within the condition. In addition to the frames of reference which have driven research on the features of DCD and related disorders, some researchers have investigated the clinical profiles of children with DCD through the determination of clusters based on clinically measurable aspects of motor performance. A study by Macnab, Miller and Polatajko (2001), which virtually replicated an earlier study by Hoare (1994) highlighted the impact that different measures have on cluster structures. Both these groups however identified five subtypes involving: (1) below average dynamic balance and kinaesthetic acuity; (2) visual perceptual competencies with poor kinaesthetic acuity; (3) visual motor deficits; (4) poor static balance and visual perceptual/visual motor functions; and (5) poor static and dynamic balance and manual dexterity. Wilson and colleagues (2000a) identified four subgroups of DCD utilizing a parent questionnaire suggesting major groupings of difficulties in fine motor skills, gross motor skills, ball skills/control during movement and complex/general motor problems. Using a teacher questionnaire in combination with a test of motor impairment, the Movement ABC Checklist and Test, Wright and Sugden (1996a) used different terminology to describe a similar number of cluster profiles. These profiles included children with generalized low scores but not severe in any, those with poor performance in dynamic (changing) environments, children with generalized poor scores across motor tasks particularly when occurring in changing environments and those with poor fine motor/speed and poor dynamic balance. Although planning problems have been identified in children with DCD, none of these subtyping studies of children with DCD incorporated specific tests of constructional praxis, motor planning ability and/or bi-manual skills to ascertain whether there may be a group of children with greater difficulty in these areas. And, in those studies by Ayres (1989) exploring subtypes of hypothesized sensory integrative dysfunction with praxis deficits, children with coordination impairments cannot be distinguished from those with more general learning difficulties (Ayres, 1971). Due to lack of direct comparability, it also remains uncertain whether these subgroups that have been defined represent distinct and replicable clusters or testing artefacts. However, it is concluded that DCD is not one discrete disorder but consists of both continuous and categorical functions.

DCD and other developmental disorders

Some studies have taken children with DCD and looked specifically for other disorders whilst others have taken children with specific disorders such as dyslexia and specific language impairment and looked for DCD. Table 5.1 lists many of those studies which have provided information about the motor status of children and the presence of additional diagnostic conditions alongside that of motor impairment. Lack of clear inclusion and exclusion criteria in these studies, particularly with respect to what constitutes a learning disability/difficulty, and inconsistent terminology and classification make it difficult to ascertain the extent to which multiple symptoms – or indeed multiple diagnoses – e.g. motor, attention, perceptual, learning, social and behavioural problems, occur (Geuze et al., 2001). As illustrated in earlier discussions, the extent to which different aspects of motor skill and control are measured may influence the type and number of overlapping 'symptoms' that may then be identified in individuals or groups of children with DCD.

DCD and attention deficits

The most comprehensive studies of attention problems in conjunction with other disorders which have included motor problems, have been undertaken on Swedish children by Gillberg's groups (Gillberg and Gillberg, 1983; 1988; 1989; Gillberg et al., 1983; 1989; Hellgren et al., 1994; Kadesjö and Gillberg, 1999b; Rasmussen and Gillberg, 2000; Rasmussen et al., 1983). Beginning in the 1980s, these studies attempted to quantify both motor and behavioural characteristics, and in the absence of definitive diagnostic criteria for coordination impairment, these researchers documented a number of behavioural as well as psychological disorders in a population cohort. Even though the measurement scales used to identify

Table 5.1 Studies reporting significant overlap of additional diagnoses with DCD/motor impairment

Reference	Motor impairment	Number of children/age	Psychopathology				Learning	Developmental
			Emotional	*Conduct*	*Attention deficit/hyperactivity*	*Social*	*Reading/scholastic*	*Speech/language impairment*
Cantell, Smyth and Ahonen, 1994	Identified at age 5 with motor delay	106 DCD equivalent and 40 controls Age 15				Clumsy children fewer hobbies and reduced social/physical activities	Reduced academic ambitions	
Cermak et al., 1986	Movement ABC/TOMI	5–8 years						40% children with SLI met criteria for DCD
Gillberg and Gillberg, 1989	MBD – perceptual-motor criteria	Population cohort 42 children with DAMP 13 years	75% children with motor difficulties had experienced school failure or were identified with emotional and/or behavioural problems					
Gillberg, Gillberg and Groth, 1989	MBD perceptual-motor criteria	Population cohort 42 children with DAMP 13 years			49% children with motor difficulties met criteria for ADHD			
Fletcher-Flinn, Elmes and Stragnell, 1997	TOMI	28 DCD 7.5–9.7 years					68% reading problems 25% >2 years below; 93% spelling problems 30% >2 years below; Most children scored poorly on phonological processing	
Green et al., 2002	Movement ABC	9 SDDMF 11AS 7–10 years				Similarities between SDDMF & AS children		

Table 5.1 contd

| Reference | Motor impairment | Number of children/age | Psychopathology | | | | Learning | Developmental |
			Emotional	Conduct	Attention deficit/hyperactivity	Social	Reading/scholastic	Speech/language impairment
Green, Baird and Sugden, submitted	Movement ABC	47 DCD children 5–11 years	70% emotional symptoms	38% conduct problems	68% attention/activity problems	51% peer problems		
Hellgren et al., 1994	Motor-perceptual criteria	45 DAMP 16 year	40% Axis I	15.5% substance abuse 4% suicide attempt	58% Axis II inc. AS			
Hill 1998 Hill et al., 1998	Movement ABC	11 DCD 19 SLI 5–13 years						60% children with SLI met criteria for DCD
Kadesjö and Gillberg, 1999b	Met criteria for DSM-IV	Population study with 55 DCD 6.8–7.8 years			47% had symptoms; 19% met diagnostic criteria for ADHD	7% diagnosed with Asperger's Syndrome		
Kaplan et al., 1998	BOTMP or Movement ABC	379 school aged 81/379 DCD 8–18 years			41%* ADHD with DCD * 28% ADHD and reading problems with DCD		55% * reading problems with DCD	

Table 5.1 contd

Reference	Motor impairment	Number of children/age	Psychopathology			Social	Learning / Reading/scholastic	Developmental / Speech/language impairment
			Emotional	Conduct	Attention deficit/hyperactivity			
Landgren et al., 1996	Criteria for motor perceptual deficit defined	Birth cohort 6–7 years 63/589 children with MBD			49% ADHD with DCD (DAMP)			
Losse et al., 1991	TOMI	34 motor impaired 15.1–17.4 yrs	82% reported to have emotional, conduct and attentional/concentration problems from school records			47% poor social self-concept	71% academic problems	
O'Hare and Khalid, 2002	TOMI/Movement ABC	23 DCD 7–10 years					Auditory processing problems associated with reading delay	
Owen and McKinlay, 1997	Motor deficits identified via Pegboard, buttoning, bead threading and graphic tasks	16 SLI 16 controls 4–7 years						SLI children were slower on speed and accuracy tasks and more likely to have mixed hand preference.
Moxley-Haegert and Ladd, 1989	Motor delay identified prior to 4 years	48 7–8 year olds			Hyperactivity associated with motor delay		Motor delay associated with later reduced intelligence	
Piek, Pitcher and Hay, 1999								

Table 5.1 contd

Reference	Motor impairment	Number of children/age	Psychopathology				Learning	Developmental
			Emotional	*Conduct*	*Attention deficit/hyperactivity*	*Social*	*Reading/scholastic*	*Speech/language impairment*
Powell and Bishop, 1992	Battery of fine and gross motor tasks	17/34 children with SLI 6–12 years						SLI group scored significantly worse on 7/19 motor tasks
Rasmussen and Gillberg, 2000	MBD criteria	15 year follow-up 49 meeting DCD criteria seen age 22 years	60% DCD with ADHD showed poor psycho-social outcome					
Rintala et al., 1998	Movement ABC	76 Dev. Language impairment 6–10 years						71% children with SLI met criteria for DCD
Robinson, 1991	TOMI	9–17 years						90% children with SLI met criteria for DCD
Schoemaker and Kalverboer, 1994	TOMI	18 6–9 years	33% STAIC			Self-report of social acceptance poor		

Table 5.1 contd

Reference	Motor impairment	Number of children/age	Psychopathology				Learning	Developmental
			Emotional	Conduct	Attention deficit/ hyperactivity	Social	Reading/ scholastic	Speech/language impairment
Sigurdsson, van Os and Fombonne, 2002	Criteria for motor impairment met at 7 years old	Birth cohort followed up at 11 and 16 years	Childhood motor impairment high risk for anxiety in males					
Skinner and Piek, 2001	Movement ABC and criteria for DCD met	8-10 years (n = 116) DCD = 58 12–14 years (n = 102) DCD = 58	Children and adolescents with DCD rated themselves as less able scholastically and athletically with lower scores for physical appearance and self-worth. Anxiety was more prevalent in the adolescent group with DCD					
Sooring-Lunsing et al., 1993	Touwens MND criteria*	Population cohort 170/346 MND				Social difficulties associated with fine motor problems	Coordination difficulties related to school failure	
Wright-Strawderman and Watson, 1992	Learning Disabled group – motor status not measured	53 students 8–10 years	Increased risk of depression in LD group (35.8% scored in the depressed range on the CDI)					

* MND = minor neurological dysfunction identified according to Touwen (1979) measuring posture (reflexes and responses), coordination; fine manipulation; and presence or absence of choreiform dyskinesia

motor-perceptual disorders varied between the studies in this series limiting direct comparison across ages, the overall results nevertheless provide convincing evidence that children with coordination difficulties are at high risk of associated attention deficits. Furthermore, the combination of motor and attentional problems in earlier childhood was found to be particularly disadvantaging with respect to additional co-morbid behavioural outcomes such as oppositional defiant disorder (ODD) or Asperger Syndrome (AS) (Kadesjö and Gillberg, 1999b).

Gillberg and Gillberg (1989) have used the term DAMP, deficits in attention, motor control and perception, to describe the overlap between perceptual motor difficulties and attention deficits. In a more recent study using the DCD diagnostic criteria, Kadesjö and Gillberg (1999b) identified moderate to severe symptoms of attention deficit/hyperactivity disorder (ADHD) in nearly half of their population of children with DCD. In a further study of Swedish children, Rasmussen and Gillberg (2000) found 60 per cent of the children in their study to have both DCD and ADHD. Figure 5.1 illustrates the high incidence of DCD with activity/attentional difficulties in a study utilizing the Strengths and Difficulties Questionnaire to identify risk of psychopathology in a small group of British children (SDQ, Goodman, 1997; 2001; Green, Baird and Sugden, in preparation).

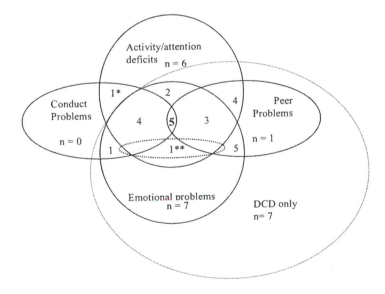

1* = one child with DCD + activity/attention + peer + conduct problems
1** = one child with DCD + emotional + peer + conduct problems

Figure 5.1 Schematic diagram of the overlap of emotional and behavioural disorders in children with DCD n = 47.

In a series of studies involving Canadian children Kaplan et al. (1998; 2001) also found high levels of overlap between children with either learning or attention problems and motor difficulties. Utilizing standardized protocols to identify DCD, these researchers identified ADHD in 41 per cent of children with DCD in the first study and in the second, 17.1 per cent of children with ADHD met criteria for DCD. The higher prevalence of ADHD associated with DCD (between 40 and 60 per cent) indicates an interesting coupling of these two developmental conditions. In their 'seminal' longitudinal study following children with quantifiable deficits in coordination over a 10 year period, although focusing on academic outcome, Losse et al. (1991) reported significant and persistent problems in concentration with behavioural difficulties in the greater majority of children who had been identified as clumsy 10 years earlier – some of the behaviour problems reported were serious enough to require police involvement. It is not known from the data presented in the latter paper whether those children with more significant attention problems were those most at risk of serious social offences. Although a number of these studies also mention conduct disorders including Oppositional Defiant Disorder (ODD), it is not possible to elucidate a distinction between ODD and ADHD to isolate a prevalence rate of conduct disorders in the absence of attentional problems or hyperkinesis in children with DCD.

Figure 5.1 shows up to 53 per cent of children with DCD to be reported by parents on the SDQ as demonstrating activity and attention problems in the study of Green, Baird and Sugden (submitted). Based on parental or teacher report, the SDQ has been found to be highly predictive of emotional and behavioural psychopathology, including inattention and hyperactivity, in children between 5 and 15 years (Goodman, 1997; Mathai, Anderson and Bourne, 2002; Meltzer et al., 2000). These results correspond to those of a UK population study in which 35 per cent of children reported as being clumsy were identified as having mental health problems following psychiatric assessment of which hyperkinetic disorders were the second most common diagnosis in this group (Meltzer et al., 2000). These studies beg the question as to whether combined ADHD and DCD constitute recognition as a separate diagnostic entity in view of the differential prognosis – reverting to the DAMP terminology of the Swedish studies.

Outcome – longitudinal studies

Gillberg and Gillberg (1989), Gillberg, Gillberg and Groth (1989) and Rasmussen and Gillberg (2000) followed a number of their original Swedish cohort from age 6 to 7 through to age 22 years. In the earlier publications, children with perceptual-motor difficulties (minimal brain dysfunction) were identified through the Southern California Sensory Integration Tests (Ayres, 1972a). Initial follow-up studies of these children at ages 10, 13 and 16 years identified motor perceptual and attentional disorders (DAMP) through operationally defined criteria incorporating neurodevelopmental/neurological examination comparable to that used by Hadders-Algra's team in Holland (Gillberg and Gillberg, 1989; Hadders-Algra, 2002; Lunsing et al., 1992b; Soorani-Lunsing et al., 1993). At age 13, two-thirds of the Swedish children originally identified with MBD no longer had obvious motor problems although there were persistently higher rates of emotional and behaviour problems and poor school achievement particularly when motor and attention problems had co-existed at a younger age. By age 22 years, those young adults who had had both ADHD and DCD (DAMP) as children, tended to have a worse outcome than either condition alone. The researchers argue that the differences in outcome could not be fully accounted for by the additional layer of difficulty (e.g. two simultaneously occurring conditions) but rather that the cumulative interaction of ADHD and DCD is particularly onerous. The persistence of difficulties in these longitudinal studies argues against the principle of DCD as a developmental delay in favour of the deficit concept incorporating a broader notion to include a range of behavioural, emotional and motor difficulties.

Specific language impairment and DCD

Children with specific language impairment (SLI) have also been found to have an increased incidence of coordination deficits (Hill, 1998; Owen and McKinlay, 1997; Powell and Bishop, 1992; Robinson, 1991). Table 5.1 outlines some of those studies which liken the motor problems of children with SLI and DCD to the performance of younger children. Those studies using standardized motor batteries such as the Movement Assessment Battery for Children (Movement ABC) or its precursor, the Test of Motor Impairment (TOMI), found between 40–90 per cent of children with SLI to experience significant coordination problems (Cermak, Ward and Ward, 1986; Hill, 1998; Robinson, 1991). Both Owen and McKinlay (1997) and Powell and Bishop (1992) found children with SLI to be slower in executing tasks with poor accuracy in a variety of fine motor tasks rather than exhibiting generalized motor difficulties when compared to controls. In a series of studies contrasting children with SLI and those with DCD, Hill (1998) and Hill, Bishop and Nimmo-Smith (1998) found 60 per cent of the children with SLI also met criteria for DCD with both of these clinical groups performing like younger children, especially in gesture reproduction of familiar postures – irrespective of the presence or extent of motor difficulty in the SLI children.

Reading and writing and DCD

From the early studies of Orton (1937), those of Denckla (1974), Gubbay (1975a), Francis-Williams and Davies (1974) and Francis-Williams (1976) through to those of Kaplan et al. (1998), Fletcher-Flinn, Elmes and Stragnell (1997), Nicolson and Fawcett (1994) and O'Hare and Khalid (2002) a strong association has been made between the development of motor coordination and academic skills, particularly reading and writing. From a population of children including 224 children with learning/attention disorders and 155 controls, 55 per cent of the children meeting criteria for DCD had a reading disability in the Canadian study undertaken by Kaplan et al. (1998). From the other perspective, whilst investigating a group of children with DCD (n = 28) Fletcher-Flinn, Elmes and Stragnell (1997) found 68 per cent to exhibit reading problems, with 28 per cent of these children having a reading age more than 2 years below their chronological age. Spelling problems and poor phonological processing were also evident in this group. These results are consistent with a number of other studies reporting links between DCD and reading and spelling problems (Henderson and Hall, 1982; Losse et al., 1991). What is not known is the nature of this relationship in terms of causality or underlying neuropsychological functions.

Perusing the referrals to community and out-patient therapy services, a large proportion of these mention poor handwriting illustrating the academic impact of poor coordination (Green, Bishop and Sugden, 2004; Peters, Henderson and Dookun, 2004). Of note in the authors' own study, is the discrepancy between referral concern regarding the presence of poor handwriting and actual writing ability as measured by a pre-read copied sample as opposed to a sample of simultaneous reading and writing. To illuminate the affect of poor literacy or reading difficulties on writing, Geuze and Kalverboer (1994), Nicolson and Fawcett (1997) and O'Hare and Khalid (2002) provide some clues to the underlying pathology of writing and reading problems in children with DCD through consideration of cerebellar processes, particularly those of timing and sequencing.

A small experimental study by Dewey et al. (1988) suggested that children with verbal sequencing difficulties also had difficulty learning limb action sequences and gesture execution. It is plausible that these children represent a subgroup whereby sequencing and timing difficulties (potentially mediated by the cerebellum) influence more generalized temporal-sequential functions incorporating language and motor control. There have been a number of studies linking academic skills in reading, writing and attention control to support this argument (Fletcher-Flinn, Elmes and Stragnell, 1997; Losse et al., 1991; Moxley-Haegert and Ladd, 1989; Rasmussen and Gillberg, 2000).

Developmental social impairment and DCD

Research has shown that children with Pervasive Developmental Disorders perform poorly on tests of motor function (Green et al., 2002; Jones and Prior, 1985; Manjiviona and Prior, 1995). The higher incidence of motor impairment (of DCD in type) in those with social impairments qualifying for a diagnosis of AS or ASD is supported by Meltzer et al. (2000), Rasmussen and Gillberg (2000), Kadesjö and Gillberg (1999b) and Hellgren et al. (1994). Albeit in UK and Swedish populations only, these researchers all found a higher prevalence of the co-occurrence of both motor and social impairments (reported to meet criteria for both DCD and AS) than would be expected by chance. To a certain extent, the Swedish group would be expected to demonstrate a high incidence of poor motor skills in those children with AS in view of the fact that the defining diagnostic criteria that these studies used for AS incorporated clumsiness. However, these longitudinal studies were instigated from a population and not a clinical base and therefore illustrate the increased incidence of social difficulties in children with perceptual motor deficits – with and without attention problems.

In the UK population study undertaken by Meltzer et al. (2000), 35 per cent of children with coordination difficulties were found to have significant psychopathology, with Pervasive Developmental Delay/ASD one of the most predominant co-morbid diagnoses. From the descriptive accounts in the school records of the children with coordination difficulties followed up in the Losse et al. (1991) study, 29 to 41 per cent were reported to have significant social difficulties and/or bizarre or aggressive behaviour.

Criterion C of the DSM-IV stipulates that a diagnosis of DCD would be ruled out in the presence of a pervasive developmental delay (APA, 1994). Children with autistic spectrum disorders, including Asperger's Syndrome (AS), would therefore not qualify for 'diagnostic' recognition of their motor difficulties in addition to their 'primary' social and communication impairments. There are however considerable diagnostic variances between professionals particularly with respect to that of AS, with some centres adopting a diagnosis of AS when there is evidence of clumsiness in conjunction with a social impairment (Howlin, 2000; Szatmari, Bremner and Nagy, 1989; Gillberg, 1998a). Subsequently some children may receive a diagnosis of DCD with social difficulties whereas alternative investigations of their social behaviour would elicit sufficient evidence to warrant a diagnosis of AS. In the study by Green et al. (2002), three of the 12 children originally entering the study as candidates for DCD were identified as having AS following in-depth interview of their early and current social development. An open debate is required to consider further the exclusionary features of Criterion C not only with respect to Pervasive

Developmental Delay but to define those medical conditions which would be expected to influence motor performance.

Emotional difficulties in DCD: are emotional and behaviour problems intrinsic or secondary?

The relationship of emotional deficits to clumsiness is indistinct. Wright-Strawderman and Watson (1992) provide convincing evidence as do Hellgren et al. (1994) of a higher incidence of depression among children with learning disability (which may include clumsiness) and DAMP respectively. Hellgren et al. (1994) followed 56 children who had been identified with motor and/or perceptual disorders (DAMP) and found 40 per cent of those children to meet criteria for affective disorders under Axis I of the DSM-III and IV (APA, 1987; 1994). Similarly, in a birth cohort study, Sigurdsson, van Os and Fombonne (2002) found a much higher odds ratio for boys who had experienced coordination difficulties as children (age 7 years) to exhibit anxiety at ages 11 and 16 years. As Schoemaker and Kalverboer (1994) concluded from their study identifying higher levels of anxiety and introversion in children with DCD it is not possible to illuminate specific risk factors, in either profile or extent of motor impairment, as predictive of emotional difficulties at a later age or whether predisposing socio-economic factors or emotional features may have been present when younger.

Links between DCD and emotional problems have been attributed to the persistence of reduced self-esteem and perceptions of competence rather than finding substance in neurological explanations. McConaughy and Achenbach (1994) have shown the increased risk of co-morbidity in children presenting to child and adolescent psychiatric services. With limited research in this area it is not possible to hypothesize as to whether depression or anxiety can be assigned to a generalized psychomotor slowing and/or disorganization or a more generalized vulnerability to a range of psychological as well as motor problems resulting from atypical central nervous system processing.

A number of researchers have explored the self-perception of children with motor impairment using the Harter's Self-Perception Profile for Children (Harter, 1985). The philosophy underpinning this measure supports a relationship between self-perception, self-esteem and global self-worth on measures of scholastic competence, athletic ability, physical appearance, social acceptance and behavioural conduct, with athletic skills and physical appearance contributing significantly to the typically developing child's self-worth. A key question at this point regards the extent to which the social deficits are considered to be intrinsic or as secondary features in DCD. Studies investigating social and/or emotional characteristics have generally concluded that children with DCD are less likely to be motivated to participate in traditional sporting activities within large groups e.g. football/baseball, with a risk of social isolation (Rose, Larkin and Berger, 1998; Smyth and Anderson, 2000). A general perusal of this literature, without systematic analysis, shows a trend for males with DCD to rate themselves more poorly on both social and motor competence (Arscott, 1997; Jongmans et al., 1996; Rose, Larkin and Berger, 1998; Schoemaker and Kalverboer, 1994; Skinner and Piek, 2001).

Although there is more evidence to support the conclusion that children with DCD have reduced perceptions of athletic ability, a few recent studies have suggested that these children may adjust the value placed on motor skills in favour of abilities such as behavioural conduct over which they have more control in their personal construct of self-worth (Causgrove Dunn, 2000; Causgrove Dunn and Watkinson, 1994; Rose and Larkin, 2002; Shapiro and Ulrich, 2001).

It may be surmised therefore that children with poor perceptions of their skills might avoid participation in tasks which expose them to public humiliation – as any external reinforcement of their difficulties may exacerbate negative self-perceptions. This hypothesis is borne out by the results of some studies mentioned previously showing reduced motivation and participation in sports of children with coordination deficits. What is not apparent from the research to date is the extent to which reduced self-perception of skill (as accurate as that may be) contributes to a risk of emotional disturbance in childhood or later life. Using the Birleson Depression Inventory, Gillberg and Gillberg (1989) found a 50 per cent greater probability of children with both motor and attention problems (DAMP) to have abnormal depression scores when compared to a comparison group without such difficulties at age 13 years. By age 16 years Hellgren et al. (1994) found persistent and highly significant evidence of depression in this same group of children who had originally demonstrated motor difficulties with/without attention problems (both DAMP and MPD children). The appendix to their paper shows three of the 11 children who showed depression at age 7 years to have continuing depression at age 16 with four further individuals showing more complex psychopathology including suicide attempt, bipolar disorder and schizoid disorder. In contrast, of the two children from the comparison group (n = 45) who had had signs of depression at age 7 years, a similar persistence of complex psychopathology was evident in only one child who had developed a bipolar disorder with histrionics and paranoia without suicide attempt. More worrying was the emergence of depressive or bipolar disorder at age 16 among a further 11 children who had experienced motor difficulties at a younger (and possibly current) age. Rasmussen and Gillberg's follow-up of the DAMP/MPD group at age 22 years, found major depression common in all groups although the only individuals (n = 3) with current depression at the time of interview were from the ADHD with DCD group. It is unfortunate that the relatively concurrent study of Kadesjö and Gillberg (1999b) in their investigations of a different group of Swedish children did not also probe for AXIS I disorders in their comprehensive analysis of behaviour and developmental (speech-language and reading problems) in younger children with DCD.

The small study by Green, Baird and Sugden (submitted) shows children with AS to have slightly more insight into their motor difficulties than children with SDDMF with neither group placing value on athletic skills in their determination of self-worth. These results and those of Causgrove Dunn and Watkinson (1994) are consistent with the 'Resilience Theory' concept with the implication that children with motor difficulties may shift the emphasis of valued attributes from motor to other skill areas to maintain a positive perception of competence and motivation. These results need to be viewed alongside the work of Segal et al. (2002) with respect to the negative 'stigmatizing' effects of poor coordination. In this qualitative study of six families with children with motor difficulties, parents felt that children either withdrew or were excluded from participating with their peers due to the negative stigmatizing effects of poor motor skills. The differences in reporting of parents and teachers and students as to the extent of any motor or social difficulties and the emphasis placed on the importance of these skills, may be partially explained by the contrast between an externally perceived 'stigmatizing' effect and the internal resilience of the child.

Importantly Missiuna (1998) considered the concept of self-efficacy and motor competency in preschoolers as potentially predictive of persistent and extensive difficulties at a later age. More recent analysis of the emotional and behavioural difficulties of children with DCD referred to local therapy services, suggests that there is evidence of significant psychopathology at a young as well as an older age (Green, Baird and Sugden, submitted). This hypothesis requires further research and follow-up; however, there is accumulating evidence that social and emotional difficulties are more prevalent in children with DCD compared to typically developing children without motor difficulties.

Qualitative differences in DCD in these studies: is the 'DCD' different in SLI, dyslexia or PDD?

Hill (1998; 2001) and Hill, Bishop and Nimmo-Smith (1998) suggest a close alignment between the motor difficulties of children with SLI and those with DCD. Similarly, O'Hare and Khalid (2002), as well as Nicolson and Fawcett (1994), connect the difficulties of children with dyslexia with those of children with DCD. The small sample sizes and specific nature of the assessments undertaken in these studies limit the ability to go beyond a general hypothesis that these conditions are closely linked. It is not possible to conjecture as to whether the profiles of motor performance are matched in these groups, however there would appear to be more similarities than differences.

More specific analysis of the nature of any social difficulties experienced by children with DCD suggests that these children also show many similarities with children with Asperger's Syndrome (AS), differing more in degree rather than the breadth of social impairment (Arscott, 1997; Green et al., 2002). The motor performance of children with learning disabilities, DCD and AS has been found to be quite similar – with the AS group tending to be worse at ball skills (Green et al., 2002; Miyahara et al., 1997). Contrasting the motor performance of these two groups of children with more qualitative analysis of movement with the study of mime and imitation, the researchers were unable to elicit a truly significant difference in the pattern or quality of motor execution between these two groups of children. Green et al. (2002) did not find significant differences between the gesture production of these children although those with DCD were found to have better performance at an older age.

To understand the nature of any functional differences between DCD and AS and again using this small but well defined group of children, an attempt was made to identify differences in self-perception and social behaviour through comparison of scores on the Harter's Self-Perception Profile for Children (Harter, 1985) and direct measurement of social behaviour during school activities. Few differences were found between these children's self-perception of either their popularity or motor skills although surprisingly the AS children were more accurate in their reporting of the extent of their motor difficulties. The teachers of these children on the other hand viewed both the DCD and AS children as being similar to each other but significantly worse in both social behaviour and motor performance than their classmates. There is some indication that the children as well as their teachers may have scored items more favourably if positive efforts were shown to overcome more obvious or 'known' difficulties with the result that the DCD children were rated more poorly than the AS on social items and the AS children considered to be worse than the DCD children on motor tasks.

Do the motor difficulties of children born prematurely differ from DCD?

The debate concerning the boundary between coordination disorder and motor disorder represented by evidence of neurological damage continues to surface, particularly in relation to children who have been born prematurely. Hadders-Algra has done a number of studies following up a Dutch birth cohort and, like Gillberg's Swedish team, developed specific criteria for operationally defining minor neurological dysfunction that in many respects represent key elements of DCD. Both the Swedish and Dutch studies do not distinguish between those children with known evidence of adverse neonatal events when analysing the profile of motor performance that may help support a cut-off of either degree or qualitatively distinct profiles representing coordination impairment as opposed to motor disorder. This creates a dilemma if deciding to exclude the diagnosis of DCD in children with negative neonatal histories despite significant coordination difficulties in the absence of measurable cerebral lesion. In practice, clinicians rarely make this distinction when determining the need for therapy services to these children, preferring to judge need through quantifiable difficulties in motor and functional skills.

The early studies of Francis-Williams and Davies (1974) have been replicated by recent studies of children born prematurely and of low birth weight which continue to support the higher risk of perceptual-motor, behaviour and learning difficulties for these children (Foulder-Hughes and Cooke, 2002; Mutch, Leyland and McGee, 1993; Samson et al., 2002). In Jongmans's (1994) study of children born prematurely, six profiles of motor impairment were identified. Excluding those children who were somewhat poor on all motor tasks when compared to their peers without coordination difficulties, the five remaining profiles are broadly similar in type to the clusters identified in the studies of Hoare (1994) and Macnab, Miller and Polatajko (2001) and, if being more expansive, using performance rather than process terminology, the variations of motor performance are similar to the clusters identified by Wright and Sugden (1996a). In the premature group, the only children to show evidence of 'minor' haemorrhagic lesions (a combination of Grade IIa haemorrhage and flares or flares present for less than 14 days) were those who showed difficulties across motor tasks. This study also explored cognitive and behavioural characteristics of these children. Again, the group with generalized difficulties across the motor tasks exhibited more cognitive and behaviour problems than other groups. However, this was not exclusive with children in other cluster groupings showing an equal if not greater range of scores in the parent and teacher questionnaires.

Of note is the alignment of those children with adverse neonatal history in Jongman's study with those without from Hoare's (1994) and Macnab, Miller and Polatajko's (2001) work – in both profile (cluster type) and prevalence. This brings us back to the 'continuum of reproductive causality'.

Explanations of overlapping developmental disorders from a theoretical understanding of motor learning and execution

The heterogeneous nature of 'clumsiness' refutes a simple theoretical model that will address the differing presentations (Hoare, 1994; Polatajko, 1999; Wright and Sugden, 1996a). Different professionals have taken varying approaches to the analysis and interpretation of specific motor difficulties often reflecting their preferred model. There have been a number of theoretical explanations for the problems underpinning the coordination deficits exhibited by children with DCD arising from the neurological foundations for motor learning. The most convincing evidence surfacing from Wilson and McKenzie's (1998) meta-analysis of research into the information-processing difficulties of children with DCD, shows visuospatial processing problems (and to a lesser extent problems with cross-modal and kinaesthetic perception) to be implicated most frequently. The relationship between visual spatial skills and coordination difficulties is epitomized by the work of Weintraub and Mesulam (1983) and Rourke (1989). Rourke (1989) defines a syndrome of 'Nonverbal learning disabilities' (NVLD) which clusters 'clumsy children' with conditions involving deficits in right hemisphere functions. Weintraub and Mesulam (1983) provided early evidence of right hemispheric deficits concurring with motor performance problems via 14 case studies. In these cases visuospatial deficits occurred together with social difficulties. Denckla (1983) further suggests that patients with Asperger's Syndrome (AS) resemble those described by Weintraub and Mesulam, presenting with clumsiness (defined as poor visuospatial motor skills), poor gestural abilities and odd/mannered speech and/or language. Reduced visuospatial processing has frequently been found in some but not all children with DCD (Wilson and McKenzie, 1998; Macnab, Miller and Polatajko, 2001; Hoare, 1994). Green et al.'s (2002) and Klin et al.'s (1995) descriptions of AS children align these children's motor difficulties more closely with DCD and nonverbal learning disabilities respectively. However, it is not known whether it is these difficulties which directly contribute to poor social perception. From what is known of right hemisphere deficits in adult onset lesions, it may be that consequent visual perceptual decrements contribute to ensuing problems orienting movements in space (Goodale, Jakobson and Servos, 1996).

There have been few studies exploring the frontal lobe contribution to movement planning and execution in children with DCD. In a small pilot study, Jongmans, Oomen and Hoop (2002) found weak links between manual dexterity and planning deficits in children with DCD which were also associated with ADHD. Frontal dysfunction in ADHD and motor planning difficulties have been intimated through studies exploring attentional control and gesture (Benson, 1991; Chaminade, Meltzoff, and Decety, 2002). Using positron emission tomography (PET), Chaminade, Meltzoff and Decety (2002) identified differential cerebral activation during goal formation versus means production in imitation tasks. Right dorsolateral prefrontal cortex was detected for both goal formation and means production – this is consistent with this area's 'executive function' role in the preparation of action based on stored information (Pochon et al., 2001). The medial prefrontal region was activated only during imitation of the means and is compatible with this area's critical role in comprehending others' intentions and may also reflect the retrieval of the goals or intention from the observation of his gestures (Chaminade, Meltzoff and Decety, 2002). Of note in these studies was the involvement of the premotor cortex when required to generate the means following the demonstration of the goal. The enhanced premotor area activation during this process suggests that goal directed action is more cognitively demanding when the (means) associated gestures are not provided. Through a series of empirical studies, Gernsbacher and Goldsmith (2000) and Hughes (1996) support the executive function hypothesis of association between motor planning problems/dyspraxia and autistic spectrum disorders.

If, as suggested by the supporting literature, frontal dysfunction theories underpin the neuropathology of ADHD, those children with pervasive frontal involvement with the co-occurrence of ADHD and DCD may suffer additional deficits in motor planning and indeed behaviour organization as a consequence of inefficiency of frontal/prefrontal systems in supporting visually prompted actions. Despite the differential outcome shown by the Swedish studies, there is insufficient evidence at this stage to argue that the coordination impairments of those children with both ADHD and DCD are distinct from those children with DCD without attentional problems.

The more recent work of Nicolson et al. (1999) and O'Hare and Khalid (2002) has implicated the cerebellum when executing pre-learnt or new sequences of movement. The former provide evidence combining positron emission tomography with behavioural signs of atypical cerebellar activity in six adults with dyslexia compared to six without. These difficulties with temporal-spatial aspects of movement control would be consistent with the findings of Dewey et al. (1988) associating the verbal sequencing difficulties of some children with difficulties in learning limb action sequences and performing gestures. As commented on earlier, one can only conjecture as to whether these children represent a particular subtype in which atypical cerebellar processing results in sequential processing problems – affecting both language (literacy) and motor execution systems.

Inclusion/exclusion criteria for DCD

It is generally acknowledged that specific learning difficulties (SpLD) have a multi-factorial aetiology to which genetics (a number of sites), sex, experience and social conditions all contribute (Hadders-Algra, Huisjes and Touwen, 1988b; Hadders-Algra and Lindahl, 1999; Kaplan et al., 1998). Hadders-Algra and Lindahl (1999) and Gillberg and Gillberg (1989) have identified pre- and peri-natal precursors which may contribute to these problems but which cannot solely account for them. These authors suggest that socio-economic class and minimal brain dysfunction interact to influence development, including children with minimal neurological involvement within either category of SpLD or DCD. Others contest that a diagnosis of DCD would be excluded in cases where evidence is present of neurological events such as prematurity or low birth weight, particularly where there are known factors contributing to these events such as foetal drug or alcohol exposure (APA, 1994; Henderson and Barnett, 1998; Hurt et al., 1995). Conditions such as Congenital Mirrored Movements, Benign Congenital Hypotonicity and Erhlos Dahnlo Syndrome, in which specific neurological or anatomical (ligamentous laxity) deficits are identified, may contribute to significant bimanual and/or more general coordination difficulties (Cohen et al., 1991; Parush et al., 1998). It is unclear whether these children also warrant a label of DCD.

The increased incidence of surviving pre-term infants may require a shift in the defining criteria of DCD to include children who may have had some neonatal insult but where overt neurological damage (cerebral palsy), learning and/or sensory impairment are ruled out. A number of studies of infants born pre-term/low birth weight have already been reported and have shown that between 30–48 per cent of these children experience persistent difficulties in motor and perceptual skills, similar in type to those experienced by children with DCD (Hadders-Algra and Lindahl, 1999; Hutton et al., 1997; Jongmans et al., 1996). These relatively 'minor' deficits have been shown to have an adverse affect on academic achievement and behaviour among pre-term infants (Botting et al., 1998; Goyen, Lui and Woods, 1998; Luoma, Herrgard and Martikainen, 1998). Gillberg and Gillberg's (1989) study, from which subjects were recruited for Hellgren et al.'s (1994) follow-up study previously mentioned, identified non-optimal perinatal factors including prematurity as a powerful predictor of persistent minor neurological dysfunction and subsequent perceptual and motor difficulties.

Hadders-Algra links the fine manipulative and coordination difficulties of those children who have experienced neonatal difficulties as well as those who have not to dysfunction of the cortico-striato-thalamo-cortical and cerebello-thalamo-cortical pathways. There are numerous problems inherent in this postulate, especially as their assessment specificity but low sensitivity with the consequence that a nu... dren developed complex minor neurological dysfunction (MND, seemingly equivalent to DCD – who would not necessarily have been predicted to do so.

Why more boys than girls with DCD?

In common with autistic spectrum disorders and speech and language impairments, more boys than girls have been reported to have DCD. The reasons for this are unknown. Kadesjö and Gillberg (1999b) found a boy:girl ratio varying from 4:1 to 7:1 when attention deficit disorder was included within DCD in a Swedish population. Clinical presentation to occupational therapy departments in the UK reveals a similar disproportionate number of males (Green and Archer, 2000; Green et al., 2002). Stephenson, McKay and Chesson (1991) found only two girls among a clinical caseload of 31 children. This is comparable for example with the autistic spectrum disorders where differences in prevalence between sexes show a discrepancy in frequency, with males more predominant than females at a rate of approximately 4:1 and female presentation more likely to be linked to the lower intellectual range (Volkmar, Szatmari and Sparrow, 1993). These studies do less to differentiate DCD from other developmental conditions at a clinical level as well as an aetiological level than bear witness to the extent of coordination difficulties in a range of developmental conditions affecting males more than females.

Implications for practice

The London Consensus (Polatajko and Fox, 1995) was sufficiently concerned regarding the prevalence of secondary characteristics – especially those of poor self-esteem, social acceptance and coping strategies – to recommend that these should be investigated during assessment of DCD. It remains unclear at what point these would be exclusive of a diagnosis under Criterion C of the DSM-IV (APA, 1994). Criterion D poses a similar problem in differentiating between cognitive potential and learning attainments.

While addressing the extent and range of co-existing disorders within DCD, the notion of DCD as a distinct condition has been revisited. It could be argued that DCD is rarely a 'pure' coordination disorder but often a feature within more pervasive/persistent developmental disorders. The notion that DCD is not only a significant impairment in itself but is additionally a marker for other possible developmental disorders of varying kinds that may be present at differing periods of a child's life is the important message from this review. Co-morbidity has been found to be more prevalent in clinically referred populations and it may be the very presence of co-existing deficits which places coordination disorders within the field of clinical concern (McConaughy and Achenbach, 1994). There is a growing body of evidence that a considerable number of children will experience significant difficulties in acquiring motor skills with the spontaneity and efficiency of their peers and that these early motor difficulties may have an impact on longer term developmental outcome. Until evidence is presented illuminating the 'specificity' of DCD, both the identification and remediation of coordination impairments should consider a greater breadth of development to incorporate emotional, behavioural and learning measures and attainments.

Perhaps the search for a theoretically coherent view of the singularity of DCD disorder and other developmental disorders defies solution. The concept of co-morbidity then becomes a question about the relationship between features, the strength of the association and the extent to which specific deficits impact on daily performance along with the 'resilience' and personality characteristics of the child – with co-occurrence more likely the more profound the functional decrement. Indeed, Whitmore and Bax (1999) cogently argue against the notion of DCD as a disorder, with so little known of the specificity and defining features of coordination difficulties.

Further to this there is the presumption that subtypes of DCD can be distinguishable from overlapping conditions. In addition, it remains unclear whether a theoretical approach to understanding the process of motor skill acquisition affects treatment/outcome. In the case of right-hemispheric learning difficulties it is difficult to conceive of a diagnostic cut-off between the visuospatial processing difficulties of a child who has dysgraphia, social impairments and poor visuo-spatial judgements and visuo-motor skills as a consequence of RHLD and the motor coordination difficulties of a child with poor visual perceptual skills associated with DCD. A similar diagnostic dilemma is evident when attempting to distinguish between the lack of coordinated bimanual skills in children with DCD and the partial hemi-syndrome without overt neurological signs of a child born prematurely. Furthermore, limited access to specialist diagnostic services for psychiatric and communication difficulties may not only reduce recognition of the motor difficulties of children with emotional and behavioural problems but also limit the identification of psychopathology in children with DCD. This is not implied to be a wish to return to more generalized terminology such as Atypical Brain Development or Minimal Brain Dysfunction in which the debilitating effects of coordination deficits are lost among an array of developmental symptoms but rather emphasize a recognition of the prevalence of co-existing developmental conditions when motor impairment may be the predominate.

CHAPTER 6

Progression and development in Developmental Coordination Disorder

MARGARET COUSINS AND MARY M. SMYTH

Introduction

Previous chapters have detailed the way in which Developmental Coordination Disorder (DCD) impacts on the lives of children and their families, and the functional and processing deficits exhibited by children with the disorder. This chapter considers the extension of DCD outside childhood, into adolescence and adulthood. Being poorly coordinated has quite different consequences for everyday activities and social life at different ages. At young ages normal clumsiness may be an 'accepted feature of childhood' (Gubbay, 1975a, p. 2), and judgements are needed as to whether motor clumsiness appears to be unusual with regard to chronological age or developmental status. However, when children are unable to carry out educational or recreational activities at which age-peers are successful, their difficulties may be noticed by parents, teachers and the children themselves. Young people and adults, on the other hand, can choose to avoid sport or other activities that expose their difficulties, and this can make it more difficult to identify ongoing problems. With less scrutiny, a disability which does affect daily living, and which may impact on employment, may not be as visible as DCD in younger children.

Opinions on the extension of coordination difficulties into adulthood are related to the understanding of the disorder in terms of developmental delay or a difference in developmental pathways. Coordination difficulties can be characterized as a delay which children will grow out of, a learning disability or 'talent deficit' in need of an educational solution (Hall, 1988), or as a medical abnormality, which might not be remediated. An editorial in the *British Medical Journal* (1962) conceptualized clumsiness as a medical problem, drawing attention to the similarities with minor cerebral palsy and with Gerstmann's syndrome.

119

However, assumptions about the long-term prognosis for children with motor coordination impairments have been made despite a paucity of research evidence to support the position one way or another. The fourth edition of the *Diagnostic and Statistical Manual of Mental Disorders* (DSM-IV; APA, 1994), for example, explicitly stated that DCD may continue into adolescence and adulthood. Few studies of adolescents, and no studies of adults had been conducted at that time. Even now, the body of research that has debated this issue is quite small.

At the present time, however, professionals who are involved in provision for children with DCD argue that DCD may persist into the teenage and adult years. Case studies of affected adults have occasionally been detailed in books aimed at parent and teacher groups (e.g. Portwood, 1999). In the UK, the Dyspraxia Foundation, a self-help organization that aims to raise awareness of motor coordination disorders in children, has an adult group. Adult members may have been diagnosed as children, or may have been referred by health professionals who believe that their symptomology is indicative of a developmental motor impairment. Others have accessed relevant literature themselves, because they believe they are unusually clumsy or 'dyspraxic'.

During the 1990s, long-term progression of DCD was an issue of increasing interest to researchers. DSM-IV terminology was widely adopted by the research community (Polatajko, Fox and Missiuna, 1995), lending some coherence to attempts to define and assess the disorder. At the same time, children who had been recruited to studies during the 1980s were in some cases available for follow-up studies. Some of these studies had recruited children with coordination difficulties in order to carry out experimental work. Some studies utilized samples referred for their motor difficulties. In others, screening procedures were instituted. For example, researchers would test large numbers of school children and select those who performed most poorly on a standardized motor test battery (e.g. Henderson and Hall, 1982; Losse et al., 1991). Other researchers originally screened whole populations, either at birth, or at school-entry age, for a selection of neurological abnormalities, learning difficulties or behavioural disorders (e.g. Gillberg and Rasmussen, 1982a; Hellgren et al., 1993). In the course of this, they selected out subgroups of children with coordination impairments, or combinations of motor and other learning problems. Models that consider motor and attentional disorders to be inherently linked are the norm in some European countries, and some epidemiological studies have reflected this. In considering issues of progression in DCD, there are already some difficulties in ascertaining that equivalent populations have been targeted in different follow-up studies.

Follow-up and epidemiological studies: motor outcome in the teenage years

To date, a small literature details the motor outcomes for teenagers who were diagnosed with DCD as children (e.g. Knuckey and Gubbay, 1983; Losse et al., 1991; Cantell, Smyth and Ahonen, 1994). Opinion is divided as to the extent children are thought to overcome their motor difficulties. The early studies were relatively optimistic. However, a major difficulty encountered by researchers working with older children with DCD is the lack of available tests suitable for use with adolescents. If older children perform poorly on tests aimed at younger children, this can justifiably be taken as an indication of continuing difficulties. It is very hard to be equally certain that adolescents no longer have motor problems if they succeed on these tests. Knuckey and Gubbay (1983) retested a group of 18-year-olds eight years after their original study, and claimed that only the most severely clumsy at age 10 still had difficulties in their late teens. However, the tests they used were a subset of those given at the earlier age. No group differences were found on threading beads, dribbling a ball, and posting shapes into a box. Significant group differences remained, however, on a clap-and-catch task and on a hole-piercing task. Knuckey and Gubbay noted that those children originally designated mildly or moderately clumsy were now performing at the level of controls; only those originally designated severely clumsy were not. In more general terms, they concluded that the outcome for clumsy children was a fairly good one.

A second 10-year follow-up study (Losse et al., 1991) gave less cause for optimism. This study re-examined, at age 15–17, children who had taken part in an earlier study (Henderson and Hall, 1982). Test batteries included a neurodevelopmental test battery, and the revised Test of Motor Impairment (TOMI; Stott, Moyes and Henderson, 1984). On the neurodevelopmental test, children with DCD seemed largely to have outgrown many of the minor and involuntary movements classified as neurological 'soft signs', but were still significantly poorer than control children on measures of dysdiadochokinesis and dysgraphaesthesia. On the motor test the index group generally continued to perform more poorly than the control group. The most discriminating items were a balance task and catching with the non-preferred hand. Eleven of the 15 children originally designated 'clumsy' were rated 'poor' or 'very poor' on the TOMI in comparison with age-matched controls. Losse et al. warned that the use of tests aimed at younger children may also have resulted in an underestimation of the degree of clumsiness in teenagers.

A major question, then, for studies of teenage participants has been whether to use an established test that is normed for younger children, or whether to use an experimental test battery more appropriate to adolescents, in the absence of performance norms. Geuze and Börger (1993) further investigated this issue. A comparison was made between the performance of clumsy teenagers on the upper age band of the TOMI and their performance on items that had been made more difficult for older children. Children who had been 6–12 years of age in the initial study (van Dellen and Geuze, 1988) were followed up five years later. Using the TOMI, half the clumsy group now appeared to perform at the level of controls, while the other half were borderline or still had serious motor difficulties. However, using the more taxing version only a quarter were classified as having outgrown their motor problems, while another quarter were borderline and half were considered to still have definite motor problems. This shows the importance of finding tasks that do reflect the appropriate age-level of the child. The results from the motor tests were reflected in responses to the parental questionnaires, all but two of which indicated that parents felt children still showed signs of clumsiness.

Cantell, Smyth and Ahonen (1994) also chose to adopt an experimental test battery designed to be more age-appropriate for teenagers. Fifteen- to 17-year-olds were followed up in a study of Finnish children with DCD (Cantell, Smyth and Ahonen, 1994). These children were originally screened at school entry and had already been followed up once (reported in Lyytinen and Ahonen, 1988) at the age of 11. Approximately 65 per cent of the participants originally designated clumsy continued to be classified as having motor problems, while the remainder were considered to have formed an 'intermediate' group, not clearly distinguishable from either the clumsy children or the controls. When Cantell, Smyth and Ahonen (1994) tested the children again at the age of 15, they selected and adapted 19 movement tasks from different motor and neurodevelopmental batteries. These included gross and fine motor tasks, ball skills, balance, timing and grip tasks, copying, imitation of gesture and kinaesthetic perception. Using these tests, Cantell, Smyth and Ahonen (1994) classified further participants into the intermediate group, leaving just under 50 per cent in the stable clumsy group. While the performance of the intermediate group was significantly better than that of the clumsy group on all measures, it remained worse than the control group on a pegboard task, on visual matching and on spatial relations tasks. This suggests that a subgroup of clumsy children may outgrow their motor difficulties, or may be in the process of doing so in their mid-teens. However, it may also indicate that clumsy children outgrow some, but not all difficulties, and that some kinds of motor dysfunction may be more intractable than others.

Following up the same cohort again at the age of 17, Cantell, Smyth and Ahonen (2003) noted that all groups had improved across tasks, and that the distinction between the intermediate and control groups had become even less pronounced, though the intermediate group was still significantly poorer than the control group at two tasks, ball throwing and the Developmental Test of Visuo-Motor Integration (VMI; Beery, 1967). The result of the ball-throwing task showed little consistency at the two different ages, and group differences here should be treated cautiously. However, the groups differed reliably on the VMI, suggesting that visuo-motor integration may be the most persistent problem for children who otherwise outgrow their difficulties.

Unlike the earliest studies, then, follow-up studies conducted during the 1990s indicate that as many as half of all children with DCD do not outgrow their motor clumsiness during their teen years, while others may have some residual motor problems. All studies agree that the most severely affected children are at greatest risk for continuing motor difficulties

Follow-up studies: academic, behavioural and social outcomes for children with DCD

As well as motor outcome, the longitudinal studies detailed above have been concerned to provide insights into the accompanying difficulties and/or potential sequelae of DCD. Most of the studies that have followed children with DCD into the teen years have also reported on various behavioural and academic measures of adolescents with motor disorders. They have shown that not only can DCD persist as a motor disorder into later childhood, but that it may be a risk factor for academic, social and behavioural difficulties. Studies vary in the degree to which they have found a relationship between childhood motor problems and poorer than expected educational achievement.

Knuckey and Gubbay's (1983) clumsy group seemed to have fared slightly less well educationally than controls, but this difference was non-significant. Clumsy teenagers did tend to be found in less skilled jobs on leaving school. Both Losse et al. (1991) and Cantell, Smyth and Ahonen (1994) looked at school records, and also gave their participants Harter's Perceived Competence Scale for Children (Harter, 1982). Losse et al. found indications that some clumsy children who had been doing well academically when first identified, seemed not to have achieved their academic potential 10 years on. Index teenagers had more educational difficulties than controls, especially with overtly motor activities, such as handwriting, art and practical science. While the clumsy children were considered to make as much effort as controls, their academic achievements were not so high. The authors noted that even those with normal TOMI or neurodevelopmental scores were often reported as having some kind of difficulty at school. Behavioural difficulties were also more common in the clumsy group.

In Cantell, Smyth and Ahonen's (1994) study, clumsy children were found to have fewer hobbies, and rated themselves less highly on the scholastic competence and athletic competence subscales of the Harter test. However, there was no evidence that they were failing to achieve their academic potential, as was found in Losse et al.'s (1991) study. The stable clumsy group had both lower mean IQ and lower aspirations regarding their future educational plans than the other groups. It is possible, again, that motivation plays some role in outcome – Cantell, Smyth and Ahonen (1994) suggested that those children who appeared to overcome their difficulties might be more ambitious educationally. In Geuze and Börger's (1993) study educational achievements were also found to be lower in the clumsy group, but this was confounded by lower socioeconomic status. The picture regarding educational achievement for children with DCD, then, is rather unclear. While achievement seems to be lower than for well-coordinated peers, some of this seems to be explainable by IQ differences or differences in socioeconomic factors. However, the relationship between motor clumsiness and academic achievement may be mitigated by feelings of self-worth and motivation to succeed.

Evidently, children with DCD become aware of their motor incompetence at an early stage. At the age of 10, low self-esteem seems to be confined to the motor domain, and tends to be a fairly accurate reflection of the actual level of motor competence (Maeland, 1994). Piek et al. (2000) noted that perceptions of competence need to be considered in the light of the importance children place on any given area of ability; self-worth is a product of these factors. While athletic competence was considered to be less important by children with DCD than those without, the opposite pertained for scholastic competence (Piek et al., 2000). In older children, where IQs have been matched, no differences in the perception of scholastic competence have been found (Skinner and Piek, 2001). Losse et al. (1991) reported that the index 15–17-year-olds in their study scored lower on both 'physical' and 'social' self-esteem subscales than controls. These studies indicate that children with DCD are realistic about their physical abilities, and that perception of other competencies, and of overall self-worth, is not lower than in other groups, although at least one study has reported poorer social self-esteem.

Epidemiological studies

As well as longitudinal studies that have specifically recruited children with motor impairments, other population-based projects have contributed to knowledge of the outcome of early motor impairment. In some cases, longitudinal studies have followed children considered to be 'at risk' for motor impairment, such as low birthweight or premature infants (e.g. Jongmans et al., 1998; Levene et al., 1992). In other cases, entire cohorts of infants or children from a prescribed area have been screened for a variety of developmental problems, and then followed up at regular intervals afterwards; two major studies based in Groningen, Netherlands, and in Goteburg, Sweden, are detailed here. While the studies conducted by Losse et al. (1991) and Cantell, Smyth and Ahonen (1994) were concerned specifically with motor problems in the population, epidemiological studies have conceptualized motor problems within a wider context of 'minimal brain damage/dysfunction' (MBD) or 'minor neurological dysfunction' (MND).

Despite the proviso in DSM-IV that a diagnosis of DCD can only be given if there is no diagnosable neurological disorder, there is a tantalizing link between incidence of DCD and minor neurological abnormality at birth. The problems of at least some children with DCD do not seem to fit with the notion of the disorder simply as a learning difficulty, that is, they do not seem to represent the low end of a normally distributed population. Certainly, numerous studies have now shown that certain neonatal populations are at higher than usual risk of later developmental disorders, including DCD. These include premature babies (Jongmans et al., 1998), very low birthweight infants (Marlow, Roberts and Cooke, 1989; Torrioli et al., 2000; Holsti, Grunau and Whitfield, 2002), and those with neurological abnormality at birth (e.g. Levene et al., 1992; Jongmans et al., 1993).

The Groningen Perinatal Project was set up to look at the incidence of neurological deviance, or minor neurological dysfunction (MND), in the full-term population. The concept of MND assumes that if a neurological abnormality is present at birth, then the child is at risk of continued neurological dysfunction, which may manifest as a variety of learning or behavioural disorders. This study followed all infants born at the University Hospital in Groningen in the Netherlands between 1975 and 1978. Neurological status at birth was ascertained using Prechtl's optimality concept technique (Prechtl, 1977). Of the 3162 infants studied, 21.5 per cent were considered neurologically 'suspect /mildly abnormal' and 5 per cent neurologically 'abnormal'. Groups of children were followed up at ages 6 (Hadders-Algra et al., 1985; Hadders-Algra, Touwen and Huisjes, 1986), 9 (Hadders-Algra, Huisjes and Touwen, 1988a; 1988b) and 12 (Lunsing et al., 1992a). Some children with a neonatal diagnosis of neurological abnormality developed overt motor handicap. Of the remaining neonatally abnormal children, the majority had recovered by the time of the follow-up studies. Nevertheless, speech and language impairments were found significantly more often in the neonatally abnormal group, and these children were more likely to have educational difficulties. At the same time, a minority of neonatally normal children were diagnosed with MND in the follow-up studies. Parent and teacher questionnaires revealed that these children were more likely to be rated 'clumsy' than their classmates.

At the age of 12, many children appeared to outgrow their MND as they entered puberty, while, oddly, a substantial proportion of normal children (22 per cent) appeared to succumb to MND. Some consideration of the course of MND during puberty and adolescence ensued. Lunsing et al. (1992a) hinted that something specific to puberty triggers signs of neurological abnormality in some susceptible individuals; however, more prosaic explanations have been put forward by other authors. Visser, Geuze and Kalverboer (1998), for example, suggested that less pathological mechanisms, such as an adolescent growth spurt, might be responsible. Visser, Geuze and Kalverboer (1998) have pointed out that

> as the metrical and biomechanical changes produced by rapid physical growth disturb the calibration, or 'fine-tuning' of the sensorimotor system, so too will the child's ability to move easily and fluently be affected. (p. 575)

The sensorimotor system is therefore in a continual state of recalibration during puberty. They also suggested that this kind of recalibration may be facilitated by large amounts of physical activity. Studying 15 boys with DCD through the adolescent growth spurt, they noted that mean amount of physical exercise was found to correlate with Movement ABC scores (upper age-band). This supports the notion that children with DCD take less exercise than those without. Though the scores of children with DCD remained significantly worse than those of controls, the difference between groups did decrease with age, boys with DCD apparently being less affected by the growth spurt. Some individuals, though, still had very poor scores at the age of 14.

Lunsing et al. (1992a) had noted that there appeared to be an increase in the incidence of MND in boys in their population at the age of 12, while there was a corresponding decrease in girls. In a further study of 14-year-olds (Soorani-Lunsing, 1993), a linear improvement was seen for girls during puberty, while boys appeared to move from 'normal' to MND groups, and back again. This might well be seen as confirmatory evidence for Visser's assertion that normal boys may be affected by the growth spurt until the nervous system effectively 'recalibrates' itself. Soorani-Lunsing noted that where MND did persist after puberty, it was associated with elevated levels of cognitive and behavioural problems. In about half the cases, however, MND symptoms disappeared between the ages of 12 and 14.

Another major population-based study was undertaken in Sweden, beginning in the early 1980s. This was intended to explore the incidence of minimal brain dysfunction (MBD) in the population. The Swedish model sees attentional deficits and perceptual-motor deficits essentially as part of the same 'syndrome', although 'pure' attentional or motor impairments are noted. In more recent years, researchers have become more wary of trying to say anything too definite about the underlying aetiology, and recent studies have adopted DSM-IV terminology (DCD and ADHD).

The background to this longitudinal study was set out in a series of papers in the early 1980s (Gillberg and Rasmussen, 1982a; 1982b; Gillberg et al., 1982; Rasmussen and Gillberg, 1983; Gillberg, 1983; Gillberg, Carlström and Rasmussen, 1983; Gillberg et al., 1983; Rasmussen et al., 1983). These detailed perceptual, motor and attentional deficits in children entering public pre-schools in Gothenburg at the ages of 6 to 7 (probably about 95 per cent of the total cohort, N = 4797). Overall, 340 children showed some degree of abnormality. As the numbers of symptoms increased, boys began to outnumber girls. A sub-set of these children (N = 61), along with a control group, were given the Touwen's neurological and psychiatric assessments (Touwen, 1979), the Southern California Sensory Integration Tests (SCSIT; Ayres, 1972a) and the performance section of the Wechsler Intelligence Scale for Children (Wechsler, 1974). Within the index group, 62 per cent of children had gross motor difficulties, and 69 per cent had fine motor difficulties (36 per cent had both). Some children seemed only to have motor-perceptual dysfunction (MPD). The importance placed on motor aspects of the disorder by the authors is illustrated by the assertion that

> In most cases of MBD and MPD the neurological picture was unspecific and could be described clinically as the 'clumsy child syndrome'. (Rasmussen et al., 1983, p. 324)

The children in this study were subsequently followed up and reported on at regular intervals, the most recent being at the age of 22.

At the age of 13 the authors defined the index groups as suffering from 'various combinations of deficits in attention, motor control and perception', or DAMP (Gillberg and Gillberg, 1989). At that age, 16 per cent of the index children diagnosed as having MBD in the original study were now considered to be free of any neurological, educational and behavioural problems. More importantly, here, the authors also concluded that perceptual-motor problems had disappeared in 70 per cent of cases; however, this assumption was based on the neurological examination given, which comprised the same items as those given at the age of 10, together with a general impression of 'clumsiness'.

At the age of 16 (reported in Hellgren et al., 1993; Hellgren et al., 1994), children in the MBD group were still more likely than the control group to have balance and fine motor problems and were significantly more likely to have been admitted to hospital after accidents, especially for fractures. Behavioural, psychiatric and personality problems were also greater in this group, and index children were more likely to be involved in substance abuse. While the range of outcomes was very variable, with some children doing well, the authors warned that there was no overall justification for the notion that children outgrow their difficulties.

This is the only study to date to follow children with developmental motor impairments into young adulthood (reported in Rasmussen and Gillberg, 2000), as a number of individuals were investigated again at the age of 22. At this stage, terminology from DSM-IV was adopted. Participants in the study were considered to have 'pure' DCD (N = 5), 'pure' ADHD (N = 11) or a combination of ADHD with DCD (N = 39). They were compared with age-matched controls from previous studies. Neuropsychiatric assessments and neurodevelopmental examinations were given, together with a reading test. These included an assessment of 'motor clumsiness' but, unfortunately, there is no further indication of what measures might have been used. Adult outcome was defined in predominantly functional and daily living measures, such as reliance on disability benefits, criminal conviction, substance abuse, or diagnosis of psychiatric or personality disorder. Of the index group cases 58 per cent (13 per cent controls) were considered to have had a 'poor outcome' based on these measures, with the figures being highest in the motor disordered groups. The index groups also had poorer educational outcomes than controls. The authors concluded that for many individuals with ADHD and DCD the outcome was worse than anticipated (Rasmussen and Gillberg, 2000).

Like the Groningen study, the Swedish study has demonstrated that early developmental impairments are not always outgrown. In this case, the functional impairments of such children have been described more fully than they were in the MND study, so it is possible to gain some measure of the extent to which motor difficulties persist and in what circumstances. Again, a wide range of outcomes was reported. Motor deficits, however, seem to be particularly persistent when found in combination with attentional ones. In young adulthood, there is also evidence that psychiatric well-being is at risk in motor disordered groups.

Clumsiness in young adults

No follow-up studies have yet been undertaken specifically with adults who have previously been diagnosed with DCD as children, though

Rasmussen and Gillberg (2000) assumed that the motor problems detailed in their study were commensurate with DCD. In the self-help and clinical literature a certain amount of descriptive information is available. Portwood (1999) for example, provides a number of case scenarios. Two studies of adult groups, though, have noted motor difficulties that appear to have a developmental origin (Shelley and Riester, 1972; Porter and Corlett, 1989). Neither looked at populations previously diagnosed with DCD or any equivalent label, though the earlier study assumed the population under consideration would fall into the category of MBD.

Shelley and Riester's (1972) study was retrospective; 16 training recruits, aged 18–23, in the US Air Force had been referred to a psychiatrist because of their difficulties in learning new motor skills, anxiety and difficulties with concentration. Psychiatric and neurological examinations were performed, and history prior to training obtained. Families had often regarded them as uncoordinated, but difficulties seemed to disappear with age until placed in a situation where a high degree of motor competence was necessary (that is, basic training). The authors noted that on removal from the training situation, all recruits became 'asymptomatic', which suggests that for the purposes of everyday living, their difficulties were not especially disabling, but that something inherent in the training situation – either the need to learn new tasks quickly, or the level of difficulty of the tasks – was problematic. The neurological examination revealed at least two 'soft signs' (which included clumsiness, poor balance, confused laterality and incoordination) in every case. Mean verbal IQ on the WAIS was 105.8, but mean performance IQ was 83.8. The recruits were given the Bender-Gestalt designs, normally completed correctly by 9-year-olds. This group of adults performed poorly on this test. A number had histories, verified by family members, of frustrated and hyperkinetic behaviour as children, which had tended to decrease at adolescence. Ten had a history of speech problems (though only three had persisting speech impairments as adults), and 12 had educational or behavioural difficulties at school. Perinatal problems were said to be 'prominent' but unfortunately the authors did not describe the exact incidence or nature of these problems. Shelley and Riester concluded that the symptoms were commensurate with a diagnosis of MBD, and that, though they had subsided, it was possible for them to re-emerge when a high degree of perceptual motor competence was required:

> Careful neurological evaluation and psychological testing indicates that all manifestations of minimal brain damage do not tend towards spontaneous remission as has been generally believed. (Shelley and Riester, 1972, p. 338)

The second study dealing with adults (Porter and Corlett, 1989) has come from a different tradition altogether. During the 1970s and 1980s there was much interest in the concept of 'accident-proneness', which stemmed from personality research and psychometrics. Porter and Corlett defined 'accident-prone' as a propensity for motoric slips and errors such as bumping into things, falling, knocking things over, and dropping things. It therefore seems reasonable to assume that they may have targeted adults with continuing symptoms of DCD (though a history was not taken). Interestingly, they targeted a student population as it was thought that a workforce might not respond accurately for fear of management bias.

Porter and Corlett's testing procedure consisted of first, six simple motor tasks, which elicited no group differences. It was then decided to use a dual task approach. The primary task was a computer-based tracking task, and the secondary task a blind reach to one of eight targets (auditorily cued) with the dominant hand. Participants had been trained on the latter task. It was found that the performance of the accident-prone volunteers was worse on the primary task alone, and in the dual task situation, though not on the secondary task on its own. Early in the dual task sessions, the index group were slower to find the centre of the target than controls. With practice, this improved to the level of the controls, but deteriorated after a 90-second break. The authors concluded that the primary task, in this case, was complex enough to give rise to group differences, and the addition of the secondary task made little difference to performance.

Adults with DCD: a retrospective approach

In a recent study (Cousins and Smyth, 2003) adults with a diagnosis of DCD or with histories indicative of the disorder were selected by questionnaire and interview and subsequently took part in motor tests. Clearly a retrospective study cannot answer questions about the proportion of young people who continue to have difficulties. However, the study does indicate that coordination impairments can continue to affect individuals across the life-span. Some respondents to initial publicity about the project were in their seventies, and felt that they were still unduly clumsy. In severe cases, participants reported that they had been adults before they had acquired certain skills said to be problematic for children with DCD; one man reported that he was in his thirties before he learned to tie his shoelaces, and others reported that they still preferred to eat with a spoon rather than a knife and fork.

Nineteen participants, aged between 18 and 65, undertook motor tests adapted from standardized child batteries such as the Movement Assessment Battery for Children (Movement ABC; Henderson and Sugden, 1992). Because such tasks have never been used before with adults, norms were not available, and so age- and gender-matched controls were also recruited. Gross and fine motor skills were tested; functional tasks included manual dexterity tests, obstacle avoidance, static and dynamic balance, block construction, handwriting and ball skills. The index group performed more poorly than control participants across the entire range of tasks, deficits being most pronounced in ball and dynamic balance tasks. There was a continuum of impairment. While many participants were clearly very impaired on these simple tasks, some participants performed close to normal levels, and possibly represented the adult equivalent of Cantell, Smyth and Ahonen's (1994) 'intermediate' group.

The index group in this study was drawn from a wider pool of 45 participants, who filled in self-report questionnaires. Concomitant problems were widely reported; 17.8 per cent of respondents had one or more diagnosed concomitant disorder (usually dyslexia and/or ADHD). Altogether, 84.4 per cent reported that they had difficulties, or had had difficulties as children, with one or more of the following: learning to read, basic mathematics, concentration and social skills. In many cases, respondents felt these were no longer problematic. The most widespread, and the most persistent, difficulties seemed to be with concentration, which may support the Swedish model of concomitant attentional and motor problems.

While adults with coordination difficulties displayed continuities in the kinds and degree of functional difficulties displayed by children and teenagers with the disorder, there were some everyday tasks that are specific to adults – such as the ability to drive a car – which many of the index group had been unable to master. While the researchers did not necessarily expect to find a correspondence between performance on simple laboratory tasks and more complex ecological skills such as driving, regression analysis suggested that the ability to drive a car was in fact strongly related to performance on items in the motor test battery. The inability to drive is a considerable disadvantage in contemporary life in the UK, and is one of the clearest indications that coordination impairment has an effect on the everyday activities of adults. Around half the index group had a higher education qualification, indicating that motor impairment need not be a barrier to academic success. At the same time, some participants were unable to maintain employment that adequately reflected their academic achievements. In a number of cases they felt they could not perform tasks quickly or accurately enough, and could not learn new systems that were introduced to the workplace after they were taken on as employees.

Individuals who are diagnosed with DCD as children, then, or who self-report as having coordination impairments, may continue to have motor difficulties into their adult years. When affected individuals are compared with normally-coordinated controls these deficits are observable on tests of simple motor skill based on extensions of child batteries. Like Porter and Corlett (1989), it was found that it was not necessary to dual-task test items in order to find group effects, although in the cases of one or two of the least affected individuals dual-tasking sometimes elucidated a problem when more simple tasks did not. Participants who were very impaired on simple tasks were more likely to have difficulties with complex tasks such as driving a car.

Difficulties of tracing developmental pathways

Linked to considerations of delay and difference in development are problems of prediction, and of understanding how developmental pathways proceed for the individual. While the tendency towards co-morbidity of disorders such as DCD, dyslexia and ADHD is widely recognized, the notion of a diffuse, low-level dysfunction affecting all cognitive systems has gradually given way to definitions of developmental disorder that have become increasingly specific. Such specificity implies a modular system. However, in a developmental context, it is likely that even very prescribed dysfunction would exert subtle effects on other functions, making the ultimate outcome unpredictable. Karmiloff-Smith (1998) outlines the complexity of transactional process, noting that

> development itself is seen as playing a crucial role in shaping phenotypical outcomes ... Thus, two very distinct phenotypical outcomes could start with only slightly differing parameters but, with development, the effect of this small difference might be far reaching. (Karmiloff-Smith, 1998, pp. 389–90)

Within this model, a host of intrinsic and extrinsic factors come into play. For example, the degree to which a child might utilize intact functions to compensate for affected ones, and the particular strategies adopted, are important factors in determining ultimate outcome (Frith, 2001). Parental attitudes, access to remediation and the child's personal motivation are other factors that are sometimes ignored in considerations of long-term outcome. The effects of the interaction of motivational factors with patterns of deficit has been noted in studies of children with a liking for a particular pastime.

Barnett and Henderson (1992), for example, investigating clumsy children with poor drawing skills, noted one child with a love of drawing cartoon characters, who developed strategies for dealing with his poor fine motor coordination. Recently, Smyth and Anderson (Smyth and Anderson, 2000; 2001) studied participation in playground activities, including football games. Some boys with DCD enjoyed the game and played regularly. However, those who scored particularly poorly on the balance subsets of the Movement ABC did not play, indicating that lack of postural control may be prohibitive. While children with DCD who wish to play football may be able to compensate for poor ball skills through practice and through motivational factors, it appears they are unable to compensate for poor balance skills.

Football is necessarily a team game, and boys in Smyth and Anderson's study who played spent longer, overall, in social play than those who did not. Here, something of the complexity of the transactional processes involved in determining outcome can be seen. Social exclusion may accompany motor problems (Schoemaker and Kalverboer, 1994), but questions remain as to the extent to which social difficulties are intrinsic to the child, perhaps because of additional impairments that affect the child's ability to interact in appropriate ways, or the extent to which reduced opportunities for social interaction present themselves to the clumsy child.

The same is true of motor skills: unusual clumsiness may demand unusual persistence at any given task. The more difficult the child finds the task, the more inclined she may be to abandon it. The consequences for lack of persistence may be long-term. O'Beirne, Larkin and Cable (1994) have demonstrated that children with DCD show poorer anaerobic performance than their well-coordinated peers, and a recent study by Flouris and colleagues (2003) has modelled the long-term effects of the increased levels of obesity and poor fitness found in children with DCD, and pointed to an elevated risk for coronary disease in later life. Coordination difficulties, then, probably do not have simple effects on motor, social and emotional outcomes in later life.

Outcome for children with DCD

These considerations of variation in developmental course serve as a reminder that outcome for children with DCD and other developmental disorders should not be seen as prescribed. The studies reviewed above that have followed up children through their teen years have identified factors that contribute to poor long-term outcome, but for an individual the suggestion that they are 'at risk' should be seen as just that. However, the longitudinal studies have pointed to a first major factor in the outcome for children with DCD; that of severity of disorder when the child is first screened. The term 'severity' of course, is open to interpretation, but it seems reasonable to assume from the way that tests are constructed that it includes both the *range* of deficits displayed by the child, and the actual performance levels. The Movement ABC, for example, tests balance, manual dexterity and ball skills; a child who falls into the lowest fifth percentile may have performed poorly across all subscales. Another risk factor is clearly the presence of one or more concomitant difficulties.

Outcome studies have shown that some children with DCD seem to recover in the teen years. However, the findings from some of these studies may be over-optimistic, given that the tests applied are usually designed for use with much younger children and some teenagers remain impaired even on these measures. In addition, different authors have reported associated behavioural, academic and emotional difficulties experienced by some children as they reach their teens. While comparatively little is known about adults, there is now research evidence that, taken together with together with clinical reports, indicates that coordination difficulties continue to impact long after the teenage years. In only one case (Rasmussen and Gillberg, 2000) is it certain that these adults come from a population of motor disordered children, but adults who report childhood coordination difficulties, or whose families provide evidence of this, are at risk for occupational disadvantages even when education has been continued to high levels. Sufficient evidence exists that the disorder should be taken seriously and that remediation measures should be available for children found to have motor coordination problems. As yet, not enough is known about the long-term benefits of different kinds of remediation technique and the mitigating effects these may have. However, the indications from consideration of the complexity of developmental pathways suggest that remediation should be flexible and should take account of more than any specific motor problem.

CHAPTER 7

Assessment of Developmental Coordination Disorder

DAWNE LARKIN AND ELIZABETH ROSE

The focus of this chapter is the identification, assessment, and evaluation of children who are considered to have Developmental Coordination Disorder (DCD; American Psychiatric Association, 1994). The movement profiles of children with this disorder are quite variable (Dewey and Kaplan, 1994; Gubbay, 1975a; Hadders-Algra, 2003; Hoare, 1994) as is the prognosis (Cantell, Smyth and Ahonen, 1994; Rasmussen and Gillberg, 2000). Children with DCD have a motor learning disability (Hands and Larkin, 2001a; Keogh, 1982) and take much longer to learn complex motor skills. When they fall behind their peers in achieving culturally appropriate skills, there are psycho-social consequences including isolation or withdrawal from social group participation (Smyth and Anderson, 2000; Summers and Larkin, 2002; Symes, 1972) and there are lifelong consequences for some (Cousins and Smyth, 2003; Fitzpatrick and Watkinson, 2003). It is important that children with these movement problems are identified and provided with movement enrichment programmes in socially supportive environments. Formal definitions of the condition are provided in Chapter 1 by Chambers, Sugden and Sinani.

A number of authors have noted the need for a multi-level approach to assessment for children with DCD (Cermak, Gubbay and Larkin, 2002; Kaplan et al., 1998; Keogh et al., 1979; Rodger et al., 2003; Schoemaker, Smits-Engelsman and Jongmans, 2003; Wright and Sugden, 1996b). This view is strongly supported by the authors and they propose here that assessment should encompass multiple sources of information in the human movement and relevant psycho-social domains. In this chapter, issues that need to be considered when assessing children's motor performance are looked at, focusing on different types of assessments that are used to identify children with DCD and those that are important for the evaluation of motor programmes and during the learning of motor skills. To further understanding of children's ability to learn and perform motor skills, the need to evaluate their physical fitness is also addressed. This aspect of motor performance can have a positive or a negative effect on how children engage in physical activity and play. Given that movement experience is essential for the development of competent motor perform-ance, an understanding of a child's movement background and participation level is also important in the overall assessment of his or her motor proficiency. Parents' and teachers' knowledge and attitudes to phys-ical activity can also play a positive or negative role in the motor development process. To this end parent and teacher questionnaires designed to identify DCD are also considered. To achieve a broad overview of the factors contributing to a child's current motor status, child self-reports of self-perceptions and attitudes to physical activity are discussed.

While looking at the different ways of identifying DCD, typical motor assessment tools essential to the identification of DCD will be discussed, such as the Movement Assessment Battery for Children (Movement ABC, Henderson and Sugden, 1992), the McCarron (1982) Assessment of Neuromuscular Development (MAND) and the Test of Gross Motor Development (2nd edition) (Ulrich, 2000). Additionally, there will be an evaluation of the use of parent questionnaires such as the DCDQ (Wilson, Dewey and Campbell, 1998) and teacher questionnaires (Keogh et al., 1979; Revie and Larkin, 1993a; Henderson and Sugden, 1992). The use of self-reports by children that attempt to get at their feelings about their movement competence (Harter, 1985; Missiuna, 1998), and movement confidence (Griffin and Keogh, 1982; Rose et al., 2000) are also addressed. These tools, discussed below, provide the opportunity to use more than one source of information about the child's movement behav-iours. The multi-level approach provides information to support intervention, as well as overcoming some of the problems associated with disagreement on the underlying or emergent causes of DCD (Cermak, Gubbay and Larkin, 2002; Gubbay, 1975a; Hall, 1988) and the varying motor profiles (Dewey and Kaplan, 1994; Hoare, 1994; Macnab, Miller and Polatajko, 2001; Parker, Larkin and Wade, 1997; Visser, 2003).

Constraints to be considered when interpreting tests

Terminology and constructs

In this chapter, the terms DCD, motor learning difficulty and movement difficulty are interchanged; this is because the primary criterion for the identification of DCD is the failure to achieve age-appropriate motor skills when there is no diagnosis of a motor disorder (APA, 1994). The current terminology, Developmental Coordination Disorder is predicated on the assumption that there is difficulty with coordination. This terminology poses a problem as the construct of coordination is not well defined and coordination is usually inferred from measurement of movement skill performances. Coordination is also viewed in a number of ways and at different levels. Coordination is seen as an intrinsic ability or as an emergent property of the system. At the perceptual-motor level, we have visuomotor coordination, hand–eye coordination, and foot–eye coordination, while at the movement level we have intralimb, interlimb and multilimb coordination. Bernstein (1967) regards coordination as

> the process of mastering redundant degrees of freedom of the moving organ, in other words its conversion to a controllable system. (p. 127)

Coordination is also conceptualized

> as the generation of appropriate spatial and temporal relations among movement-related events such that the goal of an action is successfully achieved. (Walter et al., 1997, cited in Walter, 1998, p. 326)

or as a match between an individual's internal and external environment (Parker, 1905, p. 373). Coordination is relevant to internally focused skills where the movement is essentially constrained by the individual, such as running, hopping, and tumbling or externally focused skills where coordination is constrained by environmental information such as catching a ball and/or interacting with others. Given these descriptions, poor performance across a range of motor skills could be considered to reflect a problem with coordination, but there are other constructs that could explain this outcome. For example, problems with balance, sensorimotor integration, motor timing, motor planning (dyspraxia) or low motor ability could all result in poor motor performance across a range of motor tasks. Although the term Developmental Coordination Disorder has been useful (see Henderson and Henderson, 2002, for discussion) in focusing researchers and practitioners towards the problem with movement, independent of other co-morbid or parallel problems, there is a need to recognize the difficulties and limitations inherent in measuring the construct of coordination. Terms such as movement difficulty or movement impairment focus our attention to a level of analysis closer to the items actually used to identify DCD, while the term, motor learning difficulty centres on the process that appears to be impaired. The lack of clarity, in the definition of coordination, limits test validity and leads to problems with identification and intervention.

When it comes to motor tests to assess for DCD, the emphasis has not been on 'coordination', its development, or the disorder of coordination but, rather, the tests have focused on motor proficiency (Arnheim and

Sinclair, 1979; Bruininks, 1978; Gubbay, 1975a), motor impairment (Henderson and Sugden, 1992), and neuromuscular or neuromotor development (Largo, Fischer and Caflisch, 2002; McCarron, 1982) with the assumption, either implicitly or explicitly that there is a general construct akin to coordination or more possibly motor ability. Although the construct of general motor ability guided some of the earliest tests of motor performance (Brace, 1927; Carpenter, 1942; McCloy, 1934), it has been unpopular over the last 50 years or more and the emphasis has been on skill specificity (Larkin and Parker, 2002). Nevertheless, researchers and practitioners have continued to use tests of motor ability (see Burton and Rodgerson, 2001 for discussion). Burton and Rodgerson (2001) have recently put forward a taxonomy that encompasses specificity and generality. The taxonomy includes four levels: movement skills, movement skill sets, movement skill foundations, and general motor ability in order to provide a systematic taxonomy for organizing movement assessments. Burton and Rodgerson (2001) have re-argued the case in favour of motor ability following their re-evaluation of earlier evidence. Further evidence supporting a general construct comes from research on the validity of the Movement ABC (Henderson and Sugden, 1992), the BOTMP (Bruininks, 1978) and the MAND (McCarron, 1982). Although these tests consist of items that represent different constructs or abilities and the test items are categorized in a relatively arbitrary fashion, total scores from these tests are highly correlated (Tan, Parker and Larkin, 2001). Consequently they might be considered as tests of a general construct such as coordination or motor ability. The moderate correlations found between motor tests and motor checklists are more variable (Boyle, 2003; Wilson et al., 2000b) but still provide some support for a general factor.

Measurement issues

Cut-off scores

One of the major reasons for having multiple measures is that this approach compensates somewhat for the use of cut-off scores. These are arguably arbitrary points, usually the 5th or 15th percentile, selected for determining whether a child has DCD or not. The authors' personal experience initially using the Test of Motor Impairement (TOMI; Stott, Moyes and Henderson, 1972; 1984) and then the MAND (McCarron, 1982) for entry into a motor learning programme reinforced the need for a multi-level assessment approach. Children who scored better than the 15th percentile cut-off score brought into the programme on the basis of additional information usually showed motor learning difficulties over the 10 to 12 week programme. Based on extensive experience working with children with movement difficulties, the authors would encourage the use of the 15th percentile cut-off score when using the MAND or the Movement ABC for research. In practice there is a need to be less prescriptive. With this cut-off score, it is still important to seek additional information and interpret the output of the assessment carefully. An exemplar case was of an intelligent young boy who scored 92 on the MAND, that is in the normal range. His movement profile was remarkable because of the discrepancy between his scores on the gross motor section of the MAND and the fine motor section. At the age of 8 he was unable to ride a bike like the rest of his peers and his locomotor skills were particularly inefficient. He was being isolated in the playground. From professional judgement and additional information obtained from parent interview, it was confirmed that he would benefit from a movement programme. Children like this who fit a particular subtype would not be included in research studies because they fail the criteria that is set with a cut-off score at the 15th percentile on tests that have a good balance of fine and gross motor items. However, a young child with this profile would probably be identified in a test battery such as the TGMD (Ulrich, 2000).

Identification issues

Population estimates

As the assessment tools used in the identification of DCD are explored, it becomes obvious that the tasks and taxonomic bases used are quite variable. The types of tasks included in tests have varied particularly as a function of the professionals using them. A task analysis of the items suggests that there is some confusion about allocating tasks in terms of their function or attribute (Burton and Rodgerson, 2001; Larkin and Cermak, 2002). Although there is overlap in the identification between assessment tools, there is also disagreement as to the children identified as having DCD or motor impairment (Boyle, 2003; Foulder-Hughes and Cooke, 2003; Maeland, 1992; Tan, Parker and Larkin, 2001). There has been a relatively persistent notion that about 5 to 6 per cent of the population has DCD. This is despite that fact that researchers and practitioners have not yet decided the appropriate cut-off score, the 5th or 15th percentile, on tests designed to identify children with DCD. Thus it is not surprising that studies show some lack of agreement over the percentage of the population who has DCD.

In a recent study, Foulder-Hughes and Cooke (2003) used three different types of motor assessment tools with 210 control children and 280 pre-term children in the 7–8 year age range. The assessments included (a) the Movement ABC (Henderson and Sugden, 1992) which consists of manipulative skills, ball skills and balance skills, (b) the VMI (Beery, 1997) which consists of copying shapes with a pencil on paper, and (c) the Clinical Observations of Motor and Postural Skills (COMPS; Wilson et al., 1994) which includes tasks designed to 'measure some of the skills which underlie movement and posture' (p. 1). Foulder-Hughes and Cooke (2003) found that 6.7 per cent of the control children were identified with motor impairment using the Movement ABC, 8.1 per cent were identified using the VMI, and 10.2 per cent were identified using the COMPS. With the pre-term group, 30.7 per cent were identified with motor impairment using the Movement ABC, 24.3 per cent with the VMI, and 42.7 per cent with the COMPS. These three tests come from very different taxonomic bases and use quite different tasks so that correlations were not high, however the two tests with gross motor tasks had the higher correlation (Movement ABC:COMPS $r = -.623$; Movement ABC:VMI $r = -.381$; COMPS:VMI $r = .301$). The differences in identification rates are not surprising, particularly if the tests are viewed in terms of Burton and Rodgerson's (2001) taxonomy or from a task specific framework (Larkin and Parker, 2002).

Two population studies in Australia identified quite different incidences, 6 per cent (Gubbay, 1975a) and 18 per cent (Larkin and Rose, 1999) using different tests, the Test of Motor Proficiency (TMP) and the McCarron (1982) Assessment of Neuromotor Development (MAND) respectively. The cut-off criteria for the TMP, the Motor Standard based on age and the number of failures on the tasks approximates a 5th percentile cut-off (a task failure is set at the 10th percentile cut score). The MAND neurodevelopmental index is constructed in a very different way and is less conservative than the TMP standard score, with the cut-off score approximating the 15th percentile. Thus, the cut-off scores accounted for most of the difference in identification rates. However, there are other confounding influences that could influence the identification rates. Both of these tests have items that could be classified as fine and gross motor tests, but the items differ considerably. The TMP has an orofacial skill, four manipulative skills, two locomotor skills (one involving a ball), and a complex ball skill. The MAND has four items performed while seated that involve speeded manipulative skills, three items that involve the performance of the upper limbs while standing, a steadiness item, grip strength and finger-nose, as well as two balance items, dynamic balance walking a line and static balance on one foot. The other MAND item, the standing broad jump, is used and classified in a number of ways, a locomotor skill, a test of lower limb strength and sometimes a test of dynamic balance. Although there was limited crossover in the type of motor test items (TMP and MAND) used in the two Australian studies, both school-based populations showed distribution of boys and girls with coordination difficulties.

Results from a Swedish study (Kadesjö and Gillberg, 1999b) using 7-year-olds in their first year in normal schools showed different distributions to the Australian studies. While the overall results of the Swedish study indicated that 4.9 per cent of the children had severe DCD and 8.6 per cent of the children had moderate DCD, a total of 13.5 per cent, the ratio of boys to girls with DCD ranged from 1:4 to 1:7. The method of identification was quite different for the Swedish study (see Kadesjö and Gillberg, 1999b for detail). Scoring procedures make a difference to the sensitivity of a test. If we look at the scoring on these studies that have attempted to estimate the incidence of DCD, we note that scoring procedures vary in sensitivity and probably influence the outcomes (Kadesjö and Gillberg, 1999b; Larkin and Rose, 1999). The incidence might also be influenced by the age differences of the children used in the studies. For example the Australian studies involved children aged from 5 through 12 years and all but the 5-year-olds had been at school for more than one year. The four studies reported above clearly demonstrate some of the problems with assessment related to the identification of DCD and reinforce the need for a multi-level assessment procedure. It is quite clear that cross-cultural epidemiological studies are needed to get a better estimate of the incidence of DCD, but only when a consensus is reached about some of the outstanding measurement issues.

Gender estimates

Traditionally, more males than females are referred for help with their motor skills. However, when we look at some population studies using motor performance tests in contrast to clinical referral, the number of females identified appears similar to the number of males (Gubbay, 1975a; Larkin and Rose, 1999). Even using motor performance tests, the figures can differ depending on the severity of DCD (Kadesjö and Gillberg, 1999b). Further research is necessary to explore factors that could contribute to these similarities and differences. Unfortunately there has been an assumption that during the early years, boys and girls perform motor skills in a relatively similar way. As a result many test developers have not provided separate norms for young boys and girls despite research that shows gender differences from early childhood (Hands and Larkin, 1997; Morris et al., 1982; Nelson et al., 1986; Revie and Larkin, 1995; Thomas and French, 1985). It has also been assumed that boys' and girls' motor developmental pathways are similar despite some evidence that this is not the case. Hands and Larkin (2001b) argue that the motor ability is expressed differently in boys and girls as a function of different developmental pathways that are influenced by sociological and biological factors.

Thus, it was not surprising that the study by Causgrove Dunn and Watkinson (1996) revealed that certain tasks were gender biased on the TOMI (Stott et al., 1984) and lead to differences in the identification of boys and girls. In keeping with the research on object control skills (Nelson et al., 1986; Ulrich, 2000), the catching and throwing ball skills in age bands 3 and 4 were better performed by boys. Consequently, more boys passed these tasks and more girls were likely to have a greater motor impairment score. There was also a bias favouring girls; in band 1, more girls passed the tracing task than boys. The gender-biased items are still evident in the motor section of the Movement ABC (Henderson and Sugden, 1992).

Other tests have gender biased items; for example, in the gross motor section of the MAND, the standing broad jump and hand strength scores on average are better for boys than for girls. Although McCarron (1982) has separate norms for these items starting at 14 years, gender differences are apparent much earlier. Gender-biased items are also apparent in the fine motor section of the MAND where girls, on average, perform better than boys on a timed tasks placing beads into a box. When Larkin and Rose (1999) looked at the overall score, the NDI provided by the MAND, it was more robust with no significant difference between boys ($M = 99.9$, $SD = 15.8$) and girls ($M = 101.3$, $SD = 16.7$).

More recently developed tests have started to address the gender issue. The Zurich Neuromotor Assessment (ZNA) tool (Largo, Fischer and Caflisch, 2002; Largo, Fischer and Rousson, 2003) was designed to examine basic motor function using a number of motor tasks. The authors refer to testing for neuromotor integrity and motor dysfunction. The test is designed for children ranging in age from 5 to 18. During the development of the Zurich Neuromotor Assessment, Largo and colleagues (2002) report gender differences that vary in size, depending on the task. For example, they report that boys are faster on simple repetitive movements while girls are faster on more complex tasks such as pegboard tasks and can stand for longer on one leg. These differences are accommodated in the scoring of the test. In the TGMD-2 (Ulrich, 2000), gender-based norms are provided for object control. In Stay in Step (Larkin and Revie, 1994), a short 4-item gross motor screening test for 5- to 7-year-olds, there are separate norms for boys and girls based on significant differences in performance at this age (Revie and Larkin, 1995). With the exception of the criterion referenced TGMD-2, the motor batteries discussed below have not seriously addressed the issue of gender differences in motor skill performance. This issue needs to be addressed in test construction but until such time, the experienced assessor should consider these differences when interpreting test scores.

Motor tests

There is no gold standard when it comes to the identification of children with DCD. The issues discussed above provide evidence to show that clarification of constructs and identification of gender differences are just a few of the problems that need to be solved before tests can be developed that might be considered a gold standard. In this section, three assessment batteries will be considered; the Movement ABC (Henderson and Sugden, 1992), the MAND (McCarron, 1982), and the TGMD-2 (Ulrich, 2000). All are currently used to identify children with motor problems, especially DCD. We will give a brief overview of each test and critically evaluate issues that need to be considered when interpreting the test output from these differently structured test batteries.

Movement Assessment Battery for Children (Movement ABC)

The movement assessment section of the Movement ABC (Henderson and Sugden, 1992) was designed to identify motor impairment or dysfunction. This section of the Movement ABC has a long history of use with the current form in use since 1984 (Henderson revision of the TOMI). The earlier versions were categorized into more abstract constructs including static balance, hand–eye coordination, whole-body coordination, manual dexterity and simultaneous movements (Stott, Moyes and Henderson, 1972). The Movement ABC movement assessment items are now divided into three major categories, manipulative skills, ball skills and balance skills. The Movement ABC is designed for the age range from 4 to 12 years. It provides a total impairment score, ranging from 0 to 40, that is useful for the identification of DCD. This Movement ABC was not designed for identification of well-coordinated children, that is children who have above average motor profiles, as it is not sufficiently discriminating at that end of the normal distribution. It has been widely used in research to identify children in groups designated as clumsy (e.g. Dwyer and McKenzie, 1994; Geuze and Kalverboer, 1994), motor impaired (e.g. Tan, Parker and Larkin, 2001), DCD (e.g. Mon-Williams, Pascal and Wann, 1994; Rodger et al., 2003) and controls. The cut-off score used to separate DCD in research ranges from the 5th (e.g. Mon-Williams, Pascal and Wann, 1994; Schoemaker and Kalverboer, 1994) to the 15th percentile (e.g. Dwyer and McKenzie, 1994; Schoemaker et al., 2003). Despite the discrepancy in cut-off scores, the outcome of research using the TOMI (Stott, Moyes and Henderson, 1984) and the Movement ABC (Henderson and Sugden, 1992) shows group differences on the variables of interest, adding credibility to the predictive validity of the Movement ABC. Recent research looking at the psychometric properties of the Movement ABC in relation to the check-list (Schoemaker et al., 2003) using the 5th and 15th cut-off scores shows that different patterns of results arise. Further studies are needed to help researchers and practitioners understand the implications of using different cut-off scores.

The Movement ABC has also been used as a tool in intervention research. Although it has worked in some research studies (Leemrijse et al., 2000; Pless et al., 2000; Sugden and Chambers, 2003a), difficulties have arisen in others. Thus, the researcher must be particularly careful to match the intervention to the task groupings or, in Burton and Rodgerson's (2001) term, movement skill sets. This matching was apparent in the Sugden and Chambers (2003a) study where task groupings were clearly established. The experience of the authors with the Movement ABC in a pre-test, post-test format has shown changes on the task groupings taught, with no change in task groupings not taught (Cantell et al., 2001). The overall reduction in the motor impairment score was a function of the change on the task grouping taught. Similar experiences were found with intervention programmes using the earlier version of the TOMI (Stott, Moyes and Henderson, 1972), the BMAT-R (Arnheim and Sinclair, 1979) and the MAND (McCarron, 1982). The assumption of generalizability needs systematic research in relation to the task grouping or the specificity hypothesis.

Another aspect of the Movement ABC can limit the interpretation of change over time because the task demands vary. Ball skills, which would fall into Burton and Rodgerson's (2001) movement skill set or Ulrich's (2000) object control category, provide an example of varying constraints within and across age bands that could create problems if a researcher or practitioner wanted to measure change longitudinally. For some ball skill items the environment is closed and the predominating action is projection of an object, for others the environment is open and the child must be coincident with the moving environment to be successful. In these cases, judgement of object velocity and motor timing are very important. A third group of ball skills involves both projection and reception of objects, so that control of force and direction are prerequisites if the child is going to be able to anticipate the reception of the object. The task demands change remarkably if the child does not have the ability to control force and direction. In these circumstances, the self-propelled object reception task changes from an open and predictable environment to an open and unpredictable environment, a far more complex skill. These changing task demands can add uncontrolled noise to the measurement of change. As mentioned earlier, there is also the issue of gender bias in some age bands. These issues need to be considered when using the Movement ABC in initial testing and are of additional concern if the test is used longitudinally where the bias could be apparent at one age band and not at another.

The McCarron Assessment of Neuromuscular Development (MAND)

There is good decision agreement (81 per cent) between the Movement ABC and the MAND (Tan, Parker and Larkin, 2001) for the identification of children with DCD. Both of these assessment tools revolve around a range of motor skills and are probably representative of a construct such as motor ability or coordination with a correlation between the tests of .86 (Tan, Parker and Larkin, 2001). Both batteries include manipulative skills and balance skills but differ in that the MAND does not include ball skills but does include two items that load on a strength factor, grip strength and standing broad jump. The MAND also has good concurrent validity with Stay in Step (Larkin and Revie, 1994), a gross motor screening test developed in Australia for children K-2. The test has four items, balance, run, hop, and bounce and catch and the outcome scores are time, distance and count. Despite the brevity of the test, it correlates well with the MAND ($r = .82$) and has high decision agreement (94 per cent) (Boyle, 2003). The MAND also correlates with the DCDQ parent questionnaire ($r = .79$).

The MAND yields a total score called the neurodevelopmental index or NDI. The NDI has a mean of 100, and an *SD* of 15, with a range from 40 to 155. The cut-off score for a mild motor disability is 85, while 70 or below indicates a marked motor disability. Each of the 10 items on the battery are standardized by age but not by gender. The scores range from 0 to 20 with a mean of 10 and an *SD* of 3. The range of scores provided with the MAND make it suitable for identifying well-coordinated children as well as children with DCD. The MAND also has the advantage of norms ranging from 3½ years to young adults.

The MAND works well in research and practice for the initial identification of children with DCD. The authors use McCarron's (1982) suggested cut-off score, the NDI ≤ 85 in their research. This score approximates a 15th percentile cut-off. Like the Movement ABC, research done with the MAND has yielded strong group differences on variables measuring aspects of movement (Larkin et al., 1988; Hoare, 1994; Raynor, 2001), fitness (O'Beirne, Larkin and Cable, 1994; Raynor, 2001) and children's self-perceptions (Rose, Larkin and Berger, 1997).

In practice, children with a score of 85 or less always come into the programme but the authors also take in children with higher scores based on parent interview and subjective clinical assessment. The MAND is not used during intervention as our programmes are task specific, task grouped or focus on changing particular abilities, such as balance and coordination. The MAND, with its overall NDI score, is designed to measure a general construct, for example coordination or general motor ability. There is no evidence to suggest that general motor ability can be changed with a task specific or task grouping intervention.

Assessing for intervention

Most children with DCD have a problem with motor learning as well as motor performance. Very little work has been done on the assessment and evaluation of motor learning. The assessment tools used for identification are often not appropriate as a pre-test and post-test to evaluate an intervention because they are not sufficiently sensitive or they are not focused at the same level as the intervention. A major theoretical issue when dealing with intervention is that of generality versus specificity. Burton and Rodgerson's taxonomy provides a framework that can be used to link the level of assessment with the level of intervention. If the intervention is skill specific, then the appropriate pre-test and post-test should be focused on a change in skills taught. If the intervention is focused on skill groupings or movement skill sets, then the assessment of change should match that level of intervention. Qualitative, process-oriented or criterion-referenced assessment is generally used in intervention studies where a measure of pre-test performance on the specific tasks of interest is essential. The most widely used test battery of this type is the Test of Gross Motor Development (Ulrich, 1985; 2000).

Test of Gross Motor Development (second edition) (TGMD-2)

The TGMD-2 (2000) is a criterion referenced assessment tool which categorizes gross motor skills into locomotor and object control groupings. It includes six locomotor skills (run, gallop, hop, leap, horizontal jump and slide) and six object control skills (striking a stationary ball, stationary dribble, catch, kick, overhand throw, underhand roll). The test is particularly useful as a pre-test and post-test prior to and following intervention programmes to evaluate the success of the intervention. Its use in this context has been demonstrated in young disadvantaged children in the 3–5 year age range (Goodway and Branta, 2003; Goodway, Crowe and Ward, 2003).

The TGMD has the capacity to be used in the monitoring of motor learning, although the criteria are limited with as few as three in the leap and up to five criteria in the hop and striking a stationary ball. The TMGD seems better suited to the 3–7 year age groups. To cater for older children, 5–12 years, movement analysis checklists have been constructed for a number of skills with quite comprehensive positive and negative criteria (Larkin and Hoare, 1991; Larkin and Parker, 2002). The positive criteria focus the teacher on what could be considered biomechanically optimal elements of the movement. The negative criteria draw attention to inefficient habits that the child has established already and which need to be eliminated and replaced with more efficient movement patterns. These criteria were developed using high-speed film, video analysis and subjective observation. Thus, dynamic assessment is used throughout the learning process and evaluates change both qualitatively and quantitatively throughout each session. In younger children, the dynamic assessment helps to prevent the development of 'bad habits' (Walter and Swinnen, 1994). In older children, it helps the teacher/coach adjust the movement pattern to achieve a more efficient technique. Using both positive and negative criteria provides a platform for measuring more subtle changes in movement behaviour. The limitation is that the observer needs to be very experienced in the observation of movement.

Assessing fitness

Fitness is particularly important when it comes to the assessment of children with DCD. The confound between the measurement of motor performance and fitness has always complicated the interpretation of tests of motor ability or motor skill. On the other hand, the assessment of fitness in children with DCD is somewhat confounded by the inability to perform the motor tasks used to test fitness. Children with DCD often withdraw from motor activities and are less involved in playground and sporting activities (Bouffard et al., 1996; Smyth and Anderson, 2000). However, there is, as yet, incomplete understanding of the implications of this withdrawal on the development of fitness. However, there is some evidence that the development of anaerobic power and aerobic power is compromised in this population (see Hands and Larkin, 2002 for review). Apart from the long-term health implications, low levels of aerobic and anaerobic fitness have short-term implications for motor skill production, varying according to specific task requirements. Long-term implications are predicted, in terms of neuromuscular, musculo-skeletal and cardio-respiratory development. Consequently, it is important to assess and evaluate the fitness levels of children with DCD for two reasons: (a) to evaluate the contribution of fitness to the poor level of motor performance during the initial identification and (b) to identify whether the intervention programme should include a fitness component. The limited research (O'Beirne, Larkin and Cable, 1994; Raynor, 2001) indicates that the fitness levels of children with DCD are such that this aspect of assessment is important. To this end, items from the Australian Schools Fitness test (Pyke, 1986) and the Canadian Manitoba Fitness test (1980) have been used to give us estimates of children's fitness. In summary, the movement observations necessary to give an overview of the child's motor performance should include a test of motor fitness as well as motor performance.

Checklists and questionnaires

In order to meet the DSM-IV diagnostic criteria (APA, 1994) it is necessary to identify low levels of performance in 'daily activities that require motor coordination' that interfere with academic achievement or activities of daily living. Parent and teacher questionnaires provide a useful way to access about a variety of tasks of daily living such as dressing, grooming, and eating; drawing and writing; fundamental motor skills and participation in play, physical games, and sport. In the section that follows, some checklists and questionnaires that provide information about activities of daily living, physical activities, and self-perceptions about physical activities are discussed. Questionnaires cannot replace actual tests of motor performance but they are a good source of additional information and can compensate for errors of measurement and support the information obtained from the motor tests. Some of the limitations that need to be considered when using these questionnaires and self-reports are also discussed.

Parent questionnaires

Parent information can form a substantial part of the assessment protocol. Parents' judgements provide a background about activities of daily living and social difficulties that arise from motor problems. This information cannot be gained from norm-referenced motor tests. Nevertheless, the results of studies using parent observation and questionnaires caution us to interpret the information carefully. In Gubbay's (1975a) study of children classified as clumsy, parent reports indicated that 76 per cent of the children had average to above average sporting ability and 24 per cent below average. This contrasts with the parent data from Hoare's (1991) parent questionnaire where 25 per cent were average to above average and 75 per cent were below average. The parents' estimates do not appear to be very accurate, especially in the Gubbay study. In both studies parents seemed to be more accurate for the control groups. One hundred per cent of the control group in Gubbay's study were rated as average or above average in sporting ability while 92 per cent of the control group were similarly rated in Hoare's study.

Data from the DCDQ (Wilson, Dewey and Campbell, 1998) provide a systematic way of obtaining a parent's perspective on their child's motor performance. The DCDQ has questions about a child's control during movement, fine and gross motor skills and general coordination. Wilson and colleagues (2000a) reported that there was a correlation between the Movement ABC and the DCDQ of $r = -.59$ with a group of children aged 8 to 14 years. Data from the authors' research programme with 50 children aged from 5 to 7 years, 28 with DCD and 22 without DCD, provided evidence that parents were able to make a reasonable estimate of their child's motor performance (Boyle, 2003). The DCDQ identified 22 of the 28 children with DCD giving it a sensitivity of 77 per cent and there was an overall agreement of 89 per cent. Again the questionnaire approach to identification can be helpful but should be combined with a movement test. Just as there are parents with very accurate perceptions of their child's level of motor performance, there are also parents who have little understanding of their child's movement difficulties.

Teacher checklists

Studies using teacher observations or checklists in an effort to identify children with mild motor impairment have had mixed results (Gubbay, 1975a; Henderson and Hall, 1982; Keogh et al., 1979; Morris and Whiting, 1971; Revie and Larkin, 1993a). In an early study by Whiting and colleagues (1969, cited by Morris and Whiting, 1971) only eight (26 per cent) of 50 children identified by teachers as clumsy were subsequently confirmed using a motor test. In Gubbay's (1975a) survey, teachers 'identified 25 per cent of the group identified as clumsy on the TMP as having sporting ability and bodily agility much below average' (p. 128) and a further 46 per cent as possibly falling into this category. When asked to rate the children based on being 'unduly clumsy', the teachers identified 14 per cent of the group as unduly clumsy and 39 per cent as possibly unduly clumsy. This contrasts with the 2.3 per cent and 12 per cent similarly identified in the remainder of the children and gives some credibility to teacher observation. However 46 per cent of children identified by the TMP were not identified by the teachers observation based on 'clumsiness' and 29 per cent were not included as low or possibly low on sporting ability. Other studies have also shown that teachers have difficulty recognizing many children with coordination difficulties. Teachers, using a checklist identified only 3.6 per cent of an elementary school population as poorly coordinated (Revie and Larkin, 1993a). Of the 75 children identified by teachers, only 31 (41.3 per cent) were confirmed as having movement problems when tested using the BMAT-R (Arnheim and Sinclair, 1979). In the studies where teachers were asked to identify children with movement problems, some researchers have remarked that teachers often include children with behaviour problems rather than movement problems (Morris and Whiting, 1971; Revie and Larkin, 1993a).

Some studies have shown better results. For example Henderson and Hall (1982), after providing relevant information to teachers over a number of months, found that teachers were able to accurately identify children with movement difficulties. In another survey, teachers rated the motor behaviour of children identified with and without movement difficulties based on the MAND (Hoare, 1991). The group with coordination problems had a mean NDI score of 74.6 and the control group had a mean NDI score of 107.7 on the MAND. Teachers and parents had relatively similar ratings in this survey (see Table 7.1) and over 70 per cent of the children with poor coordination were ranked by teachers as below average in most of the gross motor domains.

Table 7.1 The percentage of a group of children with DCD identified by parents and teachers as below average, average or above average on motor activities

| | Below average | | Average | | Above average | |
	Parent	Teacher	Parent	Teacher	Parent	Teacher
Draw/paint	45	62	32	25	23	12
Manual dexterity	50	66	40	25	10	9
Dressing	31	37	58	53	11	10
Ball skills	68	74	27	19	5	6
Body control	67	72	28	25	5	3
Coordination	74	79	23	17	3	3
Run	61	70	31	27	8	3
Sport	75	73	22	22	3	5

Source: Adapted from Hoare (1991).

The results from the Movement Assessment Battery for Children checklist (Movement ABC checklist) are quite variable. Junaid et al. (2000) reported a correlation of .51 between the Movement ABC and the Movement ABC checklist while Schoemaker, Smits-Engelsman and Jongmans (2003) reported a correlation of .44 between these tests. Thus these two studies identifying DCD/movement difficulties show a shared variance ranging from 20 per cent to 26 per cent. The relationship is not nearly high enough to substitute the checklist for the Movement ABC motor test as a means of screening for DCD. The hit rate agreement between the Movement ABC motor test and checklist was as high as 88 per cent for 6-year-olds using the 15th percentile cut-off point for both tests. However, this result contrasted with the 35 per cent hit rate for 7 year olds using the same cut-off points (Schoemaker, Smits-Engelsman and Jongmans, 2003). The sensitivity and specificity vary quite markedly over the age range from 6 to 9 years.

There are a number of factors contributing to these results. Some teachers can have difficulty with the identification of movement difficulties while others are very competent, particularly if they receive relevant information through systematic training or regular meetings (Henderson and Hall, 1982). Teachers have very limited time for additional observations, and accurate observation of the movement of each individual child is quite time consuming even for the experienced teacher. The ability to observe movement accurately is a skill that takes time to develop (Knudson and Morrison, 1997) and many general teachers have very little professional preparation in movement or movement observation. Physical educators, physical therapists and occupational therapists are likely to receive some formal training in movement observation but if they are unfamiliar with the motor development of young children, they may perceive that the child's motor profile is a manifestation of developmental level.

Self-report questionnaires

In order to provide appropriate intervention it also is crucial to consider the self-judgements made by children with DCD. Motivational theorists (Bandura, 1986; Deci and Ryan, 1985; Griffin and Keogh, 1982; Harter, 1981; Nicholls, 1984) have consistently emphasized the importance of self-perceptions for individuals' willingness to engage in mastery attempts in specific achievement domains. There is general agreement among these theorists that the more competent individuals feel with regard to a specific activity, the more their interest will be sustained and the more likely they will persist in a specific activity. It follows that a child who is repeatedly met by failure in the motor domain, is likely to perceive lowered self-perceptions, and as a consequence less likely to participate in physical activities. By identifying children's self-perceptions professionals and educators might be able to more accurately target movement problems that are the source of negative self-perceptions and consequent withdrawal from much needed movement experiences. While it is also important to assess children's perceptions of fear, social support and enjoyment, the central role that self-perceptions play in psycho-social health also makes assessment of the multi-dimensional self-system a prime concern.

Issues of assessment centre around which types of questions and level of specificity afford the best prediction and explanation of the child's judgement of his/her ability in particular movement situations. This issue can be more easily clarified with examples of studies that have explored the self-perception/motor competence relationship at varying levels of specificity and varying degrees of correspondence. Conceptually, this is also an issue of which types of questions children ask themselves in every-day life. There is clearly a need for more perceptive investigation of the scales in multiple movement contexts.

While early studies employing global measures of self-esteem (Johnston, Short and Crawford, 1987) succeeded in drawing attention of researchers to the plight of children with motor problems, they were limited by the generality of the instruments used. Gubbay (1975a) included child self-report in his comprehensive study of 'developmental clumsiness'. In response to a question about their sporting ability, a high 63 per cent of the children identified as clumsy regarded themselves as good or average in sporting ability. The remaining 37 per cent classified themselves as below ($n = 9$) or much below average ($n = 10$). The control group appeared to better match perceptions with competence as only 8 per cent of the control group classified themselves as below average in sporting ability. With regard to DCD, self-perceptions should be assessed at the optimal level of specificity that corresponds to the critical tasks being assessed within the domain of activity being analysed. Often no critical tasks are identified and researchers gain limited insight into the interplay among self-perceptions of children with DCD and specific motor difficulties that they experience. Thus self-perceptions will differ in their predictive power depending on the specific task they are asked to predict. The problem is that children even in domain specific measures of self-esteem are asked to make judgements about situations with no clear activity or task in mind. For example, studies employing Harter's (1985) Self-Perception Profile for Children (SPPC) have demonstrated that children with DCD have lowered perceived athletic competence (Causgrove Dunn and Watkinson, 1994; Rose, Larkin and Berger, 1997). While these domain specific measures have elucidated psycho-social difficulties faced by children with DCD, these scales do not relate to specific areas of movement. It is important that researchers are able to isolate specific abilities or tasks in which children perceive low competence and target particular motor tasks that are most in need of social support during remediation.

Some questionnaires have been specifically developed to identify children's perceptions of their physical ability (Bornholt, 1996; Missiuna, 1998) and their movement confidence (Griffin and Keogh, 1982; Rose et al., 2000). In a recent study, Boyle (2003) found that children's scores on their perceptions of drawing and motor competencies were not related to their performance on the MAND, a motor proficiency test. There was no significant difference between a group identified with motor problems and a control group on the ASK-KIDS inventory (Bornholt, 1996). Brake and Bornholt (in press) found similar results when they correlated the motor activities section of ASK-KIDS with the Movement ABC ($r = -.2$). This particular inventory asks general questions about 'motor activities' rather than focusing on specific motor tasks.

The All About Me Scale (AAMS) (Missiuna, 1998) comprises 20 items that tap children's self-perceptions of ability in specific motor tasks relating to play, games and sport as well as classroom and home activities. In addition, there are items of a more general nature about feeling competent in these contexts. As in all but four of the items there was discrimination between children with DCD and children who experience no motor difficulties, the AAMs is likely to be one of the more appropriate tools for assessing movement related self-perceptions in younger children, especially those with DCD.

Movement confidence is an issue that we deal with when working with children with DCD. Identifying their levels of confidence is particularly important for successful intervention. Based on the Movement Confidence Model (Griffin and Keogh, 1982) Rose et al. (2000) have carried out preliminary validation studies of a movement confidence scale that taps movement confidence, perceptions of competence, enjoyment and fear of harm in walking along a beam, jumping from a height and catching. Findings of a pilot study have provided preliminary validation for the catch items. An updated version of this task-specific scale of movement confidence is about to be trialled with children with DCD. In future, we plan to use this scale to identify levels of movement confidence prior to intervention in order to better target the level and pace of task teaching for children with DCD.

Summary and conclusions

In summary, many different tools are used to identify the low levels of motor performance demonstrated by children with DCD. The motor assessment tools are often focused on general constructs such as motor ability, proficiency or development. Others are more focused on fine and gross motor skills or on motor skill sets such as ball skills, balance and manual skills (Henderson and Sugden, 1992). Most tests focus on the outcome level of assessment, a few focus on the quality of the motor skill performance (Ulrich, 2000). Motor-based tests generally work to discriminate children with and without DCD, despite the different tasks involved in the particular batteries. However, most of these tests do not deal with gender differences and it is not clear how this biases selection of children for research or intervention. The issue of test difference based on test item selection needs to be further addressed to avoid sample biases in the research domain; task-based analysis and comparison of test items might be valuable. Assessment for initial identification is richer if it includes information from the parents as well as the child (this links well with the eco-development approach of intervention proposed by Sugden and Chambers in Chapter 10). Motor skill tests used in the initial identification may differ from those used for intervention. Tests used to monitor intervention should be targeted at the level of the intervention. An evaluation of a child's fitness should be included in the overall motor battery and this should be part of the motor intervention where appropriate. Questionnaires provide additional and useful information, but knowledge and beliefs of the parent, teacher, or child limit their validity. Although we recommend multi-level procedures, given the current economic and social environment that places limits on human resources, where only one test it possible, it should be a motor test administered by a movement specialist knowledgeable in motor development and learning.

CHAPTER 8

Early identification of children with Developmental Coordination Disorder

MARIAN J. JONGMANS

Introduction

It appears from the literature that the large majority of children with a Developmental Coordination Disorder (DCD) are identified after school entrance (Geuze et al., 2001). A commonly cited reason for this is that the motor demands of some school activities are so high that these children fail to perform at an accepted level (Dewey and Wilson, 2001; Miller et al., 2001a). Children in the first grades of primary education are typically engaged in a large variety of classroom and playground activities such as, for example, cutting and pasting, model building, hide-and-seek, hop-scotch etc. Although most children with DCD will have had some experience with these activities either at home, in a day-care or preschool setting before they enter school, they stand out because of exceptionally poor performance. As these children progress to higher grades, these activities become even more complex and many new skills requiring motor control, including handwriting, are introduced, exacerbating the expression of their primary difficulties even further.

The fact that most of the literature focuses on school-aged children with DCD is not to say that these children always go unnoticed at an earlier age. From clinical work there is evidence to suggest that quite a few parents recall their child to have been 'different' in some respects to other children of a similar age in the first years of life (Pless et al., 2001; Stephenson, McKay and Chesson, 1991). In particular, they may have needed more help than others to do basic self-help skills such as dressing themselves or cutting food. Similarly, day-care staff or pre-school teachers might have noticed problems when these children were trying to colour, paste or use scissors. While most parents realize that something is not quite right with their young child, most are unsure what to do about it. Some seek advice immediately and others may reason that the difficulties are part and parcel of any young child's exploration of its own capabilities or that they are of such a subtle nature that they do not (yet) have a significant impact on the child's functioning. Likewise, some professionals react to parental concerns straight away while others may take the approach of first monitoring the child's (lack of) progress for a certain period before deciding upon further action.

Early identification of children with DCD is important for a number of reasons. First, recognizing the fact that a child has motor difficulties which hinder its function in daily activities at home and in school opens the way for providing support for the child (and parents) in how to cope with these difficulties. Second, early identification and subsequent intervention might prevent children with DCD from becoming discouraged about both academic and playground activities early on in their school career. This, in turn, might prevent the development of concomitant problems such as psychosocial problems (Schoemaker and Kalverboer, 1994; Skinner and Piek, 2001).

An interesting question is what is meant by 'early' in the context of identification? Does this mean from the first moment that functional problems arise? Or does 'early' mean that the aim should be to identify children with motor problems even before these start to affect a child's daily functioning? Nowadays, identifying children with DCD from the moment their motor difficulties are apparent is regarded as the minimum standard of service provision. Identifying these children even before their lives are significantly affected would be ideal but is not yet common practice and difficult. This chapter addresses two issues. First, a brief update of selected developments in assessment is provided. This update is not meant to be exhaustive but rather meant as complementary to several other, more elaborate publications on this issue (e.g. Geuze et al., 2001; Sugden and Wright, 1998). Second, a number of issues are raised in relation to ways of advancing identification of children with DCD, including a discussion of the advantages and disadvantages of screening young children for the presence of motor problems.

Selected issues in assessment of DCD

As Sugden and Wright (1998) point out, many different formal and informal assessment methods have been used to describe the motor behaviour of children with DCD. This variety in methods reflects, in part, the heterogeneity of functional problems these children present with and also the heterogeneous background of professionals involved in identification. A review of 176 studies on children with DCD (Geuze et al., 2001) revealed that the standardized measures of motor functioning most commonly used to select children in scientific studies are the Movement Assessment Battery for Children Test (Movement ABC Test; Henderson and Sugden, 1992), Gubbay's test (Gubbay, 1975a), the McCarron test (McCarron, 1982), the Bruininks-Oseretski Test of Motor Proficiency (BOTMP; Bruininks, 1978) and the Southern California Sensory Integration Tests (Ayres, 1989). This review included studies published until 1999 but scanning the literature between then and 2004 still confirms the Movement ABC Test as the preferred measure. This is not to say that there have been no further developments in the area of assessment in the past years, with continual efforts at refining or adding appropriate tests to optimize assessment. Three examples are described below. Furthermore, a model describing the consequences of disease and condition for an individual child's functioning (WHO, 2001) has gradually been incorporated in the way children with DCD are assessed and treated, especially by paediatric physical therapists, paediatric occupational therapists and professionals working in paediatric rehabilitation. This model will be described briefly with an emphasis on implications for assessment.

Selected recent adaptations of assessments

First, for some time now the Beery-Buktenica Developmental Test of Visual Motor Integration has been used to assess the ability of children with DCD to convert a visual stimulus into a motor response (VMI; Beery, Buktenica and Beery, 2004). Originally, this ability was tested by asking the child to copy a series of geometric shapes of increasing difficulty. Children who failed the test were said to be weak in integrating visual input and motor output. However, the question remained why these children failed. Was it because they have difficulty visually perceiving shapes (e.g. visual inspection of shapes/objects or visual spatial ability) or because they have difficulty coordinating the muscles in finger/wrist/underarm necessary to move the writing implement? In order to differentiate between such difficulties the VMI has been extended to include the VMI Supplemental Developmental Test of Visual Perception (VP) and VMI Supplemental Developmental Test of Motor Coordination (MC). Kulp and Sortor (2003) administered the renewed VMI to 193 children (mean age = 8.77 years). They found that both supplemental tests were significantly related to the VMI. However, scores on the VP and MC tests only explained 36.2 per cent of the variance in scores on the VMI. In addition, of the children who did poorly on the VMI, some scored poorly on VP or MC, some scored poorly on both supplemental tests, and others scored within normal limits on both supplemental tests. In other words, there was a significant amount of variance in performance on the VMI that was not explained by performance on the tests of VP or MC alone. It was concluded that each of the three areas investigated by the renewed VMI should be individually assessed and that even children who perform within normal limits on the VMI may show a deficit in VP or MC.

Second, to be able to fulfil diagnostic Criterion C from the DSM-IV entry for DCD (American Psychiatric Association, 1994: the observed motor problems are not due to a general medical condition or to a pervasive developmental disorder) children should be examined by a general paediatrician, a paediatric neurologist or a paediatric rehabilitation doctor. He/she usually administers a neurological examination. However, there is a paucity of standardized neurological examinations suitable for clinical practice (i.e. short but at the same time reliable and valid) leaving most doctors to perform their own eclectic examination. Touwen's examination of the child with minor neurological dysfunction (Touwen, 1979) is, however, a positive exception. This examination consists of 55 items grouped under the following headings: sensorimotor apparatus, posture, balance of trunk, coordination of extremities, fine manipulative ability, (dys)kinesia, gross motor functions, quality of motility, associated movements and the visual system. Although the examination suffers from the psychometric problem that only the total score has been shown to be reliable (Kakebeeke et al., 1993), it has proven itself to be a valuable discriminative instrument in many studies. One of the reasons this examination is not widely used either clinically or in research is its lengthy procedure (approximately 45–60 minutes). Recently, Fily and colleagues (2003) have devised a shortened version of the examination. Having tried this on a group of 5-year-old prematurely born children they conclude that the concordance between the original form and short-form was excellent. Agreement on classification was reached in 169 out of 170 subjects. It is hoped that this simplified measure convinces a growing number of doctors to include it in their routine screening programme. This could lead to a more uniform approach to the operationalization of Criterion C.

Finally, a fairly recent strategy to detect children with DCD is to involve parents actively in providing clinical descriptions of their child. This follows remarks of parents that they feel their concerns are often ignored while later on their worries were confirmed (Stephenson, McKay and Chesson, 1991). Parental involvement may consist of asking them to provide appraisals of their child's motor functioning including concerns, estimations, and predictions. Likewise, parents may be asked to provide descriptions by means of both recall and report. It appears that, provided parents are properly guided by professionals and high-quality screening instruments are used, they can provide valuable insights and observations of their child (Glascoe, 2001). Moreover, it seems important to involve parents in the identification phase of children with DCD since they are often the only persons who can provide enough detail of the way the motor problems of the child interfere with activities of daily living (Miyahara and Möbs, 1995). Wilson and colleagues have taken up the challenge to construct such a questionnaire: the Developmental Coordination Disorder Questionnaire (DCDQ) (Wilson et al., 2000a). The questionnaire is suitable for children between 8 years and 14 years 6 months. It consists of 17 items divided over four factors: control during movement (e.g. throw a ball, catch a ball and run and stop), fine motor/handwriting (e.g. cutting and writing speed), gross motor/planning (e.g. team sports, rides bicycle and learns skills), and General Coordination (e.g. slow and awkward and fatiguing easily). In a study involving parents completing the DCDQ at the same time that their children were tested on the Movement ABC Test and the BOTMP it was found that the questionnaire was most accurate in correctly classifying children with DCD (86 per cent correct) in comparison with those without DCD (identified correctly as non-DCD 71 per cent of the time) and also in comparison with those whose motor skills were 'suspect' (identified correctly as suspected DCD 44 per cent of the time). It was concluded that when used as a screening instrument or together with a clinical assessment, the DCDQ could provide valuable information.

Towards a functional approach in assessment

As mentioned before, the most recent conceptual model of the *International Classification of Functioning, Disability and Health* (ICF: WHO, 2001; see Figure 8.1) seems gradually to influence the way children

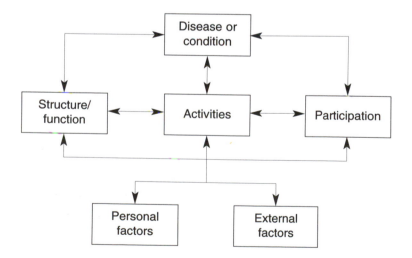

Figure 8.1 Model of the International Classification of Functioning, Disability and Health (ICF; WHO, 2001).

with DCD are assessed and treated. This model describes the consequences of diseases or conditions for daily functioning at three interrelated levels: (1) structure and function, (2) activities and (3) participation. The model also includes the influence of personal and external factors on these levels. Interactions between all components of the model determine for each individual child the current functional status.

One of the consequences of accepting this model might be that assessment of a child's motor problems encompasses all three levels. Indeed, assessment only focusing on the child's strengths and weaknesses at the structure/function level such as looking at muscle tone, range of motion, flexibility, strength and postural responses is not common practice anymore. Instead, the idea that assessment instruments should reflect a child's activities in everyday life has been widely accepted for some time now (Haley, Coster and Ludlow, 1991). This has prompted the use of instruments aimed at measuring the actual ability of the child to perform necessary daily activities during the identification process.

Two examples of such instruments are the Vineland Adaptive Behavior Scales (VABS; Sparrow, Balla and Cicchetti, 1985) and the Pediatric Evaluation of Development Inventory (PEDI; Haley et al., 1992). The VABS covers a wide range of adaptive behaviours in the domains of communication (receptive, expressive and written), daily living skills (personal, domestic and community), socialization (interpersonal relationships, play and leisure time and coping skills) and motor skills (both gross and fine). Field testing for the second edition of the VABS is currently under way. It is administered to a parent or caregiver in a semistructured interview format including a classroom form. The PEDI also is an instrument suitable for obtaining information on the child's functioning. It has been developed for chronically ill and disabled children and focuses on three content domains: self-care, mobility and social function. The aim of the PEDI is to identify children who are not keeping up with developmental expectations in functional skill development, to provide a clear description of functional status in order to identify clinical patterns of deficiencies in functional skill attainment and to evaluate change due to interventions (Haley et al., 1992). It is a judgement-based, standardized measure using parent report through a structured interview. So far, little published research exists in which functional abilities of children with DCD have been looked at in detail using the PEDI. One exception is a study by Rodger et al. (2003). They report on the motor and functional outcomes of 20 children between the ages of 4 and 8 years with DCD. Measurement at the participation level involved use of the Pictorial Scale of Perceived Competence and Social Acceptance (Harter and Pike, 1984) and the PEDI. Overall, the children rated themselves towards the more competent and accepted end of the PCSA over the dimensions of physical and cognitive competence and peer and maternal acceptance. The PEDI revealed generally average performance on social (M = 49.98, SD = 16.62) and mobility function (M = 54.71, SD = 3.99); however, self-care function was below the average range for age (M = 38.01, SD = 12.19).

The importance of including assessments like the PEDI in a standard assessment battery for children with DCD lies in the information it provides in determining treatment goals relevant for daily functioning. Such an approach toward treatment means that children are encouraged to find solutions to the motor problems they themselves want to solve most urgently without prescribing the exact way in which they should do so. In this way it is possible to fulfil the wishes of children to learn certain activities (e.g. cycling or writing). This should make it easier for them to participate in activities of daily living appropriate for their age. It is obvious that a functional approach to assessment and treatment actually fits well with the earlier described ICF model.

In sum, continual developments in assessment benefit identification of children with DCD in several ways. Adapting existing instruments or creating new instruments may provide a more detailed level of description of the child's problems. Improving the user friendliness of good, reliable and valid measures increases the chance that they are actually used in clinical practice and research. Finally, responding to the wishes of children and their parents to keep assessment and intervention as closely as possible related to actual functional problems not only increases ecological validity of assessments but is also thought to increase the impact of such services on the functioning of the children.

Advancing identification of DCD

Recently, semistructured interviews with parents of children diagnosed with DCD were held in Sweden (Pless et al., 2001). Thirty-seven parents were asked what they had observed about their child's motor ability and development, how they felt about these observations and what they had done with their feelings. There was great variability in the responses of parents to these questions. Some parents said that professionals did not listen or even seem to care about their child's problems.

> She has been examined everywhere, speech therapist, physical therapist, neurologist, EEG. But I did not give in. She will probably turn out all right in the end they said. Everyone examines the part they are specialized in and do not care about the rest. (p. 132)

Other parents had noted their child's difficulty but remarked that

> Certainly we have wondered about the motor part, but we have usually said that it will come. (p. 131)

Among the interviewed parents there were some who had not been aware of their child's problems until they were pointed out to them by a professional:

> He can't use the scissors. We were shocked when we first saw this at the speech therapist's. And I didn't know that he couldn't. I had never thought about it. (p. 132)

Taken together, it appears from these interviews that many children with DCD at a young age already show difficulties with motor tasks. Therefore, maybe one of the biggest challenges for the future is to find ways of identifying these children even at an earlier age than is currently the case.

In what follows, a number of issues will be discussed in relation to advancing the identification of children with DCD. First, the pros and cons of screening preschool children for motor problems are explained. Second, two related basic features of development, namely variability and stability, are described in more detail in order to explore the possibility that they are suitable candidates for identifying DCD before school entry.

Identifying children with atypical motor development too early or too late: balancing the scale

The time when a child's development was viewed primarily as unalterable and fixed is far behind us. Nowadays, development in general is regarded as a process of change influenced by both child factors (e.g. genes, physiology etc.) and the environment in which the child grows up (e.g. parent–child interaction, socio-economic characteristics of the family/neighbourhood, educational experiences etc.) (e.g. Bronfenbrenner and Morris, 1998). In particular, motor development is according to some best explained by using a dynamic systems approach (Thelen and Smith, 1994). This approach states that changes in development depend on the interaction of multiple subsystems. These systems include those within the child (e.g. biomechanical, cognitive and motivational), the environment (e.g. type of surface on which to walk, presence/absence of other persons/objects) and the task (e.g. complexity). For example, a child who has mastered the ability to crawl on hands and knees is now able to explore its environment even further. In this process, the child is likely to encounter a staircase at some point which challenges it to devise new movement strategies to climb the stairs once it has gained enough muscle power to do so and is allowed by its parents to do so!

Interactive approaches, such as the one described above, have strengthened the idea that the course of development might be influenced by providing support to the child and/or its environment. Partly as a result of this change in view on development, the Individuals with Disabilities Education Act in the United States of America mandates early identification of, and intervention for, developmental disabilities through the development of community-based systems. The emphasis is on screening to identify disabilities at a younger age, with the current focus being on infants and children from birth through 3 years of age. Understandably, children identified as 'at risk' for developmental problems, either because of the presence of neurobiological risk factors (e.g. premature birth), environmental risk factors (e.g. low-income families) or a combination of these two factors (children who are at a so-called 'double jeopardy'), have been the first to receive such interventions. For example, the results of randomized control trials on the effect of small-scale interventions bear a consistent message: providing intervention in the first years of life of children labelled as 'at risk' for later poor academic achievement because of poor socio-economic background or poverty improves their academic functioning at school age and beyond (e.g. the Abecedarian Project in the United States of America; Campbell et al., 2001). Similar programmes such as Sure Start were launched in the UK several years ago (see The Ness Research team, 2004). This programme aims to promote, among other things, physical (including motor) development for children aged 0–4 years from poor and disadvantaged backgrounds. Evaluation studies are currently under way to measure the impact of this programme on both the children and the environments they grow up in. Randomized control trials solely aimed at evaluating the effect of interventions for children identified as 'at risk' for later motor problems during the first years of life are currently lacking. Instead, published research on this topic involves rather small groups of children with mainly one particular risk factor, i.e. children born with a low birth weight. Whether these children benefit from early physical therapy or occupational programmes in the sense that they have no or fewer motor problems later in life still remains questionable (Rothberg et al., 1991; Salokorpi et al., 2002; Weindling et al., 1996). Nevertheless, the importance of early identification seems apparent.

Although a limited number of population studies are available to provide a reliable estimation of the percentage of children with DCD, this is commonly put at approximately 5 per cent of all school-aged children (American Psychiatric Association, 1994; Kadesjö and Gillberg, 1999b). In other words, this seems a high enough percentage to warrant early identification. Assuming that DCD is not a condition which suddenly 'appears' at school entrance it should, in theory, be possible to identify these children before that time. One of the most common methods of identifying preschool children at risk for a certain condition is to perform a population screening. Screening can be regarded as the application of quick, simple procedures to examine a presumptively normal population to find those individuals who are likely to show a particular problem in need of more in-depth assessment (i.e. screening is *not* suitable for making a diagnosis!).

There are obvious advantages and disadvantages in the process of screening young children for (possible signs of) DCD. Advantages of screening include finding 'true positive' cases at an early age. This means that help can be offered to the child in finding solutions to the difficulties it encounters and supporting parents in their attempts to teach their child how to cope with their problems. In addition, early identification may prevent the development of secondary problems (e.g. psychosocial problems; Skinner and Piek, 2001). There are, however, numerous pitfalls of screening. Many screening instruments have important limitations, including issues of reliability and validity and the lack of well-established norms. In general, a screening instrument is regarded as psychometrically sound when it reaches a sensitivity (i.e. correctly identifying children with a disability) and specificity (i.e. correctly identifying children without a disability) of around 70–80 per cent (Sonnander, 2000). The most important pitfall of screening is that of identifying 'false positives', i.e. children who according to the screening instrument are at risk for motor problems but who subsequently do not show these problems. To refer children for further assessment who subsequently do not show a problem might unduly worry parents. This concern may create a tendency to identify only markedly delayed children, denying other children potential access to needed care. Moreover, mild delays and deviations are often hard to detect. Although there is broad agreement as to what constitutes clear-cut delay or deviation in motor functioning, there is not complete consensus among professionals or between parents and professionals (e.g. physical therapists) as to the severity at which evaluation and intervention become appropriate. This may lead to under-referral (e.g. Lindstrom and Bremberg, 1997). Conversely, assuming that a screening test done at one point in time will discover all children with every type of developmental problem is also providing parents with a false sense of security. Because development is ongoing with time, and because measuring development at very young ages cannot evaluate the full complexity of the various developmental domains at later ages, it is important to continue to assess children using tools appropriate for their age throughout their entire development. A single test at one point in time only gives a snapshot of the dynamic processes of acquiring movement abilities, making periodic screening necessary to detect emerging motor disabilities as a child grows (Darrah et al., 2003; Darrah et al., 1998). This point will be elaborated on below.

Variability and stability as indicators of (a)typical motor development

If preschool children (at risk) for DCD were to be correctly identified, what should be looked for in a child's motor behaviour? One of the candidates might be movement variability. However, to date no complete agreement exists on what is exactly understood by variability nor on the precise nature of the relationship between variability and motor status (Piek, 2003). For example, both increased variability and decreased variability in infancy have been associated with later motor disability. A possible explanation for this contradictory finding might be the type of movement examined. Fluctuation of variability in the development of skilled movements (e.g. grasping) and fluctuation of variability in spontaneous motility (e.g. general movements) might not be comparable because they originate from different sub-domains of motor control. Research, especially in the latter type of movements, has generated much interest in the past 15 years. It appears that quality of so-called general movements at the (corrected for premature birth) postnatal age of 3 months is highly predictive of the presence of cerebral palsy (Prechtl, 1997). So far, just one study has investigated the association between definitely abnormal general movements and outcome at school age. In a group of 52 high- and low-risk children Hadders-Algra and Groothuis (1999) recorded general movements repeatedly and re-examined these children between 4 and 9 years of age. All children with definitely abnormal general movements developed cerebral palsy. Interestingly, children with mildly abnormal general movements were found to have more externalizing, aggressive and ADHD problems at school age compared to children with normal general movements. Mildly abnormal general movements were also related to minor neurological dysfunction in later life (e.g. coordination problems and mild abnormalities in muscle-tone regulation).

Another possible, related candidate for early detection of abnormal motor development might be stability of motor ability level throughout the first years of life. Darrah and colleagues undertook two studies on stability of serial assessments of motor abilities in typically developing infants (Darrah et al., 1998; 2003). First, intra-individual stability of gross motor scores obtained by normally developing full-term infants on the Alberta Infant Motor Scale (AIMS; Piper et al., 1992) were evaluated. The gross motor skills of 45 typically developing infants were assessed monthly from two weeks of age until they achieved independent walking. Individual infants' percentile ranks varied considerably from month to month, with no systematic pattern of change noted across infants.

Fourteen infants (31.1 per cent) received a score below the 10th percentile on at least one occasion. The results of this first study suggested that normally developing infants are not stable in the rate of emergence of gross motor skills. The second longitudinal descriptive study evaluated fine motor and gross motor ability of 102 infants at 9, 11, 13, 16, and 21 months of age. All infants were classified as typically developing at 23 months of age. Again, large variability in scores within an infant, among infants and across domains was found. For example, some infants obtained high scores to begin with and then their scores gradually declined. Others obtained low scores in the beginning and attained higher scores on each subsequent occasion while many children showed a profile of scores which went up and down. It was concluded from both studies that typical development is nonlinear, rather than occurring at a constant rate. Fluctuations in a child's score over time may therefore not always indicate deviance or the need for intervention.

Furthermore, fine and gross motor skills appeared to develop independently. Consequently, the authors recommend that screening young children for motor disabilities should include multiple domains and multiple time points before referrals are made to early intervention programmes.

In sum, there has been a shift toward perceiving development as an interactional, dynamic process between child and environment: changes in the child or in the environment both influence the course of development. Therefore, detection of young children with an atypical developmental pathway and providing them with intervention to try to adjust this pathway has gained much interest. Screening whole populations seems at first glance the most efficient way of identifying preschool children with motor difficulties. However, unless screening is performed repeatedly with psychometrically sound instruments, currently the negative effects of a large-scale screening approach outweigh the positive effects.

Conclusions

While several sources indicate that children with DCD do not 'suddenly' develop motor difficulties at school entrance, serious attempts at finding these children before the age of 4 years are currently lacking. Part of the problem of the current lack of early identification is probably that whilst severely affected children can be readily recognized, identification of children with (what sometimes is perceived as) milder motor problems such as DCD is still difficult in the eyes of most clinicians. Raising awareness among primary health care staff who deal with young children on a routine basis of the problems children with DCD encounter might over-come a possible under-referral.

Furthermore, detecting symptoms of DCD early in life implies that it is known what to look for in a child's motor behaviour. However, we seem far away from being able to do so. Fortunately, new assessment instruments keep being developed based on updated knowledge of the heterogeneity of movement problems children with DCD might present with. For example, once the Early Years Movement Skills Checklist (Chambers and Sugden, 2002), to be completed by teachers for children between 3 and 5 years of age, has found its way into the educational system, it is expected that many more children will be referred for further assessment than currently is the case. Yet, however difficult the task ahead it seems worthwhile pursuing the issue of early identification since it is known that most of the children with DCD, once properly diagnosed as such, do benefit from many types of intervention (e.g. Polatajko et al., 2001a; Schoemaker et al., 2003; Sugden and Chambers, 2003a). Indeed, the preschool years seem an ideal time to work together with the child and its family to overcome the present movement difficulties and to anticipate strategies for reducing motor problems once environmental task demands increase.

CHAPTER 9

Assessment of handwriting in children with Developmental Coordination Disorder

ANNA L. BARNETT AND SHEILA E. HENDERSON

Introduction

When discussing the problems faced by children with DCD, one is often asked whether the ability to write by hand is still necessary. Is it not becoming a redundant skill? Reduction in cost and size and increases in sophistication of both voice-driven and keyboard-driven word processors will undoubtedly continue apace. At present, however, schools do not have the resources to provide all children with a computer all the time and the demands of day-to-day lessons and examinations are such that handwriting will remain a major vehicle for the recording of facts and concepts and the demonstration of understanding in school for many years to come. Legible handwriting generated at adequate speed will therefore, continue to be required if children are to reach their full educational potential.

Handwriting as a 'motor' skill

Handwriting, as a form of language production, is a complex skill with many components. There are many different written languages, varying in the sort of units of sound or meaning represented by each elementary visual sign, the complexity of spatial design, and hence of production of these characters, and their arrangement on the page (Haas, 1976; Henderson, 1982; Samson, 1985). A recent model that attempts to capture the essential components involved in transforming an idea into its expression in visible language was proposed by Berninger and her colleagues, in the 1990s (e.g. Berninger, Fuller and Whitaker, 1996; Swanson and Berninger, 1994). Unlike models that concentrate on the mature writer (e.g. Hayes and Flower, 1980), this one also tries to account for how children learn to write. The model includes a planning component to generate and select ideas, and a translating component to clothe ideas in an appropriate linguistic structure and transcribe this through the physical act of handwriting. Finally, there is a reviewing and revising component (see Figure 9.1). In this chapter, there is a primary concern with the perceptual-motor aspects of transcription, since it is this component that the beginner writer must learn anew and the child with DCD may find impossible to master.

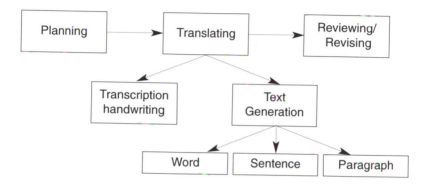

Figure 9.1 Simplified model of writing components, adapted from Berninger and Swanson (1994).

The vast majority of children learn to speak their own language fluently, without systematic instruction. By the time they reach school age, any unimpaired child can chat to his teacher and interact with peers at length (the noise in an infant school playground attests to that!). In contrast, the ability to write comes later, does not develop spontaneously and has to be taught for some time, before a fluent hand is acquired. Time taken to help children learn to write fluently and quickly is well spent, since handwriting will be required in almost every school subject, as important in science as in literacy classes.

Early in school, the focus will be on the formation, and hence legibility, of letters and words. Then speed enters as a crucial factor, particularly in secondary school where students need to take notes, write to dictation and complete written exams. Without being able to write legibly and rapidly, the ability to cope with the demands of a busy curriculum is severely compromised. Indeed, recent empirical studies have shown that if the perceptual-motor aspects of handwriting have not evolved to a level requiring little attention, then written output will be reduced in terms of quantity and quality (e.g. Connelly and Hurst, 2001; Graham et al., 1997). It is only when handwriting is fluent or 'automatic' that sufficient processing capacity can be allocated to higher level components of writing, involving planning and reviewing. Finally, the writer needs to develop the skill to the point where speed and legibility can be controlled in a flexible manner. Only then can appropriate adaptations to different task demands be made, such as the neatness required for a public wall display, the speed required in a time-limited exam or the compressed scribbling that will suffice as a personal record of a homework assignment. Difficulty in developing handwriting that is legible, fast, fluent and flexible has been shown to result in under-achievement in children, generally, not only those with DCD (e.g. Briggs, 1970; Simner, Leedham and Thomassen, 1996). Such difficulties have also been linked to poor self-esteem and relationships with peers (Phelps, Stempel and Speck, 1985).

Handwriting difficulties in children with DCD

Handwriting difficulties are extremely common in children of school age with DCD and can be devastating in their knock-on effects. Whether one asks parents, teachers or therapists, handwriting is almost certain to be listed among the most severe problems. Moreover, many of the children themselves will cite handwriting as the skill that they would most like to improve (Mandich et al., 2003; Miller et al., 2001b).

Figures 9.2a to 9.2f illustrate some of the problems experienced by six children with DCD, such as difficulties with letter formation, spacing and alignment. Comparative data on writing speed are also shown for a 14-year-old child with DCD and an age-matched peer of similar cognitive ability (Figure 9.2g).

In DSM-IV, the defining feature of DCD is specified as a 'marked impairment in the development of motor coordination' (APA, 1994). Difficulties with 'printing or handwriting' are then listed as an example of the problems experienced by children with DCD. Unfortunately, there is not yet data available that allow us to rank the problems in terms of their impact, so all of the difficulties are given equal weight in the current DSM-IV diagnostic proposal.

Although few professionals are obliged to adhere rigidly to DSM-IV diagnostic criteria in their everyday practice, most are familiar with those currently specified. With regard to Criterion A, the *essential* features of the 'marked impairment in the development of motor coordination' have yet to be identified but an impairment in handwriting might well appear on the list. Furthermore, such difficulties also guarantee fulfilment of Criterion B, which states that the disturbance satisfying Criterion A must 'significantly interfere with academic achievement or activities of daily living' (p. 55). However, the problem faced by all is how to define and

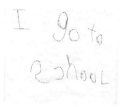

Figure 9.2a Aged 6 years, 4 months.

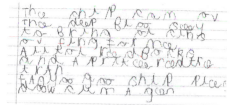

Figure 9.2b Aged 6 years, 9 months.

Figure 9.2c Aged 7 years, 5 months.

Figure 9.2d Aged 7 years, 11 months.

Figure 9.2e Aged 11 years, 6 months.

Figure 9.2f Aged 10 years.

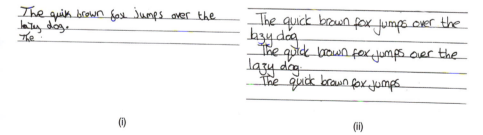

(i)

(ii)

Figure 9.2g Samples of handwriting from (i) a boy with DCD and (ii) a matched control, both aged 14. Note: each child copied text for one minute under 'normal' writing conditions. Child (i) with DCD wrote < 40 letters per minute and control child (ii) wrote > 80 letters per minute.

measure a 'marked impairment in handwriting' (see section on 'What needs to be assessed?' for further discussion).

In addition to perceptual-motor problems, many children with DCD have difficulty with spoken language, reading, attention, or social skills etc. (e.g. Kaplan et al., 1998). Sometimes these are severe enough to meet the criteria for formal diagnosis of other developmental disorders (including specific language impairment, dyslexia and ADHD). Difficulties in these domains may well impact upon various components of the writing process. Restrictions of space limit us here, to discussion of assessment of the perceptual-motor component of handwriting. In the classroom or clinic, however, this topic would, ideally, be accompanied by a broader review of writing components (for example see Berninger, 2001; Berninger, Mizokawa and Bragg, 1991).

Reasons for formally assessing handwriting

In spite of the increased awareness of DCD in schools today, the sad reality is that there are still teachers in classrooms who attribute the bright child's difficulty with handwriting (and other motor skills) to carelessness or lack of attention. Sometimes, this is because the gap between the child's reading and writing ability is so large that even the most experienced professionals find it puzzling. At other times, the child's behaviour problems (e.g. temper tantrums) interfere so much with classroom stability that the teacher simply brands the child as naughty without considering the fact that his/her 'clumsiness' might be at the root of the problem. In these circumstances, one often finds that parents are the ones who are most concerned about the handwriting problem – followed closely behind by the children themselves. Obviously, there is no way forward until family and school agree that a problem exists. Only then can an appropriate plan of action be drawn up.

On a more positive note, many schools do have policies and strategies in place for recognizing and helping children with movement difficulties. As part of the process of describing the problems in detail, most professionals involved will include handwriting in their own interviews and/or assessments and this can be a very useful starting point to record the concerns of all 'stakeholders'.

There are at least five reasons why a formal assessment of handwriting might be required:

- It may be useful to screen a group of children early in their school career in order to identify those who need help before their difficulties become entrenched.

- Screening may be employed with older children. For instance, on entry to secondary school (age 11–13 in most countries) it may be desirable to identify those who have failed to reach a standard appropriate for their age.
- Often it will be important to quantify the severity of a problem, for example in order to determine eligibility for extra support at school. In the UK, slow writing speed can be used to apply for extra time or an alternative writing medium in public examinations (QCA, 2003).
- A very detailed description of the handwriting difficulty needs to be obtained if appropriate intervention is to be devised.
- Recent emphasis on audit emphasizes the need to evaluate the effectiveness of interventions (Sackett et al., 2000).

The assessment of handwriting – some general issues

Despite the fact that handwriting difficulties are so common in children with DCD and their impact so well recognized, it is very hard to find a reliable, objective measure of handwriting skill. In contrast, the situation with regard to perceptual-motor competence generally is better, with a number of standardized tests providing useful information (see Chapters 7 and 8 for reviews). Although the latter are quite comprehensive in scope, none extends into the area of handwriting. There are good reasons for this. As noted earlier, handwriting is a skill which differs in many ways from a skill such as catching a ball or cutting with scissors. The language component alone means that it does not sit comfortably alongside other components of these tests. Another reason derives from the fact that handwriting is a taught skill. Thus the level of attainment reached will depend partly on the type and extent of initial teaching. Yet another derives from the fact that many different alphabet styles are taught in English-speaking countries. Within these, some have a national handwriting style used by all children. When this is the case, it is possible to develop a test in which prototypic exemplars can be applied universally for all children. For example, in the United States the Evaluation Tool of Children's Handwriting (ETCH, Amundson, 1995) is based on the D'Nealian, a looped cursive style taught throughout much of the USA. In other countries, such as the UK, each school is free to choose its own writing style and these may vary from a very upright 'ball and stick' type with only some joins to a fully joined looped cursive (see Figure 9.3) (Stainthorp et al., 2001). Teaching methods also differ considerably, sometimes even within the same school. In some, the teaching of handwriting is perceived to be very important and considerable time and effort are devoted to it. In others, teaching of this skill has sadly, been neglected. Such variation in styles and teaching practices makes it very difficult indeed to develop a standard measure of handwriting performance and gather norms. In the light of such difficulty, the authors have elected not to produce a detailed test by test review of available instruments, but instead to consider the problems to be faced in the design of a reliable instrument, using aspects of existing instruments as exemplars. For an impressively comprehensive review of available instruments, readers are referred to Rosenblum, Weiss and Parush (2003).

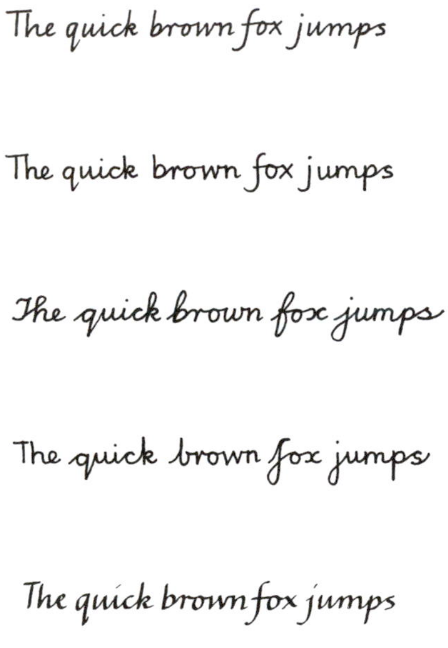

The quick brown fox jumps

The quick brown fox jumps

The quick brown fox jumps

The quick brown fox jumps

The quick brown fox jumps

Figure 9.3 Examples of scripts currently used in UK schools.

Since teachers and therapists around the world share a concern for children who fail to acquire adequate levels of skill, handwriting assessment tools have been developed for different writing systems (e.g. Chow, Choy and Mui, 2003; Tseng, 1998; Yochman and Parush, 1998). Here, however, the discussion is limited to assessment instruments designed for use with English, which employs letters of Roman origin.

What needs to be included in a handwriting assessment?

Broadly speaking, three sources of information form the basis of a comprehensive assessment of handwriting.

- The final product needs to be assessed under different demands of speed and legibility.
- The manner of production requires to be noted, especially when designing interventions.
- It is also important to determine what general strengths and weaknesses a child brings to the task. Cognitive ability, language and literacy are as essential as measures of fine motor coordination and ability to concentrate. Metacognition in the form of the child's view of his/her problem is also important as is the child's motivation to change.

In the section above, the variation that can be found from class to class, from school to school, and from country to country in the way children are taught to write was commented on. Although such variation may not matter for certain types of assessment, the planning of an intervention programme for a child cannot be well executed without knowledge of what goes on in school. Desirable information includes the prescriptions of the school's handwriting policy, the consistency with which these are applied, the teacher's attitude to handwriting, information about the child's writing history, and any additional help that has been provided.

What should a handwriting test require of the child?

The first step in the development of any test is to describe clearly the construct(s) to be measured. The second is to consider the purpose of the assessment and the constraints these might place on content. Designing a *handwriting* test poses some special problems that are not encountered in the design of other perceptual-motor tests. Perhaps the most difficult to solve involves the choice of task but close behind comes the formulation of instructions.

The choice of task

At the perceptual-motor end of the writing continuum, there are two elements with which one should be concerned – the child's ability to produce writing that is legible and the speed with which letters and words can be produced on the page. In everyday life, children are required to write under many different conditions, even though the requirements may not be made explicit. On some occasions, the quality of the output is primary and 'best writing' is required (e.g. writing a job application). On other occasions, simply getting something down that is readable by the writer will suffice (e.g. recording homework). To be fully comprehensive, therefore, any test of handwriting should include an assessment of writing under different quality and speed instructions.

To a large extent, the compass of any assessment is determined by its purpose. If the objective is to screen the entire first year intake of a large secondary school (maybe 300 pupils), what is required is a relatively short test, that yields sufficient data to permit the identification of those children whose writing is so poor that they would be unable to cope with the day-to-day demands of school. For this purpose, an analysis of a finished piece of writing must suffice. However, if the next step is to help those children who 'fail' then face-to-face observation using a more extensive range of tasks is essential.

One of the most common tasks included in published studies of children's handwriting requires the child to *copy* material over a set period of time. However, the material employed has varied unsystematically from study to study. For example, the phrase 'cats and dogs' was used by Ziviani and Watson-Will (1998), the sentence 'the quick brown fox jumps over the lazy dog' by Wallen, Bonney and Lennox (1996), Barnett, Henderson and Scheib (2002) and many others and a paragraph of running text by e.g. Blote and Hamstra-Bletz (1991); Graham, Berninger and Weintraub (1998); Rubin and Henderson (1982). Variation is found in the way the material is presented (e.g. there may or may not be difference between the style in which the test material is presented and the style of writing asked of the child). Some tests ask the child to write on lined paper, others do not. Some require the child to use a pen, others a pencil and some require the child to write for one minute, others three minutes, and others longer still. This variation greatly impedes comparison of different studies (see below for further discussion).

Critics of the copying task argue that it is rarely performed by children in everyday life. In pursuit of a more 'realistic' compositional alternative, some tests require children to write about a familiar topic, such as their favourite person. After some time for preparation they are given a fixed time to write on this topic (e.g. Allcock, 2001; Alston, 1990; Connor, 1995; Dutton, 1991; Roaf, 1998; Waine, 2001). Unfortunately 'composition', as a paradigm for assessing speed and legibility of writing confounds these two characteristics with a multitude of other cognitive activities, including the demands of composing, spelling and punctuating the text as well as the demands on working memory that are peculiar to composition tasks. These unwanted demands on the child are incalculable in their effects (which, of course, vary from child to child).

A different criticism of brief copying tasks asserts that a few minutes is unrepresentative of most classroom writing tasks. Wallen, Bonney and Lennox (1996), for example, urge users of their test to consider the possibility that a child's test score might overestimate their ability to sustain the specified writing speed. This poses the non-trivial question of what exactly it is that is required as a measure of speed. Is the 100 metre sprint event a better measure of 'speed' than the sustained 10,000 metres?

Surely the answer to the question of task is that no single task can provide all the answers. There is no doubt that a short copying task offers the 'cleanest' measure of a child's ability to write legibly, at an acceptable speed. Were we to dig deeper, for example to examine the effect of fatigue upon performance, then a much longer task must be included. Similarly, if a child seems to have other difficulties that might affect writing then other appropriate tasks must be devised. To this end, a dictation task might be included (where memory and spelling ability would be taxed) along with the compositional writing task which, of course, includes every stage mentioned in Figure 9.1, above.

Instructions

Once a writing task, or series of tasks, has been chosen and the length of writing time established, the next consideration must be the task conditions/instructions. As noted above, one of the most common contrasts to be found in existing instruments is between producing one's 'best' or 'normal' writing and writing under some sort of 'speed' instruction. However, there are instruments which do not distinguish between these two conditions clearly enough, thus creating possible conflict in the mind of the child. For example, in their test, Wallen, Bonney and Lennox (1996) ask the child to 'Write as *quickly* but as *neatly* as you can until I tell you to stop.' Now, clearly, it is essential to convey to the children that they must not write so fast that the product becomes illegible. However, the extent to which individuals will interpret the balance between the twin criteria of *speed* and *neatness* will vary considerably from child to child and will also depend on the tone of voice being used to enunciate each criterion ... 'Quickly and **neatly**' ... OR ... **Quickly** and neatly' and what does the word neat mean to the child – just legible or aesthetically pleasing? This is not an easy problem to solve. It is one which recurs in all sorts of contexts and is one which psychologists have been studying for well over a hundred years. They label it the 'Speed–accuracy trade-off' problem (Schmidt and Wrisberg, 2000). In another guise, of course, it is one which those concerned with children with special educational needs face constantly – the 'bull in a china shop child' versus the child who is too timid to really 'go for speed'.

Although the argument has been for a clear separation between tasks in which the child is asked to produce his/her 'normal' or 'best' writing and tasks in which speed is of the essence, it is often useful to know how long the child took to complete the 'normal' writing piece. This is because some children write so slowly 'normally' that their ability to keep up with the tempo of everyday classroom work is compromised. When timing a child in this condition, however, it is crucial that this is done as unobtrusively as possible so that the student is not aware that he/she is being timed.

What needs to be assessed?

Consider the boy's handwriting shown in Figure 9.2c. Without ever setting eyes on the child, it can be seen that his writing is almost unreadable. Looking at Figure 9.2g(i), it can be seen that this child has written very little in one minute. What cannot be determined, of course, from mere study of these samples is *how* the children performed the tasks. Do they know how to form letters? Is their graphic output faltering and influent? Did they struggle to write throughout the set period or spend time gazing through the window? ... and so on.

In what follows, there is a consideration of the assessment of the finished product. This may be all that is necessary or, indeed, possible if one is conducting a screening programme. It then moves on to a consideration of what new information can be gleaned from sitting down with the child and observing him write.

The finished product

Most handwriting assessments cover two aspects of performance (1) the quality of the output and (2) the speed with which it has been produced. The relative importance of these two dimensions, of course, varies with the age of the children being assessed. Although relevant, the speed with which a 5-year-old can copy a sentence is much less important than it would be if the child were just about to enter secondary school.

Quality

When looking at a piece of writing like that shown in Figure 9.4, legibility is taken for granted. Instead, epithets such as *elegant*, *fluent* and *artistic* come to mind, as do *neat* and *tidy*. However, neatness is not synonymous with legibility. When considering the basic requirement of a handwriting *assessment*, therefore, authors have tended to use legibility or readability as the key concept underlying quality, with aesthetic considerations taking second place.

There have been two approaches to the assessment of the quality of a piece of writing. The first has been to take a broad view of the quality of the penmanship, the second involves a more detailed appraisal of particular components. Instruments which employ the broad approach

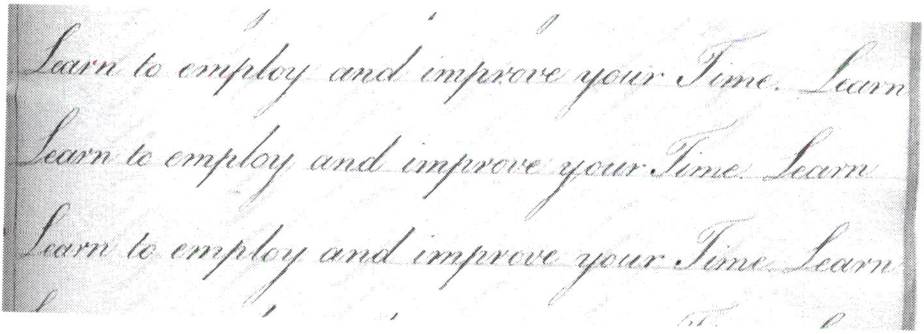

Figure 9.4 Looped, cursive script from a Victorian copy book.

usually require the assessor to rate a piece of handwriting on a scale from *good* to *poor*, with each category being assigned a numerical score (Barnett, Henderson and Scheib, 2002; Daniel and Froude, 1998; Reisman, 1999; Phelps, Stempel and Speck, 1985). This approach has been used in the analysis of individual letters, as well as words, sentences and paragraphs. Although the use of a Likert-type scale is a recognized procedure for the quantification of qualitative variables (Anastasi, 1997), it is not without difficulties. One problem with regard to handwriting is the lack of agreed anchor points. Different people may interpret the categories in different ways, especially at the extremes of the scale (Daniel and Froude, 1998). One person's view of 'good' handwriting might be very different from another's view. In an attempt to reduce the variance attributable to different assessors' concepts of 'good' and 'poor' handwriting, some instruments require examiners to match a writing sample to a set of graded specimens, which have already been assigned a score. This method, now abandoned, was used in the UK in the national literacy tests but the range of examples presented was rather limited, making it impossible to distinguish between degrees of difficulty.

Another problem with the use of this kind of rating scale concerns its suitability for longer samples of writing. In addition to the fact that judgements of legibility are likely to be influenced by semantic and syntactic constraints in writing, there may be genuine changes in legibility that make a single category judgement inappropriate. Some children with difficulties can actually write quite well initially but cannot sustain legibility beyond a sentence or two. The way round this is to divide the text into sections and rate each one separately. Even when these various problems have been addressed, however, it appears that considerable training of assessors is needed before adequate levels of inter-rater reliability can be obtained (Graham et al., 1998). Once again, however, the problem is not insurmountable and acceptable levels of inter-rater and test–retest reliability have been reported for some instruments using this procedure (e.g. Simner, 1991 quotes test–retest correlations for the Printing Performance School Readiness Test (PPRT) of 0.87 over a one month period and 0.74 over an eight month period).

Although global rating scales clearly have their limitations, their usefulness should not be underestimated. For screening purposes, it is neither possible, nor appropriate, to conduct a detailed analysis of each sample of handwriting. Yet, schools need to know how many children are failing to reach age-appropriate standards, governments need to know how many children require extra help, and auditors need to know that an attempt has been made to measure change objectively. Studies using the holistic approach report significant effects for age and gender with better legibility for girls than boys (Graham and Weintraub, 1996; Graham, Berninger and Weintraub, 1998) but there are few tests that claim to offer normative data with which all would feel comfortable.

Once a child has been identified as having a handwriting problem that requires intervention, the second approach to the assessment of quality of handwriting comes into its own. This approach is based on the notion that quality/legibility is not a unitary characteristic, but a composite of interrelated components. Without exception, instruments in this 'component analysis' category include an evaluation of how the letters are formed. The way this is done, however, varies from test to test. In the Concise Evaluation Scale for Children's Handwriting (the BHK; Hamstra-Bletz, DeBie and Den Brinker, 1987), for example, seven of the 13 items rated are concerned with how letters are formed and joined (e.g. the item names include 'ambiguous letter forms', 'letter distortion' and 'absence of joins'). Similarly the ETCH requires assessors to examine each letter of the alphabet separately and record if there is poor formation. Another common component concerns the spacing between words, and less often between letters. After that there is more variation in what is included in an assessment. However, most instruments consider, in varying amounts of detail, the consistency/uniformity with which the writing is presented on the page. This might include the overall size, the relative height of the various kinds of letter, the slope of ascenders and descenders, the alignment of the writing on the line, if there is one, and across the page, if there is not. Line quality also features in some tests, the rater being offered descriptors like tremorous, unsteady etc.

As with the global rating scales, the process of component analysis is also approached in different ways, each designed to increase objectivity and reliability of scoring. In some tests, for example, separate components are scored according to criteria presented either verbally, visually or both. Transparent overlays are also common e.g. to score the consistency of slope in a piece of writing or the relative height of the letters with and without ascenders/descenders. What is then done with the component scores varies considerably. Whereas some test authors have collected sufficient data on the psychometrics of their scales to allow the user to derive a meaningful norm (e.g. the BHK), most have not.

Since there is no gold standard against which the quality of a child's handwriting can be judged, the question of the validity of handwriting quality assessments is a complex issue. There is space to mention just two approaches. One approach has been to examine the relationship between the two types of 'quality' measure just described. For those experienced in the field the outcome of these might be unsurprising. Overall, the correlations are moderate to good and letter formation emerges as the best predictor of overall quality. After that, however, the order in which other components add to the variance accounted for varies from study to study. For instance, Graham, Boyer-Schick and Tippets (1989) found that letter formation was followed closely by neatness and spacing, with these three variables accounting for 61 per cent of the variance on an overall rating on the Test of Legible Handwriting (Larsen and Hammill, 1989). Alignment, slant and size were not significant. The second approach to validity has been to correlate test scores with a rating made by an external assessor such as a teacher or therapist. Once again, only moderate correlations are obtained e.g. Graham (1986) quotes a correlation of 0.64 between scores on the Zaner-Bloser Evaluation Scales and a teacher's estimate of quality. Very few studies take a longitudinal approach to validity, attempting to determine whether scores on a test at time 1 predict scores at time 2. However, two studies are of considerable practical relevance. Using a fairly crude 3 point rating scale, Harvey and Henderson (1997) showed that, without intervention, children whose handwriting was classified as poor at age 5 remained unchanged at age 7. Taking a longer time perspective, Simner (1991) obtained a correlation of 0.54 between children's scores on the PPRT in kindergarten and their scores on the Test of Legible Handwriting (Larsen and Hammill, 1989), six years later. In addition, Simner found that the lowest 10 per cent of children on the PPRT were also the slowest, six years later.

Speed

When compared to the problem of assessing legibility, that of assessing speed is minor. In principle, production tasks may draw upon either of two timing procedures. The time taken to complete a specified text can be measured, or the amount of specified text produced in a fixed interval can be determined. Only the fixed interval procedure is amenable to group testing and it has been adopted in almost all tests of handwriting speed. Provided that the child follows instructions to start and stop writing when told, a precise, objective measure can be obtained.

Most researchers and test designers have cited a rate of letter production corrected in some way for legibility. This correction process is often uncertain and time consuming since it requires an experienced judge to exclude from the rate count, letters that meet some criterion of illegibility. In some instruments, a very clear definition of a 'countable letter' is provided (e.g. Wallen, Bonney and Lennox, 1996). In others, much more discretion is allowed. Once a total number of letters is obtained, however, this is usually converted to a rate of production per minute.

Limited data are available on the reliability of measures of handwriting speed but the available data suggest that inter-rater reliability is very good (Barnett, Henderson and Scheib, 2002; Garmoyle, 2003; Wallen, Bonney and Lennox, 1996). Almost nothing is known about stability of the measure over time. However, there is unpublished data on 13–14-year-olds, showing test–retest correlations of 0.89 with a one week separation (Barnett, Henderson and Scheib, 2002).

Data on handwriting speed have been collected in several countries, including two substantial samples from Australia and the USA (Graham et al., 1998; Wallen, Bonney and Lennox, 1996). A few general trends emerge. As would be expected, for example, the speed with which children write increases with age. In some studies, girls have been shown to write faster than boys, suggesting that separate norms might be advisable (e.g. Wallen, Bonney and Lennox, 1996) but in others the effect is not significant. Right-handers also tend to write faster than left-handers, although this is a much less robust effect (e.g. Graham et al., 1998). In addition, it is clear that the task used has a major effect on the rates quoted. Not surprisingly, rates cited for lengthy free writing tasks are lower than those obtained for brief copying tasks.

In sum, selection procedures, age ranges and methods employed differ so much from study to study, that it would be very unwise to extract global, 'universal' norms. What is urgently required, therefore, is the application of optimal procedures to the collection of a large corpus of normative data, on clearly described sets of children, performing the same task. Speed/accuracy instructions must be explicit, carefully pondered and reflected in any correction of rates for legibility. Even then, local educational practices might have such a strong influence on performance that only local norms would be valid.

The process of writing

Although a detailed examination of a child's finished work will offer many clues to the difficulties experienced in the production process, only the dynamic information that is obtained by watching the child will provide the precision needed to plan an intervention programme. In addition, a face-to-face session allows the child to provide his/her perspective on the problem(s).

The way the written trace emerges

In the section above on component analysis, some of the aspects of a child's writing that are assumed to determine whether a piece of writing is legible or not were described – such as whether there is adequate spacing between the words, whether the size of the letters is consistent and so on. In a face-to-face session with a child, the same characteristics might well be observed but in a different way. Space will allow just two examples. In order to be able to produce joined-up writing, fluently, comfortably and fast, it is crucial that the young child learn the movements required to make each letter individually. As noted earlier, in some countries this will be the same for all children (at least initially) but in others it may vary from school to school, and even within a school. For the child with poor handwriting, the inability to learn these movement patterns often lies at the heart of the problem. Consequently, a detailed record of which letters a child cannot form easily is central to any comprehensive assessment. To do this, the assessor will need to be familiar with the style-model that has been taught to the child and aware of the start and end points of different letters for the particular script adopted. Numerous checklists are available to record letter formation when copying or writing from dictation (e.g. Amundson, 1995; Taylor, 2001), but most are informal and unstandardized. The second example concerns the spacing of words within a paragraph. There are some children who will pause when reaching the end of a word, indicating an awareness of the need for a space, but then start the next word without one. This is different from the child who produces no spaces either within or between words, perhaps being unaware of the conventions of our writing system, perhaps just not 'seeing' the problem at all (only talking about this difficulty will disentangle the options).

Pen grip and posture

Much has been written on the topic of writing implements, how they should be held and how the paper should be positioned (for a very sensible discussion see Sassoon, 1993). Most writing manuals advocate the 'dynamic tripod' hand posture, in which the pencil or pen is held between the pads of the thumb and index finger, and rests on the side of the middle finger (Henderson et al., 1999; Taylor, 2001). Although the dynamic tripod grip is usually described as the most comfortable and efficient, the extent to which it is suitable for all writing implements and all children is not clear. Moreover, there is considerable variation in how typically developing children hold writing implements and this does not seem to predict either the legibility or speed of their handwriting (Berninger et al., 1997; Dennis and Swinth, 2001; Graham and Weintraub, 1996; Schneck, 1991; Ziviani and Elkins, 1986). This seems also to be true of left-handers who need special consideration when grip is being examined. A variety of grips may be adopted in order to avoid occluding the writing, the reduction of visual feedback and the smudging of ink. Some practitioners consider a hooked grip to disadvantage the child, for example, but several research studies suggest otherwise (e.g. Athenes and Guiard, 1991; Peters and Pedersen, 1978). Many texts include photographs of the range of grips that one can see in an average primary school (Benbow, 2002) and checklists are available to document the type of grip (e.g. Taylor, 2001). What one does about it as a practitioner very much depends on the individual case, the age of the child, willingness to change etc.

Although the precise configuration of the grip may be debatable, one of the most important points to consider when dealing with an individual who has a writing problem is whether the grip is comfortable over long, as well as short periods of writing. Some children with DCD report that their writing hand quickly becomes tired or sore. This may be the result of sub-optimal location of the pen-grip along the shaft of the writing implement. For example, if the grip is too distant from the writing- tip of the implement, then the force required to generate the requisite two dimensional displacements of the tip on the writing surface will be excessive, with consequent degradation of the ability to produce finely coordinated movements of the writing tip. Conversely, some children hold their fingers too close to the writing tip, and press too firmly onto the paper. This also makes it hard to move the pen on the paper and can result in fatigue.

The question of posture is also a difficult one. Typically developing children may be able to write well using even the most unorthodox and uncomfortable postures. During the course of a school day, a child might write sitting 'properly' at a desk, lying on the floor, or even leaning against a tree during a botany lesson in the playground. For these children, such postures are stable and flexible enough to allow the child to control the hand and arm with ease. In contrast, it is generally believed that the basic postural control deficits observed in children with DCD (e.g. Wann, Mon-Williams and Rushton, 1998) make it hard for the child to develop/maintain a degree of stability that allows for fluent, fast writing. 'Ideal' sitting postures and ways to position the paper for writing are commonly reported (Henderson et al., 1999; Sassoon, 1990; Taylor, 2001).

Some of these specifications are based on ergonomic research on seating, sitting posture etc. (Mandal, 1985). Others derive from common sense observations about efficiency and comfort (e.g. the paper position for a left-hander). A number of checklists help the observer to describe a child's posture in detail (e.g. Taylor, 2001). As with pencil grip, however, it is then up to the assessor to make a clinical judgement as to how much such difficulties are contributing to the actual writing difficulty.

In sum, when the objective of an assessment is to plan a programme of remediation there is no substitute for watching a child perform a series of writing tasks in which the nature and difficulty level of the task are systematically varied. However, the data gathered from such observation are not necessarily of equal weighting. Being able to form letters using the correct pattern of movement is essential if a fluent joined-up script is the objective. How the child holds the pen may not matter so much.

Technology and assessment

Subjective ratings of neatness or legibility begin to have a serious rival, furnished by modern technology. The first stage of the necessary advances was the development of paradigms in which the metrics and dynamics of human movement could be digitized on-line so as to be entered into a computer. Two paradigms have been of particular interest where handwriting is concerned. One, widely used for the analysis of gait and reaching and grasping, involves a freely moving participant. The other has been evolved more specifically for the analysis of a person's graphic output (see Simner, Leedham and Thomassen, 1996, for detailed reviews).

Movement analysis systems have allowed human movement in 3D to be digitized by the use of reference tags attached to various body parts with multiple cameras recording the movement of these tags. The arrival of improved and much more friendly software for these analyses and reduction of the price of such systems have made them part of the basic equipment of any movement laboratory. As yet, however, such 3D systems have only occasionally been applied to the attempt to describe and quantify the movements involved in handwriting (e.g. Schillings, Meulenbrook and Thomassen, 1996). One obvious reason is fear of drowning in the vast amount of data that may be gathered but subtler and deeper torment is to be found in the problem of deciding, in a theoretically motivated way, precisely *what* to quantify.

A simpler and more tractable paradigm involves digitization of various parameters in 2D by use of a *graphic tablet* that allows 'pen' position to be recorded over time. From this can be derived measures of movement acceleration and velocity. More linguistically intelligible parameters such as variance in the slope of ascenders and descenders, or smoothness of the flow of writing, can also be extracted (van Galen et al., 1993; Rosenblum, Parush and Weiss, 2003). Within the framework of graphic-tablet analysis the dynamics of writing performance can also be analysed, by attaching force transducers to the hand in order to provide complementary analyses of pen grip or pressure on the tablet (e.g. Hill and Wing, 1998).

One must not, however, underestimate the task of extracting from the mass of data those spatio-temporal features that correspond to such disarmingly simple yet difficult to define factors as the perceived neatness or legibility of writing. However, a start has been made and results of some clinical/educational relevance are beginning to emerge (e.g. Smits-Engelsman, Niemeijer and van Galen, 2001; Smits-Engelsman, van Galen and Schoemaker, 1997; Wann and Kardirkmanathan, 1991) and by Tucha and Lange (2001). One of the interesting features of this work has been the demonstration that the quality of line production, in terms of tremor and influency detection (faltering of the velocity trace) may be very revealing. The time course of letter formation can also be recovered by the use of such systems.

Assessing the child with DCD – how does handwriting fit into the broader picture?

In the course of their lives, children with DCD undergo many types of assessment. These include formal and informal procedures, undertaken by parents, teachers, therapists, educational psychologists and other professionals. While they invariably include tests related to perceptual-motor competence, many other areas of competence might also be included, from time to time (e.g. IQ tests, speech and language tests, reading tests). Exactly when and how handwriting assessment fits into the picture will vary from child to child.

Long before a formal diagnosis of DCD is made, parents often express concern about differences between their own child and a playmate or sibling. In some cases, late sitting, standing, walking and talking might have suggested a problem. In others, a failure to show an interest in drawing and painting, doing jigsaws and using constructional toys might act as a trigger. Then, when preschool staff find that the child needs extra help/encouragement with tasks requiring perceptual judgement or manipulative ability, and does not join in with others during any activity requiring fine motor control, concern begins to grow. At this stage, a description of the young child's difficulties, formal or informal, is essential if the adults receiving such children into school are to make adequate provision for them. Since Chapters 7 and 8 in this volume deal with other aspects of assessing children with DCD, this section will be confined to addressing questions related specifically to handwriting.

One of the most difficult questions to answer is whether any of the difficulties observed in the preschool period can/should be viewed as predictive of a later handwriting difficulty. Unfortunately, the authors were unable to find any longitudinal studies which track the progress of preschool children with fine motor difficulties into school to see whether handwriting presented particular difficulty. However, what can be drawn upon are studies examining the relationship between shape copying (e.g. Beery, 1997) and concurrent handwriting skill. Although most studies report positive and significant correlations between the two (Daly, Kelley and Krauss, 2003; Tseng and Chow, 2000; Tseng and Murray, 1994; Weil and Cunningham Amundson, 1994), this is not an invariant finding in either normal (see e.g. Berninger et al., 1992), or dysgraphic children (Maeland and Karlsdottir, 1991). Moreover, even the highest reported correlation indicates that shape copying accounts for only 40 per cent of the variance in handwriting skill. Such results emphasize the fact that handwriting is not only different from other graphic skills, but also involves many other non-motor components. This suggests that being able to cut with scissors, use a knife and fork, copy or draw well does not guarantee that handwriting is easy for a child, or the converse. Compared to other areas of literacy, notably reading, we are far behind in the identification of the underlying or component skills that constitute handwriting. Compare, for example, the literature on rhyming ability as a predictor of reading ability (Goswami, 2002; Passenger, Stuart and Terrel, 2000).

As children with DCD progress through school, problems with handwriting begin to move up the priority list. In sympathetic schools, the special needs staff may perform their own assessments and set up an intervention group. In others, however, such help may not be forthcoming and this is where a standardized assessment would really come into its own. In addition, in situations where the supply of resources is tied to DSM or ICD criteria, it would be helpful to be able to specify how a child compares to his peers in the area of handwriting. At present, it is easy to say, for example, 'this 10-year-old child with a verbal IQ of 125 has a reading age of 7 and needs immediate help'. It is also relatively easy to say that a child falls below the 5th percentile on the Movement ABC (Henderson and Sugden, 1992) or test of Visual Motor Integration (Beery, 1997) but in the area of handwriting, we are very far from this point. Even if it is conceded that the nature of handwriting makes it difficult (maybe impossible) to produce a completely 'culture free' test, it might still be feasible to combine components of existing 'local' instruments to obtain the most reliable and sensitive indicators of difficulty.

At secondary level, the need for standardized measures of handwriting become ever more urgent – especially in the area of speed. In the UK at present, many children who cannot write legibly or fast enough are given concessions in examinations, being allowed extra time, the use of a computer etc. However, the criteria whereby such concessions are awarded are based on inadequate data and are not clear. The situation is similar in other countries.

Conclusion

In view of the problems discussed above, estimates of the prevalence of handwriting difficulties in a population must be treated with caution. The few studies that seem to yield fairly reliable figures, suggest a prevalence of between 10 per cent and 15 per cent (Karlsdottir and Stefansson, 2002; Rubin and Henderson, 1982). This figure should not be confused with estimates of the incidence of DCD. Handwriting difficulties are not universal in DCD and, conversely, they may be associated with other syndromes, for example dyslexia (Phelps and Stempel, 1991), Asperger's Syndrome (Henderson and Green, 2001), and Attention Deficit Hyperactivity Disorder (Tucha and Lange, 2001). There may also be children with handwriting difficulty as an isolated problem. At the moment, there is no information at all on whether the precise nature of handwriting difficulties varies systematically across different syndromes. There is, therefore, a pressing need for standardized procedures to be developed for assessing handwriting and for a reliable functional taxonomy of types of handwriting difficulty. In particular, if effective interventions for children with handwriting difficulties are to be planned, there is a need to develop tools that will allow teasing apart of the different components of the skill at all levels not just the perceptual-motor component.

Acknowledgements

We are grateful to Leslie Henderson for his insightful comments and helpful suggestions to improve the clarity of the manuscript. We also thank Angela Webb, Mary Chambers, Jane Taylor and Gwen Dornan for their help in gathering handwriting samples to choose from.

CHAPTER 10

Models of intervention: towards an eco-developmental approach

DAVID A. SUGDEN AND MARY E. CHAMBERS

Origin of approaches

Throughout the book the condition of DCD has been described, examined and analysed by a range of researchers and clinicians who bring their beliefs, background and training to their work. DCD has been shown to be a heterogeneous condition that has attracted the attention of medical and paramedical, educational and psychological professionals. If one combines the disciplines that are involved in the study and management of DCD together with the known heterogeneity of the condition, it is not surprising that a range of intervention approaches have been presented. Much of the early work involved those working in paediatrics with the discipline still attracting a variety of medical professionals including paediatricians and neurologists, as well as general practitioners who see the children through parental or school concerns. Because of the need for managing the condition, occupational therapists and physiotherapists have been at the forefront and, historically, psychologists have had an interest in the field with educational, developmental and clinical psychologists all contributing to the caucus of work in the field. The educational field, represented by teachers, have tried to deal with DCD children on a daily basis, often with a lack of knowledge in the specific area but with a good knowledge of the developing child and the advantage of seeing them on a daily basis. With the more recent emphasis on children with special educational needs, and the Code of Practice (DfES, 2001), educational approaches are beginning to become more influential as knowledge is cascaded through to the classroom. Finally, and probably most importantly, parents of children with DCD have long been requiring advice and guidance on the best way to help their children and a recurring theme throughout this chapter is that intervention of any kind must, as a first principle, accept that context and family life are a priority with success being dependent on intervention fitting into this framework and not the other way round (Bernheimer and Keogh, 1995).

Many issues and questions will be raised about intervention but as a principle it is appropriate to intervene with children showing difficulties for a variety of reasons; first because many 'do not grow out of it'; second, many show associated difficulties and third, there is a view that if a child is showing problems that are clearly causing anxiety, there is an ethical duty to ameliorate them. The conclusion reached at the end of this chapter is that effective intervention is multifaceted and multilayered; it is not confined to a single principle within one experimental or clinical framework but draws upon knowledge of the developing child, how movements are controlled and learned; additionally, it takes on board principles from cognitive psychology and is set firmly within the everyday life of the child and the family context. It is indeed an eco-developmental approach.

Approaches to intervention

The background of the individuals working with the children is very different and, although many now are becoming much more interdisciplinary in their approaches, most will bring an underlying ideology that will affect their work in intervention. The aim in this chapter is to present a brief overview and evaluation of the approaches, outline a potential working model while looking at how other disciplines such as developmental motor control and learning and ecological psychology can help us provide directions for research and practice. It is probable that all approaches are compromised in one way or another and the real trick is not only to be aware of this but to minimize this compromise and choose an approach or combination of approaches that is comfortable within the child's total lifestyle.

Here there is an attempt to place some organization on the range of approaches, while recognizing that such an attempt does lead to charges of a reductionist approach. In spite of this, a useful distinction is to separate those approaches which can broadly be labelled as *process-oriented* from those which are *task-oriented* (Sugden and Chambers, 1998; Sugden and Wright, 1998). Both of these are global categories and can be subdivided, each showing component parts and subtle differences. Other writers have made more subdivisions (e.g. Pless and Carlsson, 2000) and these are legitimate ways of examining the field. However, as more subdivisions can lead to greater overlap between them and the process–task distinction, division does contain relatively specific fundamental underlying principles, it is believed that the distinction is appropriate. In addition

to these, there are also others such as those used by physio- and occupational therapists in clinical settings which, though occasionally following
one particular approach, very often are eclectic in nature and incorporate
features of both process and task approaches. Thus, particularly with the
group labelled process-oriented approach, caution is advised in the interpretation of the underlying rationale.

Process-oriented approaches

Process-oriented approaches are broad-based and contain a number of
slightly different methods. These would include such methods as Sensory
Integration Therapy (Ayres, 1972a; 1979; 1989) and kinaesthetic
approaches (Laszlo and Bairstow, 1985a). They all aim at pinpointing the
underlying process or processes which the child has not developed adequately for his/her age and which are thought necessary for the successful
performance and acquisition of motor skills. A practical example may
serve to illustrate the general fundamental points. If a child has a difficulty in catching a ball, one can intervene by giving ball catching experiences
of various types, which would be a task-oriented approach, or one could
break the act of ball catching into its underlying processes and try to
improve these, which would be a process approach. The latter might
include trying to improve sensory functions (visual and kinaesthetic perception), memory, attention, planning and the formulation of motor
programmes. Examples of this type of approach have come from
researchers such as Laszlo and colleagues (1985a; 1988) who have produced their own strong evidence for the process approach involving
kinaesthetic training and from sensorimotor integration therapy (Ayres,
1972a). The findings of other researchers examining a kinaesthetic
approach have not always been supported by some research groups
(Doyle, Elliott and Connolly, 1986; Polatajko et al., 1995; Sugden and
Wann, 1987) while provisional support has been reported by Sims and
colleagues (1996a; 1996b) who found an improvement in children due to
kinaesthetic methods, but they were no more impressive than other methods of intervention.

In the sensory integrative therapy method, there is an assumption that
the development of cognition, language and motor skills is dependent on
sensory integrative ability (Ayres, 1972a; 1979; 1989). The children are
given help to organize sensory input by proprioceptive, tactile and
vestibular stimulation involving full body movements and training in specific perceptual and motor skills. Support for the efficacy of sensorimotor
integration therapy has been provided by Ayres many times in clinical settings and controlled independent studies, although not differentiating
between the effects of sensory integration therapy and other methods, do

provide some evidence for its effectiveness (Cermak and Henderson, 1989; 1990; Humphries et al., 1990; Wilson and Kaplan, 1994). However, Law and colleagues (1991) found no significant differences between the effects in one group of sensorimotor integration therapy and another group receiving traditional perceptual motor training on measures of reading, writing, fine motor skills, gross motor skills or self-esteem. In addition, Pless and Carlsson (2000) found little support for sensory integration or kinaesthetic methods in a meta-analysis of 13 intervention studies which she divided into specific skill (SS), general ability (GA) and sensory integration (SI) approaches. In the SI studies there was the lowest effect size followed by the GA with the best results being obtained from the specific skill studies. The authors do advise caution in the interpretation of these results and although there are great theoretical differences between the approaches, in practice in certain circumstances, there is often overlap. As a clinician has remarked, ball catching is ball catching no matter what is the underlying rationale for giving the activity.

However, there are a number of interesting and, occasionally speculative, observations one can make about these approaches. A potential theoretical advantage of process-oriented approaches is that of generalization. If one accepts that it is not possible to directly learn every task that is required, some form of generalization is needed and, by addressing the fundamental underlying processes, these may be applicable to a group of tasks. It is not simply one task that is being learned, but the processes that will transfer across situations. Logical as this is, the difficulty lies in deriving the true underlying processes together with devising activities which directly address them. In addition, process approaches that break down tasks into subcomponents are susceptible to the criticism of not setting the intervention in an appropriate ecological functional context, with the apparent paradox that the nearer one approaches this context, the more task-oriented the approach becomes.

Task-oriented approaches

Task-oriented approaches contain a range of methods all involving a concentration on functional tasks or group of tasks without an emphasis on underlying processes. As such, the intervention strategy focuses on the tasks that are causing the child difficulties (Henderson and Sugden, 1992; Larkin, Hoare and Smith, 1989; Revie and Larkin, 1993b; Wright and Sugden, 1998). The term 'task-oriented' covers a multitude of approaches united by their emphasis on teaching the skills that are absent or deficient. The intervention strategy focuses on the tasks that are causing the child difficulty with some emphasizing task-specific instruction (Revie and Larkin, 1993b), some knowledge-based (Wall et al., 1985), others involving more cognitive and motor control processes (Henderson and Sugden, 1992; Polatajko et al., 2001b; Wright and Sugden, 1996b) while some recent ones link these and, additionally, emphasize the importance of the context in which the child is moving (Sugden, in preparation; Sugden and Chambers, 2003a).

A management plan devised for intervening with children with DCD is the cognitive motor approach advocated in the Movement ABC manual (Henderson and Sugden, 1992). The approach involves an eclectic programme based on principles derived from the motor learning and motor development literature and is built upon the idea that the cognitive, affective, and motor competencies of the child interact in a dynamic manner. The emphasis is on children performing functional tasks in settings which are as near as possible to everyday life. The approach conceptualizes the acquisition of movement competence as a problem-solving exercise involving action planning, action execution, action evaluation. These are not discrete and separate entities but interact dynamically with one another according to the environmental circumstances and manner of presentation. This type of approach has been taken forward by Polatajko and colleagues with their Cognitive Orientation to Daily Occupational Performance (Polatajko et al., 2001a; 2001b) which is described in a later chapter.

There is also a recognition that learning takes place over a period of time and that distinctive features will emerge at various times in the learning process. For example, the early part of any skill learning is dominated by the individual trying to understand the demands of the task: what the objective is, how it is to be performed and what strategies to use. At this time, the individual must begin any task by learning the most relevant aspects. As a broad picture of the objective of the skill is built up, the serial or sequential organization becomes apparent and the component parts become clear. This phase of learning is experimental and children need to discover, or be taught, the 'rules' of the task. The role of the teacher/therapist is to help the child by pointing out the relevant and distinctive features of the task; by relating the task to previous experiences the child may have had such that it becomes meaningful; by encouraging the child to make his/her own connections to previous experiences. As the child starts to understand the task, the reduction of errors is of primary concern. There are two types of error to be eradicated or minimized: errors of planning, i.e. the individual makes an inappropriate plan for the intended movement, and errors of execution, i.e. the individual executes the movement in a different manner to what was intended. Initially, these errors are large and performance is characterized by inaccuracy and variability. As the individual progresses, both types of error are systematically reduced. Actions become more effective and movements become more consistent as better control is achieved. Variability of performance is an initial characteristic but over time this is reduced (Henderson and Sugden, 1992).

Using a task-oriented approach in Singapore, Wright and Sugden (1996b) based their intervention on a cognitive motor programme (Henderson and Sugden, 1992). In this study, the children's teacher, with assistance from a researcher, helped the children with their specific difficulties during the normal lesson time. Wright and Sugden (1996b; 1998) report significant differences between pre- and post-test assessments for all children, with anecdotal evidence from teachers available as confirmation. Other studies using the same task-oriented approach and finding similar results have been reported by Larkin and Parker (2002), Pless (2001), Polatajko et al. (2001a), Polatajko et al. (2001b), Revie and Larkin (1993b), Sugden (in preparation) and Sugden and Chambers (2003a). Chapter 12 in this book by Mandich and Polatajko illustrates how a comprehensive programme is built up and cascaded using this type of approach. In their meta-analysis of the various approaches, Pless and Carlsson (2000) do advocate a specific skills approach reporting an effect size of 1.45, which translates into a real improvement in children's performance and which was substantially more than a general approach or one involving sensory integrative methods.

Task-oriented approaches do have a face validity that is difficult to counter; if a child has a difficulty with a particular task, it is logical to try to teach that task. However, just as a potential advantage of process-oriented approaches is the promise for generalization, albeit rarely tested even in experimental conditions, the opposite is true in task-oriented approaches. Paradoxically, Pless and Carlsson (2000) give this as a reason to use task-specific methods, almost as though they believe transfer is not possible thus recommending teaching specific tasks. Attempting to teach for transfer using functional skills is a necessity, because simply stated, there is not enough time to directly teach all the skills that are required and, thus, attempting to teach for transfer is obligatory and, in many cases, this is simply ignored in most task approaches. The possibility is that it can be addressed by using the concept of variability of practice derived from Schmidt's Schema Theory of Motor Learning (1975). In this, transfer is achieved by presenting practices that are varied around a central class of movements. For example, if a child has difficulty with intrinsic manual movements such as manipulating objects by the fingers, a range of tasks surrounding this difficulty is presented rather than extended practice on just one or two activities. In this way, the child builds up a 'schema' of this class of events which he or she can draw upon when confronted by a novel movement situation. Guidelines for teaching for transfer are provided by Sugden (1988; in preparation).

Finally, and in a different vein and possibly pointing the way to new directions, Wilson, Thomas and Maruff (2002), have shown that children assessed as displaying motor clumsiness can improve their motor skills through motor imagery training. The children in the study were randomly assigned to one of three groups: imagery training, traditional perceptual-motor training and a control group. Results showed that the imagery protocol was equally as effective as the perceptual-motor training in facilitating the development of motor skills in the referred children; both groups showed significant pre–post-test gains while the control did not. Additionally, Wilson and colleagues note that continued gains in motor performance were observed six weeks after the intervention ceased. Correlational analyses revealed that the effects of the imagery intervention were most pronounced for children with greater motor impairment.

The intention has not been to describe a set of studies that is comprehensive in nature but select ones that provide examples of different approaches to intervention. This sample represents some different approaches and some supporting evidence demonstrating that many approaches do provide positive results. Differences between control and experimental groups have been consistently shown, as have pre- and post-treatments. What has not been shown are identifiable and consistent different effects of the different approaches. The question remains as to why different approaches produce similar results. From those advocating underlying perceptual or motor processes, an explanation would rest in these areas and, similarly, those supporting task-oriented methods would point to the face validity of this logic. That they all show an effect, although sometimes small, raises important issues and three factors are useful to consider.

First, it is known that children coming under the generic title of DCD are not a homogeneous group. The different studies identify them using different instruments and different criteria. A simple example is the difference between a referred group of children at a developmental centre and one identified from a non-referred group selected through a mainstream school. More standardization is required before effective comparisons can be made across studies. It may also be advisable to concentrate less on group data and focus on individual cases using multiple base line designs and linking to characteristics of individual children (Sugden and Chambers, 2003a; 2003b). Second, many of the studies have used 'experts' in the intervention process and this expertise may be effective, no matter what method is used. Studies which control for the effect of specialist expertise are required. Finally, are the specific intervention methods more or less important than general learning and intervention principles? There may be some common elements in intervention that run across a range of developmental disorders while others may be peculiar to DCD. In autism, for example, intervention is guided primarily by a pragmatic concern for what is useful in promoting development and adaptation. The primary locus for intervention is almost always educational and the central professionals involved in intervention are educators (Cohen and Volkmar, 1997). Researchers and practitioners have made significant progress in improving language skills in autism and from this a number of principles emerge which it is felt could be useful in the development of a theoretical basis for the management of children with DCD. These principles include an emphasis on natural contexts, accurate assessment of need, setting priorities and goals, and the involvement of parents. A logical extension of this would be to set some common agreed principles followed by an examination of specific methods.

Fundamental principles: ecology and motor development

Ecological context

For a number of years an ecological perspective has had a presence in developmental psychology that fits neatly into our proposals for intervention. From this perspective, the relationship between the development of the child and the environmental context is inseparable from any intervention process. Bronfenbrenner (1977) describes human development through a series of successive and reciprocal interactions and relationships with the environment and how these affect an individual's understanding of the world and their subsequent development. From this angle, any intervention is inextricably linked to part of the child's development and how this interacts with his/her total lifestyle, particularly in the context of the family. Bernheimer and Keogh (1995) stress that interventions should be embedded in the business of everyday life, which begins with a family-based approach to assessment and incorporates an ecocultural approach to intervention.

The basis for this approach lies with Brofenbrenner (1977) who proposed a number of structures that build up the environment in which the child develops and these structures are composed of different levels of interactions. The microsystem involves the relationship the individual has with their immediate or physical environment such as home and school, with the major players in established roles being parents, siblings and teachers. The mesosystem refers to the relationships between the most important settings for the child at a particular point in life and for a school aged child involves interactions among family, school and friends. The exosystem refers to other social structures of both an informal and formal nature which, while not specifically involving the child, do have an influence. Examples of these would be the school system, voluntary agencies, community groups, media and management in the Local Education Authority. Finally, the macrosystem takes the ideology that is present at the time and includes political, social, legal and educational systems. This would comfortably fit with the social model of disability (e.g. Oliver, 1996) that describes how society disables people with impairments and is at the root cause of the problems they encounter. This contrasts with the more medically based model which views disability as residing within the child. Fundamental to a social model of disability is the movement for social change, where disabling barriers are removed so disabled people are included in all activities and aspects of society. The multilayered dynamic model of Bronfenbrenner (1977) could fit a social model, is adaptable to many aspects of development and appears particularly appropriate for developmental disabilities such as DCD, where children's difficulties are identified within their everyday functioning at home or at school.

The Bronfenbrenner model has been portrayed as a series of concentric circles with the child at the centre moving outwards from the microsystem through the exosystem and mesosystem to the macrosystem (Bailey and Wolery, 1992). From this, principles for intervention can be derived drawing upon both the ecological context together with how the child develops and performs motor skills.

Dynamic motor development

In recent years, the focus of attention has moved away from models of maturation and an information-processing approach towards those that are more dynamic and ecological in nature. Explanations have been offered by those who are promoting dynamic systems as the theoretical underpinnings for how babies and infants perform, learn, and change in their motor behaviour (Thelen, 1995; Turvey and Fitzpatrick, 1993). A dynamic systems approach examines the interaction between the demands made by internal constraints, such as body mechanics and the external environmental requirements and, as noted by Clark and Phillips (1993), it is a theory that specifically offers a set of principles for studying the emergence and evolution of new forms and one that seeks to explain change.

Details of a dynamics systems approach is explored in detail in Chapter 4 by Wade, Johnson and Mally but, here suffice to say, that the fundamentals were originally derived mathematically to examine properties used in the understanding of systems with large numbers of interrelated elements such as ecosystems in the natural sciences, cities and regions, industries and businesses and biological systems. Researchers such as Turvey, Kugler, Kelso and Thelen (Kelso and Tuller, 1984; Kugler and Turvey, 1987; Thelen, 1995; Turvey, 1990) have offered a replacement for the cognitive/ information-processing model of motor control with one which does not search for a top-down, hierarchical model driven by some executive in the brain but uses the total resources of the individual set in the context in which the action takes place. Development is dynamic and patterns of movement emerge from particular constraints with preferred patterns of behaviour that are self-organized. The dynamic systems explanation of development emphasizes that the infant explores and finds solutions to new environmental demands. It is not simply a matter of maturation driving the infant; it is the task that motivates the infant, interacting with the child's resources and producing the driving force for change.

This approach has a number of fundamental principles; a first one being that the end result in any action is a result of multiple subsystems. Thus, it is not a central executor that drives development, it is not simply maturation that influences an activity such as walking but action is the result of multiple variables combining together, often in non-systematic ways. The approach emphasizes

> the multicausal, fluid, contextual, and self-organizing nature of developmental change, the unity of perception, action, and cognition, and the role of exploration and selection in the emergence of new behaviour. (Thelen, 1995, p. 79)

Behaviour emerges spontaneously from these subsystems with the system open to information flow leading to a perception–action interaction.

Another principle is that behavioural changes are not specified a priori but are self-organized. A problem that confronts motor control scientists is how the organism organizes the multiple joints, muscles and motor neurons into smooth, coordinated, purposeful movements without invoking an executor with the movement already stored. To do this would require such a massive and cumbersome system that it would be unwieldy and impossible to work. This has become known as the degrees of freedom problem (Bernstein, 1967); how are the variables that are free to vary in any movement controlled? Part of a solution that comes from a dynamical systems approach has been called coordinative structures which are defined as groups of joints, muscles and limbs that are softly assembled and constrained to act as a single unit. Movements are not programmed in detail a priori but planned at an abstract level and honed and refined by the demands of the task.

A major principle of a dynamical systems approach is that multiple subsystems can be constraints and these constraints can be intrinsic or extrinsic in nature. Any action, therefore, is the result of the interaction between the resources of the child, the context in which the action takes place and the manner in which the activity is presented. All of these three contain constraints. Thus, child resource constraints might be anthropo-metric variables as Thelen (1995) has shown in babies walking – variables such as fat content, strength in the leg or neural integrity; motivation and arousal are also constraints which serve to affect movement, as are the environmental supports when the child is learning a task. The task itself is a constraint, as is the context in which the task is performed. The developmental process, thus, becomes a confluence of interacting variables that are present in the developing child's daily life.

A further characteristic of a dynamic systems approach is that the changes seen are non-linear; the progression is not a steady increase but abrupt non-linear leaps are seen after a plateau period. Preferred patterns of behaviour, or attractors, are involved in the change process by being constantly replaced through a destabilization of the system, forcing the system to look for alternatives. For example, the increase in strength and control of the head during gaze will influence locomotor changes in the first year of life. The emergence of new behaviour takes place and becomes stable but one part of the system starts to change again, having a step change effect on the rest of the system.

Supporting principles: motor control and learning

The discipline of motor control and learning has been an important area of study for a century and within the last 40 or 50 years has provided us with both a theoretical base and practical implications in fields as diverse as teaching individuals to use military equipment, stroke rehabilitation, operating machinery at work and in the area of sports activities. From this work there are a number of principles which have become established, each one containing a huge literature base (see Schmidt and Lee, 1999, for a review).

Activities

If we start at the micro level, that is the level of the child practising particular activities, we should first examine what kind of activities to give to the child. This is fundamental and at the heart of the micro level. From research and clinical observations, it is clear that movements with no purpose and not set in context will not be as successful as those that are (Schmidt and Lee, 1999). Thus, goal-oriented, purposeful organized actions should be the ones that are used. We have always argued for providing functional skills for children to learn and earlier in the chapter we make a stronger case for these, rather than those which purport to address underlying processing difficulties.

As noted earlier in the chapter, criticism has always been made that teaching specific functional skills does not properly address the problem of transfer but transfer has to be an aim when teaching life skills. A potential solution to this is to group like-tasks into a class of skills and teach to this group, an idea that has been an offshoot of schema learning theory (Schmidt, 1975). Thus, if the aim is to improve manual skills a set of tasks are grouped and these are learned together, stimulating transfer to any skill that is within the group and to others that are closely similar. The trick here is how to group the skills. For example, one could use the distinction between intrinsic and extrinsic manual skills (Connolly, 1998) with the former involving those actions that take place in the hand – i.e. an object is manipulated and moved with the hand such as turning a coin or fastening a button using both hands, and the latter involving activities which require reaching and grasping an object outside of the hand involving visuospatial placement of the hand and arm. Occasionally, an action will require both of these processes, such as reaching for a coin, picking it up and placing it elsewhere. It is believed that teaching a variety of related tasks within a class of skills provides the best compromise between teaching isolated skills which have been shown to be difficult to transfer and teaching the more underlying processes which may offer the lure of transfer but are difficult to identify. There is the additional problem of teaching them in context, making the process method difficult to support if one is looking for the most parsimonious, yet effective, methodology.

Practice conditions

There are strong steers in the area of practice conditions from motor learning specialists who outline many of the variables that make for effective practice (for a review see Schmidt and Lee, 1999). Children with DCD have not developed or learned the appropriate motor skills that face them in their day-to-day lives and the motor learning literature concentrates on how individuals learn skills, providing a theoretical background to practical implications. Thus, the proposal is that teaching children with DCD is about teaching them to learn motor skills; it is not about rectifying some unknown speculative brain disorder or perceptual disturbance but it concerns directly addressing the problems that are shown.

A fundamental principle, and the one Schmidt and Lee (1999) stress, is one that in their words 'dwarfs' all others; *namely, that all other things being equal, the more practice a person engages in, the more learning will occur*. Thus, in structuring the practice sessions, a child should be engaged as much as possible and the number of deliberate practice attempts maximized. The independent variables that are operating during the practice sessions and that will affect learning include pre-practice preparations such as helping the learner recognize what it is that needs to be done, often through a problem-solving methodology. The structure of the practice sessions themselves is of importance with the balance between massing and distributing practice having an effect, with distributing practice being more beneficial to short-term one-off performance but no discernible difference in more long-term learning. Variability of practice, where each practice is slightly different, seems to be more effective than a constant task, and randomly ordered practice is detrimental to performance but again is better for learning and retention. Mental practice is useful when it is not possible to practise physically though it is not as effective as the physical act. We have noted the recent opportunities for this in the DCD area (Wilson, Thomas and Maruff, 2002). A very common practice is to task analyse a skill and break it down into its component parts. This has proved to be successful but only where the task naturally lends itself to this process and care needs to be taken not to change the nature of the task (Magill, 2001; Rosenbaum, 1991; Schmidt and Lee, 1999).

Feedback

Feedback is at the heart of the motor learning literature and it is unclear why this topic has been rarely studied in detail in the learning approaches of children with DCD. Augmented feedback is that which is provided by a source other than the task itself; that is a parent, teacher or other professional. It can be divided into two categories – knowledge of performance (KP) which is information about the form of the movement, and knowledge of results (KR) which is information about the performance outcome. Both can be given verbally or through technology such as film or motion analysis, and research shows us that precision of both KP and KR is of great importance to the learner. Put more simply, the learner needs to know exactly what is wrong or right in order to change, modify or consolidate a particular skill and the provision of accurate, understandable KP and KR should be in every professional's repertoire. Augmented feedback through KP and KR not only provides information to the learner in the form associating intent with the resulting action but also as a motivator providing targets and goals to the learner. Of course, the real trick for the skilled clinician/educator is to pick out which piece of information is most useful at a particular time for a specific child, taking into consideration the nature of the task and the resources of the child.

Phases of learning

Learning is a process that is continuous and involves varying degrees of rate of improvement and different variables at different stages in this process. The early stages have been labelled the cognitive phase whereby the learner has to recognize what is needed in the skill; this is followed by the associative phase in which the perfecting of the action, through practice, is the primary goal, finally leading to the autonomous phase when the person can perform the task with apparently little attention to it or can perform two tasks at once (Fitts, 1964). Although it is difficult to empirically separate these phases into discrete partitions, they are something that can be recognized in the clinical setting and any professional working in the DCD area should be cognizant of these possibilities. As the child moves through these phases, the abilities required for further success appear to change, making prediction very difficult. Most of the changes involve less cognitive and more motor involvement as the skill progresses, again requiring recognition by the professional working with the child.

Teaching methodology

The literature evidence is also strong in the area of teaching methodology. When a child cannot perform a particular task, the two related actions of task analysis and task adaptation can be used to help. Put simply, task adaptation involves changing the nature of the demands of the task such as changing the equipment – different pencils with easier grips, larger balls, differently shaped to catch and different types of implements with which to strike a ball. The rules of any game can be changed and, together with the above, help the child participate in the skill learning. Task analysis involves breaking down the task into smaller component parts such that they can be more easily learned. There is often a fine line between task adaptation and task analysis but together they allow the child first to participate in skill learning and then they aid the learning process. Both appear to be crucial actions and are very much dependent on the skill of the professional. Task analysis from an ecological point of view is strongly recommended as it involves examining the totality of the learning context (Davis and Burton, 1991).

The term 'expert scaffolding' is used to describe the part of the teaching methodology which involves the teacher or parent providing big, initial support for the child and then gradually withdrawing it as the child becomes more competent (Brown and Campione, 1986). This can involve physical guidance, physical support, simplifying the task then building it back up, putting it into a game situation and relating it to previous experience. Thus, scaffolding can be the adding of something which is more complex or the withdrawing of support; both actions seek to give support in the first instance and then gradually make the task more difficult as the child becomes more competent.

Very often a child with coordination difficulties has problems in the area of planning, such as the inability to follow a series of instructions or difficulties in matching or imitating actions. Many children showing these attributes have been called 'dyspraxic'. In these cases, a child's problems seem to be more in knowing what to do rather that in the doing itself and providing activities that demand decision making or problem solving would appear to be a good way forward. Simple games like 'Footprints', where the child has to use different coloured stepping stones to walk on and make a colour sequence as they walk, are activities that are often given.

Only a small proportion of the literature on motor control and learning is included here, but attention is drawn to the great contribution it can have in teaching children skills that they are lacking. The principle is that if it is known how children learn and control movements, this information will be useful in the teaching of these skills. Thus, intervention approaches do need to be informed by the vast amount of available literature in this area, and it becomes part of the multifaceted approach that is proposed.

Context, routines, ecoculture and the developmental coach

It is an obvious statement that the more meaningful and enjoyable the activity, the more the child is likely to engage and pay full attention and for this to occur, activities ought to be set in an appropriate context. Bernheimer and Keogh (1995) note that many interventions designed by professionals fail to be implemented by parents and this gap between good advice and practice should give food for thought. They argue that we should move the concentration from the child to the family and build upon family strengths so that interventions are designed to best meet the needs of the child in the context of the everyday business of family life. This is very much in line with both an ecological approach described earlier using the Bronfenbrenner model and the dynamic systems approach which looks at the totality of a child's development incorporating interacting variables or constraints from all parts of daily life and not simply the intrinsic ones within the child's resources. Figure 10.1 shows how the variables or constraints of the child's resources, the nature of the task and the environmental context interact and transact to influence the outcome.

This figure is similar to one used by Newell (1986) who, employing a dynamic systems framework, talked of 'constraints' which can be used to either hinder or encourage a particular action. These constraints arise

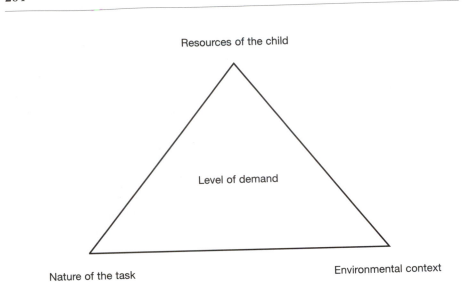

Resources of the child

Level of demand

Nature of the task

Environmental context

Figure 10.1 Interacting variables in motor skill performance.
Source: Keogh and Sugden (1985).

from the child, the environment or the task in a similar manner to the model above, and both models are in agreement that action is a result of these multiple interacting variables.

Within the environmental context, whether it is named ecological, eco-cultural or dynamic, there is an emphasis on the family unit constructing and giving meaning to their lives and, thus, any part of it such as a child with DCD will have a dynamic effect on their routines. How this takes place and with as minimum change as possible should be an aim for professionals who are working with the family. According to Bernheimer and Keogh (1995), families construct their daily lives and they reflect functional activities which are a mixture of personal and cultural values, together with constraints, pressures and resources and an understanding of these routines is important for professionals when working with parents to devise an intervention programme. From these, a better understanding of the child's functioning in the context of daily life is available and there is less chance of interventions failing because they do not fit into everyday routines or are incompatible with the goals, values and beliefs of the parents.

The proposal is that it is not enough to emphasize the traditional variables of cognitive, motor and other developmental variables when devising an intervention routine. Families do not develop their routines to scores on a test; they respond to the effect the child has on their daily lives with it being set in the ecoculture of family. For this reason, the idea of a 'developmental coach' is raised; this is a person who looks at the child's life and helps decide upon the bigger decisions as well as the micro ones that deal with DCD. Obviously, the recommendation is that the parent is the developmental coach, with support from professionals with help and training schemes for the child; this involves the parent at all levels and so decisions on management are made with reference to family routines. This type of approach has great implications for the professional working with the child. It is now not enough to provide an intervention programme that is well thought out and backed by research that does not involve the family, the routines of that family, how the child fits into these routines and how any intervention is delivered, taking these variables in mind.

The role of parents and teachers

From the above it is not simply a case of what is the most appropriate method to use with children with DCD but, often, how any method is put into practice and how it fits in with the rest of the child's and the parents' daily routines. Some approaches have been shown to be relatively successful, even if the most stringent evaluations have rarely been employed. But the questions surrounding which approach to use go beyond whether that particular approach is successful or not. For example, if it is suspected that through occupational therapy, there is a strong chance of successful intervention, how is the occupational therapy delivered? In many major health trusts in the UK there is a waiting list for occupational therapy and OT visits are infrequent. If a decision is taken to intervene through the educational system, how is the specialist knowledge obtained by those engaged in the intervention process?

One of the strong guidelines for intervention is one that is common in all motor learning literature, that successful learning of a skill is very much dependent on the amount of practice undertaken by the individual. Thus, a major aim is to try to ensure that children can receive appropriate intervention three to four times a week for up to half an hour each in duration. When one looks at who could provide such a schedule, parents and teachers are obvious choices. Parents and teachers generally have few specific skills with children with DCD but they are either professionals used to working with children or individuals with a huge vested interest in the outcome and know their children well; both qualities which go a long way to successful intervention. It is hypothesized that with support these individuals could provide another intervention route for the children. In Leeds, our recent work has been supported by two grants from Action Medical Research and from the NHS. The two grants from Action Medical Research cover a project which neatly splits into two interrelated, yet distinctive phases. The first deals with the role in intervention by parents and teachers and asked three major questions. First, whether parents and teachers, with help can be successful in providing intervention for children with DCD. Second, whether children with DCD can be helped in this way. Finally, whether there are children who do not benefit from such intervention and require a more specialized approach. The results so far provide a qualified yes to each of these questions and from these results a model is tentatively proposed that could be used in some education and/or health authorities.

The project was intended to be a careful blend of controlled and structured research methodology together with an ecological validity that is often lacking in tightly controlled experimental research projects. With an approach like this there are a number of inherent dangers, particularly the one of striking a balance between controlling those internal variables that can have a biasing effect on the results and being so tight and restrictive such that the dynamics that normally interplay in real life are missing. The first of the studies was designed in such a way as to try to achieve this balance and initially involved group analysis but with an emphasis on single subject design and individual profiles, linking the actual amount of intervention to any improvement that was seen, together with an analysis of why and how the intervention took place (Sugden and Chambers, 2003a).

For the sample of children an age group of 7–9 years of age was selected, representing a time when the children were established in school, with difficulties that had been identified and a time that we believe is an appropriate one for intervention. First, the teachers were asked to identify those children they believed had difficulties in the movement domain. This was followed up by testing the children on the Movement ABC using the guidelines suggested by Wright and Sugden (1996b) in their two-step approach to identification and assessment. This procedure resulted in 31 children identified, with 23 in the bottom 5 per cent and the remaining eight within the range of the 5th to the 15th percentile. Originally, it was only planned to work with children in the bottom 5 per cent but once the other eight had been identified, a group normally labelled 'at risk' or 'borderline', there was an ethical obligation to intervene. Following testing on the Movement ABC and parent and teacher interviews, the children were left alone for eight weeks before being tested again. This was done to examine the stability of their scores and to ensure that there was little effect on the scores through maturation. Following this second assessment, the children were randomly split into two groups; one a teacher group and the other a parent group. Each child had a profile of their motor behaviour, identifying both strengths and weaknesses and from this profile, priorities were set and a programme of work developed. This programme of work was given to the teachers and parents and each week a set of activities, including ways in which to presents activities and methods of teaching were taken to them. These were carefully constructed and involved feedback from previous weeks and the success or otherwise of the child. The guidelines were based on 'A Cognitive Motor Approach' (Henderson and Sugden, 1992) updated to engage recent thinking on dynamics and the effect of context (Sugden et al., 2003). Both the teachers and parents were asked to work with the children for a minimum of three to four times a week for a period of time not less than 15–20 minutes in each session. Of great importance were teachers and parents noting the number of sessions they had with the children and making observations.

Following the division of the children into the two groups, parents and teachers worked with them for eight weeks after which they were assessed again. The teacher group then switched to the parents and the parent group to the teachers where again eight weeks of intervention took place followed by a fourth assessment. Finally, there was a period of eight weeks followed by a fifth assessment; this period being to determine whether any effects of the intervention could be sustained following a period of no intervention.

The results of this first study were encouraging. If a score of 13 is taken as an indicator of motor impairment, at Test 1 there were 23 in this category and by Test 5 there were only four. In addition, all those scoring between 10 and 13 (n = 8) on Test 1, scored a maximum of 7.5 by Test 5. Recognizing that growth and development may have occurred and influenced some scores, progression between Tests 1 and 2 and Tests 4 and 5, when there was no intervention, was examined using the same cut-off criteria. By Test 2 the 23 who scored above 13 increased to 26 with one child moving out of this category and four moving in. By Test 4, when the two intervention sessions had been completed, six children remained in the plus 13 group and by Test 5 this had reduced to four. Using a broad brush categorical analysis, it suggests that no improvement took place between Tests 1 and 2 but improvement did take place between Tests 2 and 4 during the intervention phase, and that this improvement was maintained to Test 5 during a period of no intervention. Statistical analysis confirmed that no improvement took place between Tests 1 and 2 when there was no intervention and improvement did take place between Test 2 and Test 4, during the intervention phases, and that this improvement was carried over from Test 4 to Test 5, when there was no intervention.

Individual profiles placed the children in categories according to the amount of intervention they received and the amount of improvement they have displayed. Category 1 consists of 22 children who received a moderate amount of intervention or more and who showed improvement; Category 2 consists of two children who, despite receiving moderate or more intervention, showed little or no improvement; Category 3 consists of six children who received only a small amount of intervention and yet showed improvement; Category 4 consists of 1 child who received little intervention and did not display improvement. Each child in the project has a detailed individual profile detailing all aspects of the programme and assessments.

Figure 10.2 shows a child who, following the period of rest, improved immediately in the first intervention session followed by a small gain during the second session. After that, however, there is decline in the scores, until the last testing points. It may be concluded that this child improves during intervention but requires some form of practice in order to maintain the gains. Figure 10.3 shows a child over a period of time and who clearly demonstrates very little improvement. This is one of the very few children who showed this profile and may indicate that more specialist help is required. Figure 10.4 is an example of a child who improved greatly during the second period, from a score of 16 to below 6, and this gain was maintained throughout the whole monitoring period.

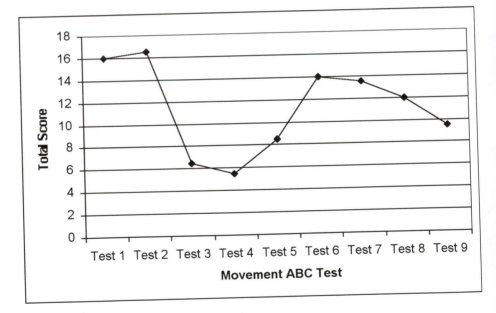

Figure 10.2 Movement ABC Test scores for Child 8.

Concluding comments

In proposing a model or an approach to intervention, it has been emphasized that there are multiple components to successful intervention. It is clear to us that parents and teachers need to be part of any scheme. They are the ones who see the child on a daily basis and can form some

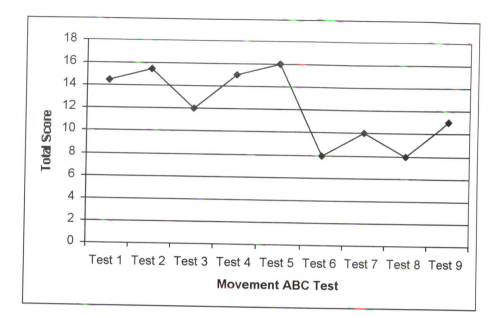

Figure 10.3 Movement ABC Test scores for Child 26.

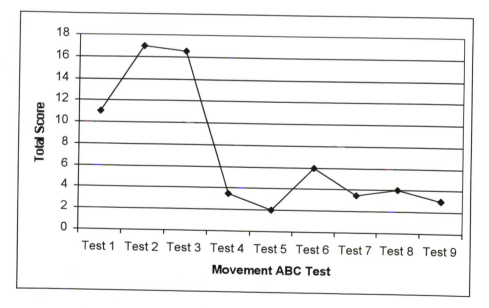

Figure 10.4 Movement ABC Test scores for Child 4.

assessment about how the intervention is incorporated into the daily life of the family. It is stressed that there is a need for professionals to provide specialist help. This specialist help, often involving health professionals, will range from detailed assessment of the child through to intervention methods. Just as important as this is the advice and guidance the professionals can give to parents to make their own decisions in the context of family life. With help, the parent can become the developmental coach and all that implies about decision making. There is a bias towards a specific task approach because of its face validity, its relative ease to cascade the teaching method and its research support. It is believed that any intervention is firmly set in the developmental progress of the child and informed by the work in not just motor development but also motor control and learning. If these guidelines are to be translated into some form of action, a possible scenario is as follows.

Stage 1

Someone is showing concern that the child has difficulties in the coordination of movement and this is having an effect on their daily living, their work at school or is seen in combination with other difficulties, such that together they present a problem. This concern can be from the teacher, parent, significant other or the child themselves. This concern is reported via the school through the SEN procedures or through health through GPs and paediatricians.

Stage 2

The child is professionally assessed, all strengths and weaknesses noted and a profile developed. A variety of methods can be used for the assessment with our main instrument being the Movement ABC (Henderson and Sugden, 1992). From this profile, general priorities are set. The professional should have expertise in working with children with DCD and should be familiar with the assessment tool that is being employed. Parents and children should be engaged in discussions about outcomes and possible ways forward.

Stage 3

The profile and priorities for the programme form the basis of an intervention programme, which is designed and developed professionally in consultation with parents and involving the child as much as possible and based on weekly or fortnightly timescales. This programme has to be sound with respect to what the parents can do with respect to their daily family lives. The programme should include a statement about the areas to be addressed, the activities to work on and the manner in which they can be taught. The programme needs to be revisited at regular intervals to ensure that it can be comfortably run by parents. In addition, if school-based programmes are being followed, they should be in conjunction with the parents who with help are in overall control – they are the 'developmental coach'.

Stage 4

The programme is enacted by parents and/or teachers and should involve at least 3–4 sessions per week of 20–30 minutes' duration. Ideally, parents and teachers should keep a record of sessions and should be in regular contact with the professional devising the programme.

Stage 5

Both the professionals and the teachers/parents monitor the programme using standardized instruments, checklists, notes and observations. This should not simply be the progression of the child but will include the relevance of certain activities, the ease of teaching, problems encountered and the fit with daily life. Certain time frames can be set as targets for evaluating the success or otherwise of the programme.

These are the basic essentials of our programme with large amounts of details surrounding the programmes, assessment and monitoring. This type of model has a number of advantages: first, it utilizes the skills and motivations of the teachers and parents, and takes advantage of the daily contact with children; second, it uses the skills of occupational therapists and physiotherapists and others specializing in DCD work in a more economical manner; and third, it directs the limited resources of the educational and health systems; finally, it empowers parents to be skilled in working with their child in an environment that is determined by them and their children, thus promoting an intervention approach that utilizes the best research evidence set in a family lifestyle context.

Chapter 11

Neuromotor task training: a new approach to treat children with DCD

Marina M. Schoemaker and Bouwien C.M. Smits-Engelsman

Introduction

Over the past forty years, various treatment programmes have been developed for children with Developmental Coordination Disorder (DCD). These treatment programmes can roughly be divided into two categories: the so-called process-oriented approaches and the task-oriented approaches (Sugden and Wright, 1998). The process-oriented approaches concentrate on the treatment of deficits in processes assumed to underlie poor motor coordination. Task-oriented approaches, on the other hand, focus directly at the functional skills with which a child experiences problems.

Examples of process-oriented approaches are kinaesthetic training developed by Laszlo et al. (1988) and Sensory Integration Therapy developed by Ayres (1972b). Laszlo et al. (1988) attributed a prominent role to kinaesthesis in the control of movement, and assumed that the motor coordination problems of children with DCD were the result of a deficit in kinaesthetic awareness. Sensory Integration Therapy (SIT) is based upon the assumption that children with learning disabilities in general, and those with motor problems in particular, are deficient in integrating perceptual information from various modalities. Treatment is directed at stimulating the tactile, vestibular, visual and other sensory systems so that children learn to integrate sensory information into adequate (motor) responses. Among physical and occupational therapists, SIT is one of the most popular approaches (Mandich et al., 2001a).

However, despite its popularity, there is not much evidence that SIT or other process-oriented approaches are effective. Pless and Carlsson (2000) conducted a meta-analysis regarding the effectiveness of treatment approaches for DCD. A rather small mean effect size of .21 for process-oriented approaches was found. In line with these results, Mandich et al. (2001a) found no support for the effectiveness of process-oriented approaches in a review of effect studies.

During the last decade, various researchers started to advocate a task-oriented approach to treatment. In Australia, Revie and Larkin (1993b) developed a task-specific intervention programme to increase motor competence by teaching functional motor skills. More recently, Polatajko and co-workers (2001a; 2001b) developed the 'Cognitive Orientation to daily Occupational Performance' (CO-OP) in Canada. In this programme the focus is on motor skill learning, but skill learning is enhanced by teaching problem-solving strategies. Children learn to ask questions about their own performance and to find solutions for these questions. By applying these strategies to other motor problems, the authors aim to enhance transfer of motor learning outside the therapy programme. Although the task-oriented approaches to treatment are relatively new, the first results regarding their effectiveness are promising. Pless and Carlsson (2000) found an effect size of 1.46 for these approaches in their meta-analysis.

Simultaneously with the development of CO-OP in Canada, a task-oriented training programme called 'Neuromotor Task Training' (NTT) was developed in the Netherlands for treatment of children with DCD by paediatric physical therapists (Smits-Engelsman and Tuijl, 1998; Smits-Engelsman, Reynders and Schoemaker, 2001). In this chapter, the characteristics of NTT will be described, and guidelines for clinical practice will be given.

Neuromotor task training: no general recipe but a tailor-made programme

Children with DCD referred for intervention are a heterogeneous group. Geuze et al. (2001) conducted an extensive analysis of publications regarding children with DCD to obtain a profile of the population characteristics and an outline of the criteria used for diagnosing the condition. The referral criteria of DCD in clinical practice vary from a simple note by the school doctor or general practitioner to an exhaustive report of poor scores on tests of neurological, perceptual-motor, social and cognitive development. Since the introduction of a standard diagnostic category for children with DCD in the DSM-IV (American Psychiatric Association, 1994), clinical diagnostic criteria are increasingly derived from the DSM-IV criteria (Geuze et al., 2001). However, this does not imply that children who meet the criteria form a homogeneous group. Not only do these children differ greatly in their perceptual-motor profile, the clinical picture becomes even more complicated because of frequent co-morbidity for other developmental disorders (Dewey and Wilson, 2001; Geuze et al., 2001; Henderson and Barnett, 1998). It can probably be stated that the child with pure DCD is more the exception than the rule.

Both clinicians and researchers seem to agree on the heterogeneity of the group of children diagnosed as DCD with respect to the profile of perceptual-motor problems as well as co-morbidity. This has prompted a search for subtypes to gain a better understanding of possible underlying mechanisms of dysfunction and to provide clues for effective therapeutic intervention (e.g. Macnab, Miller and Polatajko, 2001; Schoemaker, Smits-Engelsman and Kalverboer, 1998; Smits-Engelsman, van Galen and Schoemaker, 1997). Moreover, it is essential to note that according to present knowledge the observed motor problems in DCD do not have a common and well-defined aetiology. Although there is evidence that complex visual spatial tasks involving a motor component are most often affected (Wilson and McKenzie, 1998) it can by no means be suggested that visual spatial processing in DCD plays a *causal* role in poor motor performance.

Few treatment methods so far have pursued a systematic intervention from a consistent theoretical motor control viewpoint. However, NTT is based on motor control and motor learning principles but also takes motor teaching and motivation principles into account. Treatment of children with DCD must be based on an understanding of the functional nature of the impairment. Interventions may then be tailored to the unique combination of symptoms and problems exhibited by the child. Although an individualized approach is needed in each treatment, some general guidelines for intervention will be described.

The NTT becomes tailored to the individual needs and constraints of the child because it is based on a neuromotor assessment and a task analysis of the skills the child experiences problems with. Research findings on motor control, lead to the choice of this specific *skill-based approach*. In the treatment, priority is given to those skills a child or his or her parents particularly want to master, as they bear ecological value for the child, and as it will increase the motivation of the child to practise. This is mandatory since skilled motor performance is not something a child only learns by thinking or talking about it but mainly by a lot of practising.

Motor control, motor learning and motor teaching theory

Application of neuromotor control theories

Recently, neuromotor control models, with each adding its own emphasis, are clinically applied in the development of treatment approaches (Mulder,

1991; van Galen, 1991; Smits-Engelsman, van Galen, Schoemaker, 1997; Smits-Engelsman and Teulings, 1992; Cools and Smits-Engelsman, 1998; Smits-Engelman, Steenbergen and van Galen, 2001). Cognitive neuroscience, which provides a framework for many developers in the field of motor control therapies, distinguishes the following steps for the processing of motor task related information: encoding the information from internal and external sources, stimulus recognition, response selection, action planning, motor programme preparation, movement parameterization and muscle initiation. Several processes have to be run through bottom-up and top-down loops after a decision to move has been made, including the retrieval of an action pattern from long-term motor memory, parameter setting (i.e. the step by which the overall force level and tempo of the task performance are regulated) and muscular initiation (the process of neurological recruitment and initiation of the motor units which are appropriate for a task in a given biomechanical context) (van Galen, 1991). The latter process is thought to be responsible for the striking constancy of motor acts in a changing biophysical environment. Each of the subprocesses, differentiated within the motor control models, contributes to the manner in which the act may be steered. The sequence and degree in which certain subsystems contribute to a specific action depends on the type of action and the consequences thereof, on the situation and on the stage the learning process is in.

Compare, for example, the manner in which a service during a final at Wimbledon is controlled with the manner in which it is controlled during the first tennis lesson. In the first instance, it may be assumed that the movement has been learned to perfection, making full use of the biomechanical characteristics of the body and the characteristics of the racket, that are attuned to each other to the maximum extent and whereby the processing capacity is mainly used for perceiving the environment and the opponent. With respect to the beginner, however, the action consists of various sub-patterns that have to be tuned to each other from the point of view of time–space coordination and that still lack the necessary adjustments in posture and relocation of weight. The attention will be fully aimed at 'how do I have to move?' (motor programme) rather than on 'in what direction shall I hit the ball and what effect shall I give to it?'

How is the knowledge derived from neuromotor control theories translated into therapeutic actions within the NTT approach? After the intake the physical therapists continue with the assessment of the strengths and weaknesses of a child's functional motor performance. Therapists will also analyse which process might be involved within deficient motor skill performance. For instance, a child may fail to learn a specific motor skill due to attentional problems, fear of failure, lack of motivation, or lack of understanding of how to execute a particular skill. In addition, other motor control processes might hamper successful performance such as timing of components of a motor skill, motor planning or parameter setting (the execution of a motor act with the required speed and force). In NTT, the functional exercises are designed in such a way that the therapist can analyse which motor control processes are deficient within the specific task to be trained (see Table 11.1). For instance, if giving a secure and supportive surrounding improves ball catching, task training will aim at more psychological processes. If however a child can catch the ball only when standing still and warned beforehand, ball catching in complex and attention demanding situations will be trained. If the child hasn't developed a throwing pattern yet, the opportunity of merely throwing a variety of objects (size, weight, material) will be given. Later, a demand on parameter setting will gradually be introduced by propelling the object over various distances or by aiming the objects at targets of different sizes. Through this approach, functional skills are trained in such a way that they tap the specific motor control processes that are thought to be involved in the motor skill problems of a child.

Table 11.1 Learning in relationship with motor control processes

Motor control process	Motor learning
Perception	Gaining experience in various circumstances with increased information-processing load
Action planning	Learning to make choices under changing stimulus/response conditions (if/then)
Movement planning	Execution of the skill with increased complexity and longer sequences
Motor programming	Learning certain coordination patterns and sequences, and loading the level of movement deflection
Parameterization	Training variations in adjusting the necessary extent, speed and direction of the movement, learning how to make use of the biomechanical characteristics
Initiating force	Training fine-tuning by making choices (type/number) of motor units in different exogenous contexts

Source: Smits-Engelsman, van Galen and Meulenbroek (1996).

Application of motor learning and teaching principles

Another important characteristic of NTT is that learning principles derived from motor control research are applied. Treatment approaches generally describe in detail the theories on which an approach is based, while information about the best way to teach a particular treatment approach is discarded. Moreover, a common view within some treatment approaches is that merely providing the opportunity for children with DCD to practise all kinds of motor skills during treatment without formal tutoring will lead to improved performance (Schoemaker, 1992). However, research findings demonstrate that children with DCD have difficulty learning and generalizing motor skills because they are less able to select the right motor response and they appear to continue the same task again and again, whether it was successful or not (Missiuna et al., 2001). Through trial and error, they attempt to master a skill but without the desired result. This may be caused either by their lack of ability to reflect on their own actions (explicit learning) or by the fact that they do not spontaneously engage in information processing while practising (implicit learning). Consequently, it seems unlikely that children with DCD will actually learn motor skills by just providing the opportunity to practise. Therefore, formal tutoring is used in the NTT approach to reach the ultimate goal of treatment, which is not only to improve functional task performance during treatment but also the transfer of learned skills to daily life performance.

Motor learning principles

It is well known from research that explicit motor learning in general and transfer in particular can be enhanced by applying the most effective motor learning principles. In literature, research concerning motor learning has concentrated on three distinct subjects: (1) how to instruct people; (2) how to practise skills; (3) how to provide feedback. In NTT, the results from studies on motor learning about the most effective method to instruct, practise and provide feedback are applied in the treatment sessions.

However, the most effective method of practising or providing instructions and feedback depends on the learning stage a child has reached. When children try to acquire new motor skills, they go through several distinct stages. Several models have been proposed to describe these stages, but the three-stage model by Fitts and Posner (1967) is still one of the most influential (Magill, 2001). In the first stage of these models, the beginning level, children are more engaged in cognitive activities to detect what movement coordination pattern will be required to achieve the goal of the skill. For instance, they need to solve problems such as 'what is the goal of this task?'; 'which limbs do I need to achieve this goal?'; and 'in what position do I need to hold my limbs?' During the second stage, the intermediate level of motor learning, children are able to master the basic coordination pattern of the skill but still need to refine their performance. They still make errors in this stage but their errors are fewer and less variable. Only after much practice, children will reach the third stage of skill learning, the advanced level. In this stage, children are able to perform a skill almost automatically, without conscious attention. Therapists trained in NTT guide children with DCD through these stages by applying the most effective learning principles (see Table 11.2). In order to do this they need to assess which motor stage a child has reached for each skill.

Studying the literature on motor learning processes, one notices three consistent findings which are important in relation to practising motor skills within the NTT approach for children with a coordination disorder: The low level of transfer from one acquired motor skill to the next; the large contextuality of the acquired motor functions and the 'time on task principle'. Differences as regards these principles between treatment approaches and their application within NTT will be discussed below.

Table 11.2 Phases in motor learning and teaching principles

Motor learning phase	Therapeutic action
Beginning level of motor learning	Introduce major aspects only Provide demonstration or model Permit try out Provide time for exploration and (guided) self-discovery Compare new movement with a familiar one or situation Provide immediate, precise and positive knowledge of performance (results not yet important) Stop when patient gets the general idea
Intermediate level of motor learning	Provide ample opportunity to practise Provide supportive non-threatening environment Give short practice sessions with frequent breaks Provide constructive feedback Let patient correct himself (find out what went wrong) Stimulate intensity Increase demands (speed and accuracy)
Advanced level of motor learning	Promote enthusiasm Provide encouragement and motivation Provide feedback on specific aspects Use many relevant contexts of increased difficulty (transfer) Increase complexity (sequentially and temporally) Provide suggestions for other strategies

Source: Smits-Engelsman and Halfens (2000).

Transfer of motor skills

In bottom-up approaches to treatment, such as Sensory Integration Therapy, treatment is directed at the remediation of just the underlying processing deficits. Once these processing deficits have been 'cured', the child will be able to perform all kinds of motor skills. However, it is well known that transfer effects across tasks, even when they seem to be very similar, are rather small. This fact is explained by the 'specificity of motor abilities hypothesis' (Henry, 1961). According to this hypothesis, the performance of each skill requires many specific motor abilities, which are relatively independent. Research findings support this hypothesis, as correlations among tests of different motor skills are often low. As a result, it is not expected that improvement in skills, which are trained during treatment, will transfer to untrained skills. Transfer will only occur between skills that are made up of the same underlying abilities. The specificity hypothesis might explain why the claim of bottom-up approaches that once processing deficits have been cured, daily life motor performance will improve, is not justified by the research of effectiveness studies (Pless and Carlsson, 2000).

Consequently, a task-oriented approach is advocated in NTT. In this approach, those skills are taught in a methodologically appropriate manner, which the child needs, without first teaching or practising a wide range of assumed conditions that do not form part of that specific skill. For instance, it is not the selective improvement of mobility or muscle strength that is regarded as proper therapeutic goals for improving motor functions; it is creating therapy-oriented interactions between the client (as adaptive system) and his environment (context) at a skill level that will result in acquiring new or improved motor functions. NTT as a task-specific approach focuses directly on teaching the skills a child needs in daily life. The higher the resemblance between skills and the circumstances practised during treatment and skills needed in daily life, the more transfer can be expected.

Task-oriented training is in concordance with a recent theory about neural development, the Neuronal Group Selection Theory (NGST; Sporns and Edelman, 1993). According to this theory, during development, neuronal groups or networks are formed consisting of large amounts of strongly interconnected neurones. The structure and function of these networks are selected by development, behaviour and contextual factors. Children are born with primary neuronal repertoires. These repertoires, determined by evolution, consist of multiple neuronal groups. During development, selection occurs as a consequence of behaviour and experience, with behaviour becoming less variable. However, variability soon returns due to the enormous amount of information to which a child is exposed. As a result, the connectivity within neuronal groups changes (secondary repertoire), which allows for situation specific motor behaviour (secondary or adaptive variability). According to Hadders-Algra (2000), children with DCD might show deficits in secondary variability which means that they are not able to adapt their motor behaviour to the specific demands of the situation. In her opinion, intervention should provide active practice in the skills that are deficient, in order to enhance the right selection of neuronal groups which will lead to an increment of adaptation of motor behaviour (Hadders-Algra, 2000). Also Ulrich (2000) states that patterns of movement that are repeated frequently generate stronger neural pathways that support the movement pattern. Therefore, task-oriented interventions such as NTT, which concentrate on active practising of the skills a child experiences problems with, may increase secondary or adaptive variability.

Contextuality

The ultimate goal of treatment is the ability of a child to transfer the skill acquired in the treatment situation to his or her daily life situation. Next to active practising of motor skills, research findings have emphasized the importance of practice variability, which refers to the variability in movements and context characteristics, as close as possible to real life situations a child encounters while practising a skill (Magill, 2001). A common idea of the relationship between contextuality and transfer to novel contexts is that the more variants of a specific task are met in training, the greater the likelihood that any future variant will be one previously met.

Especially in the second phase of motor learning, the intermediate level, variability of practice within the same skill is important as it provides the child the opportunity to vary task performance. In this way, task performance may be refined and adapted to the specific demands of the task situation. In terms of Edelman's theory, a child will reach secondary or adaptive variability (Hadders-Algra, 2000). It is hypothesized that variability of practice will enhance transfer of learning during treatment to daily life motor skill performance (Magill, 2001). Variability of practice might involve practising the task by loading the spatial or temporal demands of the tasks, by changing speed–accuracy demands or by performing the same skill such as ball catching, with balls of different weights or sizes. During the first phase of motor learning, constant practice is required as the goal of treatment in this phase is to acquire a basic coordination pattern and this goal is better reached by practising the same skill without much variety.

Schmidt and Bjork (1992) cite several experimental demonstrations of how transfer works. One involves teaching children to play 'beanbag', a game that involves throwing a beanbag through a hole in the wall. One group was trained on a single version of the task, with the hole always 3 feet away from them while the other was trained with the distance randomly varied between 2 and 4 feet. The random group took longer to reach criterion performance but then was significantly more accurate in their shots; not only at their training distances but also at novel distances for which they were not trained, including their competitors' 3-foot distance. The transfer effect may be explained in terms of a cognitive process called 'schema induction' (Schmidt, 1975). A schema consists of the elements shared between the motor activities seen apart from their unshared elements. Of course schema induction proceeds with further experience of variants of the same skill and takes quite some time to develop.

Time on task principle

Different parameters of the learning process have different time constants. For instance getting an idea of how to perform a task can be a matter of minutes. Increasing time related parameters of motor performance may take weeks but they still change faster than magnitude related (accuracy) parameters. So, depending on the process of learning (and the constraints of the child) more time on task training is needed. The NTT focuses on learning a task within a variety of contexts, meaning that in the example of beanbag throwing the distance, the angle, the target size or even the weight of the beanbag may be varied. Although the parameterization process is trained this way, which might look like a mere process-oriented approach, it is done within a task specific training paradigm, namely a goal directed throwing or aiming task a child can use in everyday life.

Motor teaching principles

Instructing children

Research findings indicate that motor learning in children may benefit from some kind of model like a demonstration of a skill during the early phases of skill learning, whereas verbal instructions may be more helpful in later phases of skill learning (Magill, 2001). Although research is limited, our own work has shown that demonstrations are seldom used in treatment of children with DCD by physical therapists (Niemeijer et al., in press; Schoemaker, 1992). However, the work of Bandura has pointed out that children, in general, learn by observing others (Bandura, 1986). In particular, during the first phase of motor learning when a child needs to acquire a basic coordination pattern, model examples may convey information about how to perform a skill such as the invariant characteristics of a movement pattern (Magill, 2001). These examples can be complemented with verbal instructions or questions to direct the attention of the child to specific components of a skill. During the intermediate phase of skill learning, when children learn to implement new parameters for the new coordination pattern through much practice, verbal instructions and dialogue are more useful in general, such as by providing information about the objects used or the speed or accuracy with which the skill has to be performed (Magill, 2001).

Table 11.3 Motor teaching principles

	Therapeutic actions
Ways of teaching the child	Instructing
	Improving insights
	Give feedback (appropriate to developmental level, increase error detection capability)
	Explore mechanical principles (through guided discovery)
	Give knowledge of performance (spatial and temporal)
	Give knowledge of results
	Correcting
	Supporting
	Watching
	Helping (including manually)
Ways of motivating the child	Making task important: goal setting
	Giving locus of control: attribution of success and failure
	Giving efficient practice and time on task
	Using variability of practice
	Using variety of practice
	Taking retention into account
	Showing transfer and generalizability
	Be interested, stimulating, reinforcing
	Keeping the child alert
	Diverting attention from other problems (in case of co-morbidity)
	Reacting and adapting to child behaviour
	Reward, withdraw (or punish)

Providing feedback

As children with DCD are often not able to reflect on their own performance of a skill, augmented feedback, such as knowledge of performance or knowledge of results may be essential for skill learning (Missiuna et al., 2001). Providing adequate feedback may enhance motor learning, particularly for children with DCD. Physical therapists trained in NTT learn to implement feedback in clinical practice. In the beginning of the learning process of a new skill, the therapists will provide positive feedback about the movement. The provision of feedback may be complemented with a technique called 'sharing knowledge', in which the therapist attempts to stimulate the explicit learning process by asking all kinds of questions about the performance of a skill. In the intermediate learning phase, the nature of the feedback will move away from the movement itself to the outcome of the performance. Information will be given or questions will be asked whether the goal of the performance has been reached and/or what needs to be done to improve performance in future attempts at the task. Next to the informational role of feedback in the learning process, feedback may also serve to motivate the child to continue practising (Magill, 2001). By providing positive feedback, a child will experience success, which will motivate the child to engage in the treatment exercises (see Table 11.3). Motivation in general is an important factor of treatment effectiveness. The next section will describe how therapists trained in NTT attempt to induce motivation in children with DCD.

Motivation

Motor learning when suffering from DCD requires a lot of extra effort. If the objectives are unrealistic or thought to be unrealistic, the child's cooperation will suffer and hence the effectiveness of treatment. For this reason, it is not sufficient to merely practise skills. The child will also have to be taught that s/he is responsible for the effectiveness of treatment and consequently take pleasure if the efforts are successful.

Due to their motor problems, children with DCD often have a history of failure in all kinds of motor tasks when they enter a treatment programme. Whereas most of their peers seem to learn all kinds of motor tasks rather effortlessly, children with DCD fail the same motor tasks, even though they try very hard to perform well. As a consequence, their perceived competence of their physical abilities is often found to be low (Schoemaker and Kalverboer, 1994; Cantell, Smyth and Ahonen, 1994; Skinner and Piek, 2001). A low perceived competence for physical abilities may have consequences for the way children perform future motor tasks, because they attribute their successes and failures to different factors than children with high perceived competence for physical abilities. Children with high perceived competence in general attribute their successes to internal, stable causes such as their ability in physical tasks, but their failures to unstable, external factors, such as luck. However, children with low perceived competence tend to credit their successes to more unstable, external factors, such as luck, and their failures to internal stable causes, such as lack of ability. They believe that success is beyond their control. This attribution style has direct consequences for their motivation. Children who believe that they lack the ability to perform well in motor tasks are either unwilling to try new motor tasks or show a lack of effort to do well in motor tasks (Haywood and Getchell, 2001).

When children with DCD enter a treatment programme, therapists assess their actual competence level. NTT therapists learn to take into account the perceived physical competence of the children because of the consequences a low perceived competence may have for the motivation of the child to do well during treatment. If children with DCD show evidence of low perceived physical competence, therapists can help these children by retraining their attributions (see also Table 11.3). Retraining of attributions in children with low perceived physical competence has been a successful approach in sports (Horn, 1987). Instead of attributing failure to lack of ability, therapists can emphasize that improvements in motor tasks can be reached either through more effort or through continued practice. Therapists can provide the child with progressive learning experiences, such that they experience success. They also provide the children with accurate feedback about their motor performance, so that they know how to improve their performance. In this way, children with low perceived physical competence learn that successes are not just a product of luck, but that they are personally in control of reaching success. It is expected that the effectiveness of treatment will be enlarged if children with DCD learn to credit their successes to their own ability or effort, because they will be more likely to try new motor tasks in daily life when they believe that success experiences are within their control.

Implications for clinical practice

To be able to take motor control and motor learning principles into account, the NTT approach uses a wide-scope and theory-based examination of children with DCD symptoms, before setting the individual treatment goals. It goes without saying that taking into account the broadly defined diagnostic category of DCD, which includes a heterogeneous variety of motor disorders, no predetermined motor training programme can be prescribed and a broad assessment is necessary. The purpose of a broad assessment protocol is twofold. First, differentiating primary DCD from normal age-related variations in motor skills. For this purpose, General Motor Performance and Fine Motor Performance Tests are used in the assessment protocol (Table 11.4).

Table 11.4 Summary of the assessment protocol

1	Neuromotor assessment
1.1	Quantitative examination
1.1.1	General motor proficiency tests
1.1.2	Fine motor proficiency tests
1.2	Qualitative examination
1.2.1	Fundamental motor patterns
1.2.2	Manipulative movement patterns
2	Questionnaires and reports on associated problems (ADHD; PDD-NOS; LD)
2.1	Motor behaviour (in context)
2.2	Classroom behaviour
2.3	Academic achievement, learning problems
2.4	Behaviour at home
3	Self-reports on personality traits
3.1	Fear of failure
3.2	Attributions

More general inventories are included as well to evaluate co-morbidity. A detailed examination of individual items that contribute to the motor (dys)function profile should provide us with the means to decide whether the reported problems are supported by norm referenced standardized testing. Validated questionnaires for teachers and parents on the child's motor performance, classroom behaviour, academic achievement, learning difficulties, and behaviour at home, as well as self-reports to assess personality traits like fear of failure and personal attributions, are utilized. The second goal of the assessment is to find the level of motor learning in the skill and the neuromotor process that is causing the majority of the problems within this specific skill. Potentially relevant information is obtained through a qualitative examination of fundamental (gross) and manipulative (fine) movement patterns by loading on specific task constraints (see Table 11.1). Once the learning stage and motor process are assessed, to which the motor problems of a specific task of a child with DCD are predominantly related, the therapy programme can be designed according to the above mentioned learning and teaching principles (see Tables 11.2 and 11.3). By assessing this way, the therapist uses the neuromotor control and learning theory as a basis to find out at what stage of motor control the motor problems occur and what level of skill acquisition is already attained.

Effectiveness of NTT

The effectiveness of NTT for DCD children was examined in two studies. First, a pilot study was conducted with a group of ten children with DCD (Schoemaker et al., 2003). A general motor test, the Movement ABC (Henderson and Sugden, 1992), was used to evaluate improvement in both gross and fine motor skill performance. As children with DCD often experience problems with handwriting, which hinders academic functioning at school to a large extent, the effectiveness of NTT on a scale measuring dysgraphia was also investigated (i.e. the Concise Assessment Method for Children's Handwriting, or BHK (Hamstra-Bletz, De Bie and Den Brinker, 1987)).

Fifteen children with DCD, nine boys and six girls (7 to 10 years of age), participated in this study. Ten children were included in the intervention group and five children were included in a no-treatment control group. All children in the intervention group were referred to a paediatric physical therapist by their general practitioner because of motor coordination problems. The children in the no-treatment control group were either referred to physical therapy (n = 3) or were recruited from schools because either their parents or teachers were concerned about their motor skills (n = 2). Children in the intervention group were tested three times on the Movement ABC and the BHK: before the start of intervention, after nine intervention sessions, and after a final nine intervention sessions. Intervention was provided once a week for 30 minutes. Children in the no-treatment control group were tested twice with a period of nine weeks without any intervention in between in order to measure spontaneous improvement.

Although a relatively small group of children was included, a positive effect of NTT was found. Children with DCD improved on both gross and fine motor skills after 18 treatments with NTT, whereas the no-treatment control group did not improve at all during nine weeks without intervention. When examining the relationship between the kind of motor skills that were practised during treatment and the improvement on those particular skills, it became clear that children with DCD specifically improved on those aspects that were practised. If ball skills, manual dexterity or handwriting were practised, children did improve on these skills, and they did not improve when these skills were not practised. These findings demonstrate the task-oriented character of NTT: only skills that have been practised improve, whereas non-practised skills do not improve (Schoemaker et al., 2003).

In a second, as yet, unpublished study, the effects of NTT were evaluated on a larger scale. Two groups of children with DCD were formed; an intervention group of 26 children who were referred for paediatric physical therapy because of motor problems, and a no-treatment control group of 13 children recruited from schools. All children were diagnosed with DCD according to the criteria for DCD in the DSM-IV. Children in the intervention group received nine intervention sessions once a week, children in the no-treatment control group did not receive any form of intervention. Both groups were tested at the start and end of the nine-week interval. The Movement ABC and the Test of Gross Motor Development (TGMD-2; Ulrich, 2000) were used to evaluate treatment effectiveness.

Again, positive effects of NTT were obtained. The intervention group improved their performance significantly on both the Movement ABC and the TGMD-2, whereas the performance of the no-treatment control group did not improve at all on the Movement ABC and even deteriorated on the TGMD-2.

In two further studies in which only children with fine motor deficiencies took part, poor writers received NTT. In the first study, 12 children in elementary schools received treatment over three months. Their proficiency in handwriting was assessed after three months of therapy and again after nine months without therapy (Smits-Engelsman, Niemeijer and van Galen, 2001). After the three-month treatment period their mean score for quality of handwriting had improved from 25 to 21 on the Concise Assessment Method for Children's Handwriting (Hamstra Bletz, DeBie and Den Brinker, 1987). After a nine-month period without any further therapy the quality of their handwriting had improved further, resulting in an average score of 14. As to writing speed improvement, before treatment they wrote on average 132 letters in five minutes, in contrast to 149 letters after the treatment period. After nine more months, they wrote 212 letters in five minutes, i.e. 80 letters more than before therapy. In the second study children with both DCD and learning disabilities participated. In this study a group-wise variant of NTT was used and also led to positive results (Jongmans et al., 2003).

So, it is possible to conclude that the initial results regarding the effectiveness of NTT are, up to this point, promising. More research is needed to confirm these results and to investigate whether NTT is more effective than other treatment approaches.

CHAPTER 12

A cognitive perspective on intervention for children with Developmental Coordination Disorder: the CO-OP experience

ANGIE D. MANDICH AND HELENE J. POLATAJKO

He decided he wanted to learn how to ride a bike and, yes, this is something he was determined to do for whatever reasons for comparison reasons with his friends, his sister, whatever. And when I first saw him trying to do it at home and we took off the training wheels and I thought, oh I don't know, 'keep trying James'. And he came here and I saw him falling over, and he couldn't even get the pedals started and I thought there's just no way. This kid is going to be really disappointed because he's, for whatever reasons, he just isn't, it's not clicking. And even half way through, I still thought, I don't know, he's learning to think about what he's doing and why he's doing it but is he going to be able to do it? And now it's like he's been riding a bike forever. It's like everything just came together, him thinking about it, and implementing all that stuff. Even the examples, like feet on the pedals are like a Ferris wheel, okay one person gets on and then quickly another person has to get on. And then it just comes. Amazing. He's so proud of that. He tells all his friends and I'm going to get a new bike and I accomplished this, because he knew. He set his own goal; 'I want to learn how to ride my bike. Dad if I learn how to ride my bike what do I get, what's in this for me? I'd really like a new bike, Dad. I'd really like a bike.' So that's what he's getting. He worked towards his goal and he accomplished it and he's happily looking already [forward to his new bike].[1] (James's Mom, Polatajko and Mandich, 2004, p. 47)

Engagement in the everyday activities of childhood is integral to normal child development and well-being. Research findings have demonstrated that a child's participation in the typical activities of childhood influences not only development but also self-esteem and social adjustment (Macnab, 2003). For many children, skills such as tying shoelaces, riding a bike or handwriting are acquired incidentally. However, for a subgroup of children, those with Developmental Coordination Disorder (DCD), learning a new skill is difficult (Polatajko, 1999). For these children, learning new skills is often so difficult that they become frustrated, needing to expend excessive amounts of effort to learn a new skill, and frequently abandon the skill. Alternatively, some children are referred for intervention.

Approaches to intervention for children with DCD

When parents seek support for their children with DCD a number of options become available, depending on the professional the therapist consults and the orientation that professional has to this group of children. The understanding of the disability and its causes dictates the choice of intervention for professionals. DCD is a motor impairment known to significantly affect a child's ability to perform the everyday activities of childhood. Since little is known about the specific aetiology of the disorder, interventions are based on the perspectives of motor-based performance the professional holds (Mandich and Polatajko, 2003).

Two competing perspectives on the motor problems experienced by children with DCD dominate the field: the reflex-hierarchical model and the dynamic systems model.

Historically, the reflex-hierarchical model predominated the approaches to intervention for children with motor performance problems. This model views performance problems from a deficit perspective, therefore the interventions that evolved from this view are focused on remediation of the underlying defect, for example perceptual motor training. For the most part, the interventions based on the reflex-hierarchical model either remain untested or have focused exclusively on demonstrating changes in specific motor components (Kaplan et al., 1993; Kavale and Mattson, 1983; Mandich et al., 2001a; Polatajko et al., 1995). However, no evidence has emerged to demonstrate that improvement at the impairment level leads to measurable improvement in the specific motor skills that the child needs to perform (Mandich et al., 2001a; Sigmundsson et al., 1998).

The more contemporary view is performance oriented and has emerged from a theoretical shift towards a dynamic systems perspective on motor performance (Thelen, 1995). The approach, based on a systems model, points to the importance of learning in the acquisition of motor skills (Mulder, 1991; Shumway-Cook and Woollacott, 1995). Motor learning is considered to be a multistage process of interaction between the individual, the environment, and the task, with motor control emerging as the individual becomes efficient and effective at performing the task (Schmidt and Wrisberg, 2000). Driven by these theoretical underpinnings, a variety of new performance-oriented approaches have emerged. Unique among these is Cognitive Orientation to Daily Occupational Performance (CO-OP).

CO-OP is unique among performance-based approaches because of its emphasis on the role of cognition in skill acquisition. Experience gained from using CO-OP with children with DCD has provided a new understanding of the nature of performance problems experienced by these children. It is the purpose of this chapter to discuss these new insights. In this chapter we will first introduce the reader to CO-OP and then discuss how this approach has highlighted the importance of cognition as a mediating factor in facilitating the learning of new motor skills and how this has informed our understanding of DCD.

Cognitive Orientation to daily Occupational Performance (CO-OP)

CO-OP is a client-centred, performance-based, problem solving, approach that enables skill acquisition through a process of strategy use and guided discovery. (Polatajko and Mandich, 2004)

Embedded in a learning paradigm, CO-OP breaks from traditional, deficit-based views on motor performance and adopts a contemporary, learning-based perspective on motor skill acquisition.

CO-OP embraces the shift of the World Health Organisation (WHO) from a disability model to a new framework for health and disability, the *International Classification of Functioning, Disability and Health* (ICF) (WHO, 2001). CO-OP is compatible with the concepts of ICF and focuses on improving motor performance, thus, it is nested in the health context at the level of activity and participation. Intervention is focused at activity and participation, not at disability and impairment. As such, the focus of CO-OP is on improving the motor performance of the child in his environment by discovering strategies to eliminate barriers and create supports that enable activity and participation. Developed within a research context, CO-OP draws on the knowledge of a number of disciplines, including behavioural and cognitive psychology, health, human movement science and occupational therapy, to achieve its objectives (Polatajko and Mandich, 2004).

Objectives of CO-OP

Cognition forms the foundation of CO-OP and enables the achievement of the four objectives of CO-OP:

- skill acquisition
- cognitive strategy use
- generalization
- transfer of learning.

The primary objective of CO-OP is motor skill acquisition. Congruent with the ICF model, CO-OP focuses at the level of activity and enables the child to learn to perform three specific motor skills over ten intervention sessions. The specific motor skills learned by the child are those identified by the child, in collaboration with his parents, and may include activities like riding a bike, handwriting, tying shoe laces or cutting. Cognitive strategies are used to solve motor performance problems and acquire motor skills. Consequently, the second objective of CO-OP is to teach the child how to use strategies to achieve their motor goals. Children are actively taught a problem-solving strategy and are enabled to discover additional strategies that will support their motor skill acquisition. The third objective of CO-OP is to facilitate generalization, i.e. use the skill at other times or in other settings such as home and school. (A skill is considered to have generalized when it can be performed under different stimuli conditions than it was learned, i.e. at a different time, in a different place or with different people. For a discussion of generalization of learning, see Martin and Pear, 1996.) Once the child has acquired the desired motor skill, the focus of therapy shifts to facilitating generalization of the learning beyond the therapy situation. The final objective of CO-OP is skill transfer, i.e. using the skill as a basis for learning other, similar, skills. (Transfer of learning is 'the gain or the loss of a person's proficiency on one task as a result of previous practice or experience on another task' (Schmidt and Wrisberg, 2000, p. 179); for a discussion of transfer of skills, see Schmidt and Wrisberg, 2000.) Since only three skills are addressed in the course of a CO-OP intervention, it is important that the children learn to adapt their skills and strategies to the demands for new skills that they encounter in everyday life. The aim of intervention is for the child to leave therapy with the ability to generalize and transfer the problem-solving strategies and skills that have been learned in therapy into everyday life.

Research evidence to support CO-OP

CO-OP was developed over the course of ten years as an alternative to the traditional approaches for the treatment of children with motor-based performance problems, especially children with DCD. Developed by Dr Polatajko and colleagues, within an academic research setting at a university clinic, CO-OP was the result of the work of a number of graduate students under the supervision of Dr Polatajko (Polatajko and Mandich, 2004; Polatajko et al., 2001a; Polatajko et al., 2001b). The decision to develop a new approach to the treatment of children with motor-based performance problems came as a result of Dr Polatajko having conducted a number of trials with various colleagues investigating a variety of treatment approaches based on traditional thinking; all of which yielded negative results (see Kaplan et al., 1993; Law et al., 1991; Polatajko et al., 1991; Polatajko, Kaplan and Wilson, 1992; Polatajko et al., 1995). One of those trials (Polatajko et al., 1995), however, provided evidence that these children could improve their performance with direct teaching. Noting this finding and drawing on her background in behavioural and learning theory approaches to skill acquisition, Dr Polatajko undertook to apply a learning paradigm to the treatment of children with motor-based performance problems, children with DCD.

A number of studies were conducted in the development and testing of CO-OP. The first study, a single-case experimental design with nine direct replications, demonstrated that children with a primary diagnosis of DCD, aged 7 to 12, could improve their performance of a variety of skills with the assistance of cognitive strategies (Wilcox, 1994; Wilcox and Polatajko, 1993; 1994). In a second study (Martini 1994; Martini and Polatajko, 1998), also using single-case experimental design, a systematic replication of the first study was carried out. Martini demonstrated that another therapist could successfully replicate the results of the first study.

In a third study, Mandich (1997) examined Wilcox's and Martini's treatment sessions to fully understand how cognitive strategy use promoted skill acquisition. In her analysis of the video tapes of the CO-OP treatment, Mandich found that in addition to Meichenbaum's global problem-solving strategy, task knowledge had been provided to the children and a number of domain specific strategies had been used (Mandich, 1997; Mandich et al., 2001b). Mandich identified eight domain specific strategies that were directly related to the specific problems the children were experiencing in task performance. It became clear from Mandich's investigation that the approach was much more than the simple use of verbal self-guidance in applying a global problem-solving strategy. In other words, inherent to the approach were tailor-made strategies that were divined from a careful task analysis of the performance issues the child was experiencing. Accordingly, a new name was coined. The approach was named Cognitive Orientation to Daily Occupational Performance (CO-OP) to capture the essential components of the approach, i.e., that it involved the use of cognitive strategies applied to specific issues of performance.

A number of other studies have been conducted to investigate the efficacy of CO-OP (Polatajko and Mandich, 2004; Polatajko et al., 2001a; 2001b). The most significant of these was a randomized clinical trial (RCT) (Miller et al., 2001b). A number of approaches can be taken to examine the efficacy of a treatment approach including single-case experimental design studies, direct systematic replications and clinical replications

(Ottenbacher, 1986). However, the randomized clinical trial (RCT) is considered to be the gold standard, and hence the most important type of evidence. Initially intended as a pilot study, the purpose of the RCT was to identify the size of the CO-OP effect (i.e. how much improvement could be expected) so that power calculations could be made and a larger randomized trial could be undertaken. Twenty children with DCD were randomly assigned to one of two groups; ten received CO-OP treatment while another ten received the typical treatment approach. For each child in the typical treatment approach (TTA) group, the treating therapists were encouraged to carry out the treatment they felt was the most appropriate for the child. The only caveat was that these therapists could not use CO-OP techniques. The actual treatment given to the children in the TTA group was a combination of approaches, mostly focused on treating component skills, typical of the traditional approaches discussed earlier. The findings indicated that even with groups as small as ten, the CO-OP treatment was shown to be significantly more effective in promoting skill acquisition and skill transfer than the typical treatment approach. Finding a significant difference between treatments with a group size as small as ten indicates that the effect size for CO-OP is considerably larger than that for the typical treatment approach, essentially making a larger trial unnecessary. Thus, findings of the RCT indicated that CO-OP was more effective than the typical treatment approach.

Evidence for the effect of CO-OP has also been gleaned from several qualitative studies that have been conducted to explore the impact that DCD had on the lives of children and their families (Polatajko and Mandich, 2004). During interviews for these studies, parents inadvertently offered commentary on the efficacy of the CO-OP approach and its broad impact on the lives of their children (Mandich, Polatajko and Rodger, 2003; Segal et al., 2002). Parents indicated that CO-OP was not only effective in having their children reach their goals, but more importantly, from their perspective, CO-OP had far-reaching effects. Not only did the children's skills generalize beyond the therapy room to natural settings and transfer to other skills, but it also made the children generally more open to new learning and more willing to participate.

The studies providing evidence regarding the effectiveness of CO-OP both quantitative and qualitative, indicate that a new approach had been found for the treatment of motor-based performance problems in children: an approach that (1) meets the demands of parents, in that it is effective in helping children succeed; (2) meets the demands of therapists, in that it is client-centred and performance-based; and (3) meets the demands of administrators, in that is cost-effective, efficient and evidence based (Polatajko and Mandich, 2004).

The key features of CO-OP

Essential to the effectiveness of CO-OP is that the child and therapists are fully engaged in the approach as it has been specified in the intervention protocol. The CO-OP protocol, described in detail by Polatajko and Mandich (2004) comprises seven key components, referred to as key features (see Figure 12.1).

The key features of CO-OP are:

1. client-chosen goals
2. dynamic performance analysis
3. cognitive strategy use
4. guided discovery
5. enabling principles
6. parent/significant other involvement
7. intervention structure.

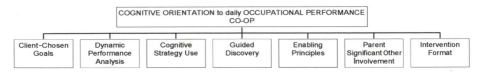

Figure 12.1 Key features of CO-OP. Source: Polatajko and Mandich (2004).

Each of the key features addresses one or more of the four objectives of CO-OP. The first key feature is the identification of child-chosen goals; that is, the goals are set in collaboration with child and family and focus on activities the child wants to, needs to, or is expected to perform. The child is actively engaged in the goal setting process to ensure motivation. In the CO-OP approach, the child's perspective is of central importance, beginning with the process of setting child-chosen goals, and continuing throughout the intervention. Once the child has chosen the goals, the therapist observes the quality of the child's motor performance, and begins a dynamic process of analysis.

The second key feature of CO-OP is dynamic performance analysis (DPA) (Polatajko, Mandich and Martini, 2000). Developed specifically for use in CO-OP, DPA is a dynamic, iterative process that is applicable to any performance situation. DPA is based on the understanding that performance is the product of the interaction of person, environment and activity, and thus highly individualistic. DPA is carried out while observing performance; points and sources of performance problems or performance breakdown are noted. This requires careful attention to various aspects of the fit between client abilities, skills and actions and the task and environmental demands and supports. The focus of CO-OP is on performance, and correcting performance problems or breakdown, not underlying skills. The DPA process supports this by focusing the analysis on the observed actions of the child, the observed demands of the skill, and the environmental variables that affect the performance. Underlying skills are only considered as background information to help identify potential solutions. Once the therapist has identified the initial performance breakdown points, the therapist uses cognitive strategies to bridge the gap between ability and skill proficiency.

Cognition strategies, the third key feature, are used to support skill acquisition, generalization and transfer. Cognitive strategies are cognitive operations over and above those that are inherent in the task itself (Pressley, Borkowski and Schneider, 1987). The CO-OP approach uses strategies to facilitate this process. The strategies help the child engage in problem solving a performance issue and monitoring the outcome; in other words the strategies promote metacognition, thinking about one's thinking (Flavell, 1979). In CO-OP, two types of strategies are used to facilitate the use of metacognition in solving performance problems and promoting competence, generalization and transfer; namely global and domain.

The child is specifically taught the CO-OP global strategy and is guided to discover domain specific strategies. The global strategy used in CO-OP is the GOAL-PLAN-DO-CHECK strategy developed by Camp and colleagues (1976) and used by Meichenbaum (1977, 1991). In CO-OP, the child is taught to use the mnemonic GOAL-PLAN-DO-CHECK, to support the solving of performance problems. In the very first session after goal setting, the child is introduced to the GOAL-PLAN-DO-CHECK strategy and is directly taught to use it. While this can be done in a number of ways, in CO-OP, the child is generally taught the strategy through the use of a puppet. The global strategy remains at the centre of each intervention session. Initially, the therapist takes the lead in using the GOAL-PLAN-DO-CHECK strategy. As the child becomes familiar with the strategy, the child gradually begins to initiate strategy use.

The second type of strategies used in CO-OP is called domain specific. Domain specific strategies (DSS) are strategies that are specific to a particular task or part of a task, such as the Ferris wheel strategy in the opening quote. Domain specific strategies are embedded in the global strategy; are task, child, and situation specific; and are often used only for a short time. The child is taught the global strategy, whereas domain specific strategies emerge in the context of skill acquisition. In CO-OP, the DPA process is used to identify the need for a DSS and the therapist's knowledge about task performance is used to identify potential DSSs that will solve the particular motor performance issue. Table 12.1 describes the various types of DSS that are used in CO-OP.

Table 12.1 CO-OP Domain Specific Strategies*

Strategy	Definition	
Body position	Any verbalization of attention to, or shifting of, the body, whole or in part, relative to the task.	Verbal Guidance
Attention to doing	Any verbalization to cue attending to the doing of the task.	
Task specification/ modification	Any discussions regarding the specifics or modification of the task, or parts of the task, or any modification of the task or any action to change the task, or parts of the task.	
Supplementing task knowledge	Any verbalization of task specific information or how to get task specific information.	
Feeling the movement	Any verbalization of attention to the feeling of a particular movement.	
Verbal motor mnemonic	A name given to the task, component of the task or body position that evokes a mental image of the required motor performance.	
Verbal rote script	A rote pattern of four or five clear concise words that are meaningful to the child to guide a motor sequence.	

Source: Adapted from Polatajko and Mandich (2004).

All DSSs are nested in verbal guidance. Early in the intervention, all the verbal guidance (talking through a performance sequence) is given by the therapist. However, the goal is to lead the child from early reliance on the therapist's verbal guidance, to the independent application of cognitive problem-solving strategies through self-talk. Therefore, as the intervention progresses, the therapist encourages the child to talk himself through a sequence, i.e. to use verbal self-guidance. Each of the DSSs is expressed in terms of a verbalization. Verbalization of strategies is a hallmark of the CO-OP approach, as has been said above, CO-OP is a highly verbal approach. Verbalization ensures that the cognitive mechanisms that distinguish it from other approaches are used; that the strategies are brought to the attention of the child, that the child understands the role of the strategies; and that the child can use the strategies independently, in the absence of the therapist. Once the child and therapist have identified the strategies, the therapist reinforces their use during the intervention sessions.

The next key feature of CO-OP is guided discovery. Guided discovery is the process whereby the therapist guides the child to discover answers to problems. In CO-OP, the process of guided discovery is closely entwined with the process of strategy use. It is used in conjunction with the DPA process primarily to identify when the child becomes 'stuck' and elucidate the plan and within the GOAL-PLAN-DO-CHECK problem-solving process. Guiding the child to discover the PLAN and the DSSs increases the likelihood that he will attribute the success of the PLAN to himself, positively impacting his self-efficacy.

In conjunction with guiding discovery the therapist uses four enabling principles to facilitate motor skill acquisition. The enabling principles, the fifth key feature, are an integral part of the approach, and are used throughout the intervention. CO-OP has its foundation in the client-centred philosophy of occupational therapy, which focuses on enabling people to perform the occupations they want to, need to, or are expected to perform. Four enabling principles have been identified for use in CO-OP to support skill acquisition, strategy use, generalization and transfer. The principles are in addition to guided discovery, which, in essence, is also an enabling principle. The enabling principles are an integral part of the approach, and are used throughout the intervention. They are captured in four imperatives:

- Make it fun!
- Promote learning!
- Work towards independence!
- Promote generalization and transfer!

The next key feature is the involvement of parents or significant others. The primary role of parents or significant others is to support the child in the acquisition of new skills and to facilitate the generalization and transfer of these to the home and other settings. Throughout the intervention, the therapist shares information with the parents or significant others, so that they can celebrate successes with the child and support the child's use of newly learned skills and strategies in environments beyond the intervention sessions, as James's Mom describes in the opening quote.

The experience of being involved in CO-OP has benefits beyond helping the child acquire the desired skills (Mandich et al., 2003; Polatajko and Mandich, 2004; Segal et al., 2002). By enabling their children to succeed, parents or significant others change their perspective on the child. In the same way that the children learn the relationship between strategy use and outcome and learn to attribute the lack of success to failure of the PLAN, rather than a personal failure, so too, successful strategy use alters the parents' perception of themselves and their child. Parents can see that failure can be attributed to an ineffective strategy, as opposed to personal factors. This awareness often results in a new appreciation of the factors that contribute to their child's performance and the realization that there are strategies that can help.

The final feature of CO-OP is the format of the intervention sessions. The CO-OP programme involves ten intervention sessions. In the first phase of the CO-OP process, the child identifies three goals to address during intervention and then the therapist baselines the child's performance on these chosen goals. Subsequently, the therapist teaches the child the GOAL-PLAN-DO-CHECK strategy and then it is applied to the child's three goals. The GOAL-PLAN-DO-CHECK strategy is then used to identify the DSSs. Once therapy is complete the therapist re-evaluates the child's performance.

CO-OP: where cognition and motor meet

As indicated at the outset of this chapter, experience with CO-OP has provided a new understanding of the nature of motor-based performance and, in particular, the performance problems experienced by children with DCD. A distinguishing feature of Cognitive Orientation to Daily Occupational Performance (CO-OP) is the emphasis on the role of cognition on skill acquisition. The discovery and verbalization of cognitive and metacognitive strategies are fundamental to CO-OP. The success of CO-OP points to the important role that these cognitions play in mediating and facilitating the learning of new motor skills.

Historically, therapy has often focused on remediating or fixing motor performance problems by focusing on the neurodevelopment of the child. Little attention was given to the other dimensions of the child, including the use of the affective and cognitive aspects of performance (see Figure 12.2). CO-OP incorporates the theoretical work of Fitts and Posner (1967) who describe a model of motor learning where the first stage of learning is the cognitive stage. During this stage, cognition can be used to guide the motor performance. The child learns to develop and verbalize cognitive strategies that form the bridge between the innate abilities and skill level (see Figure 12.3). CO-OP also utilizes the affective and motivational aspects of the child by allowing the child to choose their own goals, goals that are ecologically salient for the child. This triad forms the foundation of intervention (see Figure 12.4).

Practice informs theory: a new perspective on DCD

The cumulative results of the research on CO-OP challenge the traditional assumptions regarding how children with DCD acquire motor skills and indicate that cognition is a mediator of motor performance. Indeed, the data from CO-OP studies demonstrate that cognitive and

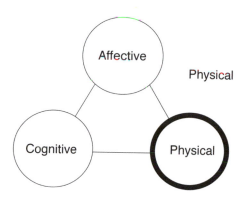

Figure 12.2 Foundations for CO-OP, focusing on the physical.

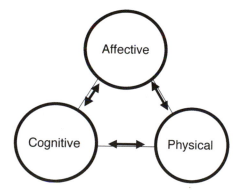

Figure 12.3 Foundations for CO-OP, incorporating the cognitive and affective with the physical.

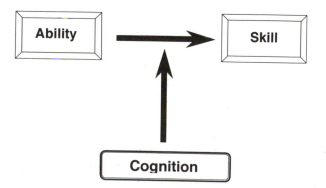

Figure 12.4 Where motor and cognition meet.

metacognitive strategies improve the performance of children with DCD and may indicate the origin of the difficulties experienced by these children.

The motor learning literature indicates that typically developing children learn new motor skills by watching and imitating others (Schmidt and Wrisberg, 2000). They often use trial and error learning to develop and refine motor skills. However, for children with DCD the scenario does not appear to be the same. The literature reveals that children with DCD do not learn by imitation and repetition and that left on their own they simply practise the same errors over and over again. This can be seen in a study by Marchiori, Wall and Bedingfield (1987), who investigated the movement patterns of physically awkward boys during the performance of slap shots in hockey. Results indicated that even after practising 1200 slap shots with direct instructions, the children continued to display extreme variability in their performance. The children did not learn from observation, direct teaching or trial and error.

Historically, such motor difficulties experienced by children with DCD have been explained by an underlying deficit in foundational skills such as midline crossing or bilateral coordination (Mandich et al., 2001a; 2001b). If a child with DCD came to therapy with the goal of learning to ride a bike, the therapy would focus on identifying the underlying deficits in such foundational skills as balance, righting reactions, postural adjustments, or bilateral coordination, and 'fixing' those deficits before ever placing the child on a bike. Research has shown limited effectiveness of that type of approach and often the child outgrows several bikes while waiting for the therapist to fix the underlying deficits.

In contrast, in CO-OP, once the child has chosen the goal (e.g. bike riding) the therapist draws the child's attention to specific performance breakdown points in the task to create an awareness of the behaviour, and then guides the child to discover strategies that work to solve the performance problems. The physical components form the background of the intervention and other components such as cognitive and affective factors are used to facilitate skill acquisition. The task, bike riding, becomes the foreground and the child is guided to discover strategies to improve motor performance. In the opening quotation, James learns to pedal by developing a strategy: 'like feet on the pedals are like a Ferris wheel, okay one person gets on and then quickly another person has to get on. And then it just comes'. Once James was able to find a strategy to bridge ability and skill he was able to progress in mastering bike riding and learned to ride his bike just like the other kids. CO-OP research has demonstrated that the experience with James is not unique; that children with DCD who have specific motor goals, like learning to ride a bike, can be taught to use cognitive strategies to solve their performance problems. More importantly the CO-OP data have indicated that children with DCD can achieve success in acquiring motor skills without any direct attention being given to the remediation of so called underlying deficits.

The CO-OP results challenge the traditional assumptions about skill acquisition in children with DCD. It would appear that the remediation of deficits in such underlying skills as balance and bilateral coordination is neither necessary nor sufficient in helping children with DCD acquire motor skills. Rather, cognitive factors including attention to the salient features of the task, task knowledge, identifying the point where the task performance breaks down or task knowledge is deficient, become the mediators of performance. These data would further suggest that DCD may not be a coordination problem, per se, but a learning-based motor problem. Although this research is promising, further research is needed to investigate this hypothesis.

Summary and conclusion

Experience gained from using CO-OP with children with DCD has provided a new understanding of the nature of motor performance problems experienced by these children. The success of a cognitive approach in solving the motor performance problems of children with DCD suggests that these children have unique learning needs when it comes to the acquisition of motor skills, and that the problems they exhibit are not neurodevelopmental in nature stemming from deficits in underlying foundational skills such as balance. Rather, they stem from an inability of the children to learn motor skills by imitation or trial and error. It seems that children with DCD need to have their attention directed to the specific aspects of task performance that give them difficulty; they need to have their task knowledge augmented and to develop idiosyncratic strategies for success. In short, that DCD is a learning-based motor problem. In general, the findings from the application of a cognitive approach to motor performance problems suggest that skilled performance arises from a dynamical interaction of a variety of factors, one of which is cognition; and that cognition can be a mediating factor in facilitating the learning of new motor skills. Further, these findings suggest that cognition ought to be given a more prominent role in the design of interventions that are based on a dynamical systems perspective.

Note

1. In the tradition of qualitative research, all the quotes in this book that are from participants in qualitative studies are presented verbatim, no editorial corrections have been made.

CHAPTER 13

Overlapping conditions – overlapping management: services for individuals with Developmental Coordination Disorder

AMANDA KIRBY

DCD and management

In order to consider the management of the child with Developmental Coordination Disorder and overlapping difficulties it is necessary to consider a number of elements.

What does management mean?

Is it about seeking cure, seeking strategies for the child, family or school or seeking first the cause of difficulties being experienced?

Who or what are we trying to manage?

Is this the child, the family, the school or the system?

Once we have considered what is meant by management, it will be possible to consider how help is given at present to support the child and consider the barriers in place to improving services for children with DCD and other related conditions.

at's in a name?

derstanding a label

revious chapters have described evidence from Gillberg (1998b) and other esearchers to show the overlap of DCD with other neurodevelopmental disorders and that the 'pure' DCD child is indeed rare. However, managing the whole child with a range of functional difficulties remains a challenge for the parent of the child and for health and educational professionals working with the family. There is inconsistency with treatment programmes and few randomized controlled trials in the biomedical and psychological literature comparing one type of treatment programme with another.

Labels, at times, are used inconsistently by health professionals; Peters, Barnett and Henderson (1999) showed that health and educational professionals use different labels to mean different things with regard to DCD, clumsiness and dyspraxia. A recent study looking at the knowledge of general practitioners' understanding of labels used to define specific learning difficulties and showed that 96 per cent of general practitioners did not know the term DAMP, another 36 per cent could not define or gave incorrect definitions for Asperger's Syndrome and 71 per cent could not define DCD (Kirby, Davies and Bryant, in preparation). This was compared with teachers' knowledge who similarly did not know the term DAMP (96 per cent). However, fewer teachers had difficulties defining Asperger's Syndrome and DCD than general practitioners studied (15 per cent and 46 per cent respectively). This lack of knowledge on the part of the health professional, who may be seen as the gatekeeper to services, combined with compartmentalization of provision, may leave parents feeling both frustrated and confused.

Does labelling help the parent?

Case AS

'I have a seven-year-old who has low muscle tone, gross and fine motor problems, speech articulation issues, severe handwriting difficulties, (he tape records his homework and we scribe for him), visual tracking problems, balance issues, sits on special cushion in school, has work printed out so that he doesn't have to read or copy from board, has seat in front of blackboard, has attention difficulties. Yet no-one will diagnose him with dyspraxia. No-one will statement him. His paediatrician prefers to 'describe' his difficulties individually because he is 'improving'. Since when did you have to be not improving to have a diagnosable problem? His brother has speech issues and is diagnosed with dyspraxia, and my son is not daft. What is the big problem with having a diagnosis?'

■ *www.dyscovery.co.uk message centre (2003)*

Parents are often anxious to seek out the label, often believing that once it is given, support and treatment will follow. In the current system, for many children there is a need to label in order to access help and support. However, many, if not most, children with a developmental problem qualify for more than one diagnostic label and this can cause confusion for educational professionals deciding on the type of support required. For example, a population study showed that 23 per cent of children showed signs of DCD, 8 per cent met criteria for ADHD, and 19 per cent were categorized as dyslexic (Kaplan et al., 1997). Nearly 25 per cent of the affected children were found to have all three, while 10 per cent had both ADHD and DCD, and 22 per cent had dyslexia and DCD. One label may be more socially acceptable than another and gain greater support and remediation for the child.

A conceptual framework developed by Kaplan and colleagues (1997) called *atypical brain development*, which is an umbrella term to encompass the overlap, may help to explain developmental disorders and their relationship to each other. This harks back to the days where minimal brain dysfunction described some of these difficulties. One positive implication of this newer framework is to emphasize more the individual's strengths and weaknesses, with individualized treatment programmes based on the child's profile rather than on any one diagnostic category. However, this label may not be a very popular one with parents. It is important to consider the context that it may be used in. If used to describe the child having an 'odd or atypical' brain, the child and the parents may find this a less acceptable label to use with others to describe the difficulties.

Parents may have to wait months to access services then may need to go from one professional to another, first trying to find out what's wrong and then what to do. The wait may also increase the feeling that once the label has been given all help will follow and until it is given little can be done. Children with DCD by definition, using DSM-IV (APA, 1994) criteria, have difficulties in activities of living and learning on a daily basis. Many of these difficulties have functional impact and could often start to be addressed with or without a label at school or home with little risk of harm.

Case DS

'My son has recently been diagnosed with dyspraxia [*term generally used for DCD in the UK*] and basically school just do not want to help. I've had a comprehensive report and school have been given a copy of it. They say that they have taken it on board, but last week my son was made to stand on a chair in the classroom and recite his times tables. When I went in to see his teacher – she stated that he was perfectly safe!! This year he was put in the skipping race on sports day – he was getting so stressed out and upset that I kept him home that day. School has told me that there are no funds available for dyspraxic children. I just want to help my son and help him to achieve to the best of his ability – I just don't know where to get the help that he needs. I have been told that he would be helped by occupational therapy and physiotherapy – but he is currently not getting either.'

■ *www.dyscovery.co.uk message centre (2003)*

In recent years there has been an increased recognition of DCD by health, educational professionals and parents in the UK. However, there remain barriers to delivery for appropriate support. One of the barriers is long waiting times, as reported in the 'Doubly Disadvantaged' Report (Dunford and Richards, 2003) from the College of Occupational Therapists and the National Association of Pediatric Occupational Therapists in the UK. This is partly due to shortages of professionally trained staff. Disparity in management models also causes confusion where in one area the health authority may provide the dominant lead with occupational therapists providing, for example, a sensory integration therapy approach to 'treat' children with DCD but in another area the local education authority may take the lead by providing 'motor pro-grammes' delivered within a school setting.

Who labels a child?

There is a debate in many areas over who should undertake both the ini-tial screening and assessment and the subsequent support and whether this should be placed in the hands of education or in the health arena. In the past there has even been an element of competition and territory set-ting with regard to who should undertake this. Is this the key domain of the occupational therapist where there remain long waiting times or should services be set within an educational setting where the child spends most of the time and has most of the functional difficulties? While this debate continues and shortages in allied health professionals prevail, there are pragmatic management issues that need solutions, otherwise children remain having difficulties with little or no support. This is espe-cially true for children with overlapping difficulties who may end up going from service to service.

Case CJ

'My six year old daughter has just had an assessment done by the educational psychologist and she's written for the teachers to try for one to one help but got turned down. She sees a paediatrician, a physiotherapist and a speech therapist. The psychologist also states that she has a moderate learning difficulty but because she got turned down I don't know what to do next as she's still not reading etc. Her doctor has said that she's got autistic spectrum disorder tendencies and dyspraxia and ADHD tendencies but their still doing tests and she also has epilepsy which is controlled. I don't know what I should do next.'

■ *www.dyscovery.co.uk message centre (2003)*

Children given the label of DCD, although all having the same diagnosis, when looked at closely, are a heterogenic group. Hadders-Algra (1999) referred to the 'aspecificity' of the term DCD and Barnett and colleagues (1999) also discuss the difficulties in applying the DCD diagnosis.

Clinical work from the Dyscovery Centre

The case series shown is of 31 children; all scoring below the 5th percentile on the Movement ABC and fulfilling the DSM-IV (APA, 1994) criteria for a diagnosis and label of DCD. Figure 13.1 (Kirby, Davies and Bryant, in preparation) shows Movement ABC scores for 31 children broken down into the Test components of fine motor skills (manual), ball skills, and static and dynamic balance. These cases highlight differences

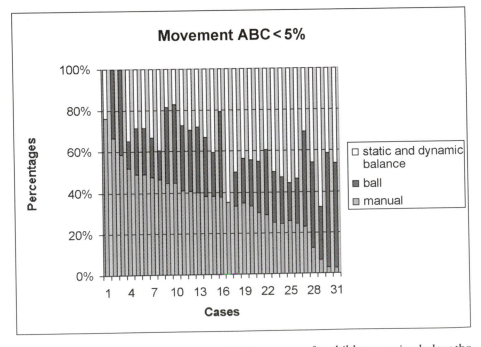

Figure 13.1 Breakdown of Movement ABC Test scores for children scoring below the 5th percentile.

within a group of children with a label of DCD. One end of the scale shows children with difficulties with fine motor tasks and having little difficulty with ball skills, at the other end of the scale children show difficulties with ball skills but show few difficulties with fine motor tasks.

The following are four cases from this cohort of 31 children and demonstrate how children may present with their different profiles of difficulties. Information was gathered from structured questionnaires to parents and teachers prior to the assessment and through semi-structured interview as well as using standardized assessments and observation.

Case MG

MG is female; she was born at 42 weeks' gestation, did not crawl but walked at 13 months. She wears glasses for visual acuity correction and has astigmatism. She was noted to have increased ligamentous laxity and pragmatic language difficulty when assessed by a physiotherapist and speech and language therapist. She has also been given a diagnosis of dyslexia by an educational psychologist.

Main educational concerns: Difficulty following and understanding instructions, poor fine motor skills, and difficulty working independently.

Main parental concerns: Poor motor skills, her ability to concentrate when working, low self-esteem, getting tired more easily than her peers, difficulty controlling her emotions with peers and adults. She was also reported to have difficulties understanding verbal instructions.

Hobbies: MG likes to swim.

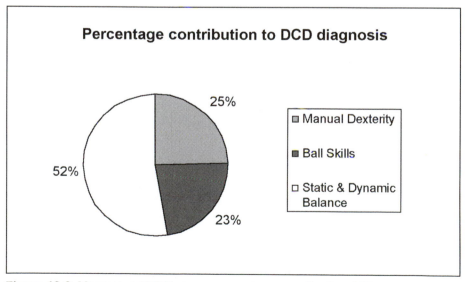

Figure 13.2 Movement ABC Test scores as percentages for Case MG.

This first case demonstrates the wide range of difficulties in a number of domains including communication and coordination and how this impacts on her self-esteem. She also shows on the MABC a contribution to the total score from static and dynamic difficulties. This may be because of her increased ligamentous laxity. It exemplifies the need to consider the child as a whole and how an assessment looking at one aspect could potentially miss out on essential information when choosing and planning the type of intervention for her.

Case JD

JD is male. He was born full term. He was a bottom shuffler and walked at 13 months. He was reported to have increased ligamentous laxity on examination by the occupational therapist. JD also showed pragmatic language difficulties when assessed by the speech and language therapist. He did not show any visual perceptual difficulties.

Main educational concerns: Difficulties with clarity and organization, difficulty in organization of his books and papers such as mislaying tools and exercise books, difficulties in PE.

Main parental concerns: Writing is practically illegible to himself and others. He has unclear speech and finds it hard to remember instructions. He has difficulties concentrating when working. He is easily discouraged from things he is not very good at and has low self-esteem.

Hobbies: He likes to play on PlayStation games.

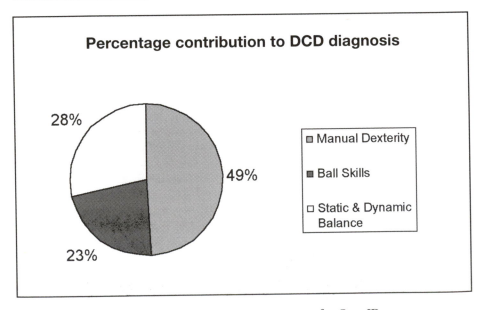

Figure 13.3 Movement ABC Test scores as percentages for Case JD.

This second case on the surface seems similar to Case MG. However the main educational concerns are the child's organizational skills, whereas the parents are more concerned about his ability to record work and concentrate on tasks set for him, and his low self-esteem. This case demonstrates the need for gathering evidence from multiple sources as discussed by Crawford, Wilson and Dewey (2001) to ensure a full picture of the child's difficulties.

Case LR

LR is a male, born full term, crawled and then walked at 16 months. He has also pragmatic language difficulties.

Main educational concerns: Difficulties with mathematics. He is reported to be overactive and impulsive. He has been bullied in school. He has particular difficulty with writing and scissor skills. He has no specific difficulties with PE and rugby.

Main parental concerns: Difficulties dealing with anger and frustration with consequent behavioural difficulties at home. Inconsistent work in school linked to an inability or unwillingness to concentrate in school. He shows a lack of self-esteem. He is also reported by his parents to have irrational obsessions and concerns starting from arrival at new school.

Hobbies: He likes to go to scouts, rugby, and play on computer games, and watch comedy shows.

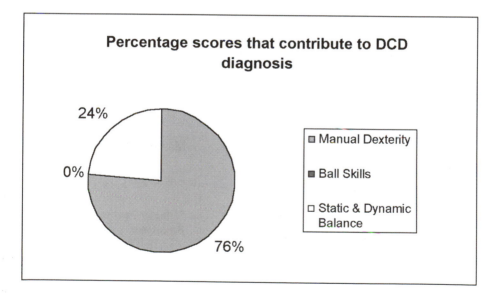

Figure 13.4 Movement ABC Test scores as percentages for Case LR.

This third case shows a child again with a diagnosis of DCD, but who mainly has difficulties with fine motor skills and social use of language. He is also demonstrating additional difficulties with attention and concentration, with his parents also reporting irrational obsessions. This case demonstrates the need for children with DCD to be seen in an interdisciplinary team as his needs are not confined to motor difficulties. It also demonstrates a child who has predominantly fine motor difficulties contributing to his score on the Movement ABC battery, and little or no difficulty in the area of gross motor difficulties. This is reflected in his choice of rugby as a hobby.

Case DF

DF, male was born full term by Caesarean section. He crawled at 10 months and walked at 14 months. He has expressive, receptive and pragmatic language difficulties.

Main educational concerns: Lacks concentration and unable to carry out instructions. He is reported to fidgets, and be restless and have difficulties remaining on task. He has poor gross and fine motor skills. He has difficulty with throwing and catching balls.

Main parental concerns: Inability to record academic work. Poor social skills and has low self-worth. He is frustrated by his own inadequacies, leading to aggression and unhappiness.

Hobbies: He likes to swim, likes wildlife and watching videos.

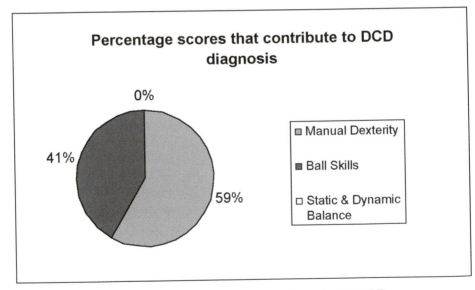

Figure 13.5 Movement ABC Test scores as percentages for Case DF.

Finally, this last case demonstrates a child with difficulties in both fine and gross motor skills as well as having difficulties socializing. It is of interest to note that the parents' main concerns were his low self-worth and behaviour. This case highlights the social and emotional impact of having difficulties for the child and the family.

These four cases demonstrate how different children are in a clinical setting and the range of functional difficulties displayed at home and at school. For example, MG's score for balance makes up 52 per cent of the overall score, whereas for DF it is zero. Similarly, LR's score for manual dexterity makes up 76 per cent of the total score, while MG's score for manual dexterity makes up 25 per cent of the total score. Other differences can be seen between these children. Many of the children, however, have similarities of low self-esteem and difficulties with attention and concentration and associated pragmatic language difficulties impacting on their social skills. The children show a variety in the type of hobbies they choose to undertake, and this may be related to their differing profiles.

It highlights the need for an interdisciplinary approach to assess the whole child and exemplifies that in clinical practice the 'pure' DCD child is a rarity. If a holistic approach is not taken deficits may be missed and the child may then be insufficiently supported. There is great value in gathering information from a number of sources, including the parent and teacher and, where appropriate, the child and the use of questionnaires is one way of gathering information as to where the child's difficulties lie and to consider potential assessment that may need to be undertaken (Phillips et al., 1999).

Managing the services

Barriers to entry

Professional shortages There is currently a national shortfall of allied health professions across the UK, in particular occupational therapists, speech and language therapists and physiotherapists. The need for training more professionals has been recognized for some time and was reported in the Department of Health paper 'Meeting the Challenge: A Strategy for Allied Health Professionals' (2000). This shortage has a knock on effect with even fewer people available to train others in suitable programmes of support. It also has implications for the development of interdisciplinary working.

In the past, children with physical difficulties, such as cerebral palsy and those with multiple disabilities, have been perceived as having greater need. DCD has been seen as limited to childhood and a relatively mild disorder and this has not always allowed for sufficient attention to be paid to service provision for this group.

Knowledge shortages At the present time, the responsibility and understanding of the needs of the DCD child will vary from one health and education authority to another. Often support is related to the motivation or interest of individuals in a particular school, or driven by a personality often with a personal interest in the field. Hamilton (2002) discusses the need to recognize the significance of what are seemingly minor motor difficulties and the need for the family physician to be aware of this condition, as well as the associated coexisting deficits. With shortages of trainers and lack of standardization in models of training, knowledge can vary from one area of the country to another. Training programmes are often developed at a local level and the information may influence local approaches and may not always be evidence-based. Training is usually separated by profession, e.g. different training for teachers and health professionals and even separation in developmental disorder training; for example, training in ADHD separated from DCD and other related difficulties. This may add to the confusion in how to best manage the child within the classroom setting when the teacher has to deal with a real child in the classroom who may have several labels.

In order to resolve the training gaps, an example of an alternative delivery mechanism to enable information to reach further across the UK and internationally has been developed by the Dyscovery Centre in Wales, in partnership with the University of Wales. This is an online (Internet-based) certificate as a part of a Masters Degree (SEN) programme along with additional materials to demonstrate assessment processes and to describe a range of children and their management delivered using CD-ROM. This approach provides the possibility for a mix of professionals to interchange their views as a part of the course process. Umble, Shay and Sollecito (2003) have shown that similar distance learning programmes showed high acceptability among learners and offered the opportunity for interdisciplinary training. This is a new course and evaluation in terms of learning and transference into clinical practice remain to be measured.

Development of other e-learning approaches such as CD-ROM/DVD materials may also allow training to reach out further and be a cost effective route where trainers may not be available on the ground. This cannot be a substitute for experience but may support training at a local level.

Waiting lists Increased awareness has led to increased referrals into services. The staff shortages have exacerbated the long waiting lists for both assessment and treatment. In a survey carried out by the College of

Occupational Therapists (Dunford and Richards, 2003), high priority children were seen between immediately and 16 months with a mean of seven weeks, in comparison with children with DCD, who waited from one week to 2–4 years with a mean of 46 weeks.

Compartmentalization of service provision

At the present time the usual referral route for the child is that he or she is referred into a community paediatric service. Little triage takes place at this stage to assess the level of urgency for seeing that child, in terms of how the child's difficulties are impacting on their ability to be integrated into school, home life or ability to maintain his or her self-esteem.

Assessment and intervention delivery are often compartmentalized, with either occupational therapy or physiotherapy taking a lead for the child with a potential diagnosis of DCD; speech and language therapist for the child with pragmatic language difficulties; the psychologist for ADHD etc. with inter-professional working being limited, often because of staff and time shortages. Lack of communication because of lack of time exacerbates the difficulties of good inter-disciplinary working. The assessment often achieves a diagnosis but does not always supply to the parent the pragmatic suggestions for supporting the child or how to translate these suggestions into the curriculum.

This more uni-disciplinary approach may also lead to duplication of limited resources as one child may end up seeing several professionals separately and has implications for health and education authorities in terms of economy, efficiency and best value. Ultimately, service inefficiency has an impact on the child and the family, leaving parents frustrated due to having to go from one service provider to another, repeating their 'story'. This may also act to increase the already long waiting lists where children are sitting on several waiting lists at a time. Parents, while waiting, may be left in limbo with little practical help or general advice. Schools are often also waiting for the diagnosis in order to decide on the type and amount of educational support required.

Growing waiting lists mean that some children may not receive any assessment or therapy. This is especially true for older children as health services for this group are often very limited beyond the age of 11 years and some areas even as young as 8 years. This presents a difficulty, as a study by Parr, Ward and Inman (2003) recently showed in the assessment of children with ADHD where the mean age for diagnosis was 8.3 years. Delay in supporting the child may mean that the child's self-esteem and confidence may decrease and secondary, negative, behaviours start to develop. Skinner and Piek (2001) showed that in two groups of children, one in the 8–10 year age group and the other 12–14 years with DCD, both groups had lower self-worth and greater anxiety than the control group. In addition, the older group saw themselves as less competent and had less social support than the younger group, implying that delay may have an impact on self-esteem as the child with difficulties gets older.

It is of interest that a paper by Greydanus and colleagues (2003) states that

> Management of ADHD should include a multi-modal approach, involving appropriate educational interventions, appropriate psychological management of the patient (child or adolescent), and judicious use of medications. Parents, school officials, and clinicians must work together to help all children and adolescents with ADHD achieve their maximum potential. (p. 1049)

This is as true in the area of DCD. Occupational therapy and physiotherapy should not be the sole service providers for a child with DCD; what is needed is a range of services, each offering a part and combining to provide a holistic approach.

Current mechanisms for referral

Interdisciplinary working should be the gold standard, where teams work effectively with one another, passing information and discussing outcomes. This should include all the professionals (Health, Education, Social Services, Voluntary and Independent sectors) and importantly, the parents and child. The Department of Health in England, published a consultation document (December 2002) discussing the development of Children's Trusts. This proposed structure would enable organizations to join together in local partnership and assist them to commission and directly provide services for children, in particular those with a combination of health, educational and social care needs. It would also enable partner organizations to formally integrate management and budgets in order to improve the coordination and quality of service provided to children. This model may see pilots emerging, clearly demonstrating that joint planning, commissioning and delivering services can be centred on the needs of the user and some evidence of real partnership working between health, education and social services ideal for this scenario. A Government Green Paper 'Every Child Matters' (DfES, 2003) discusses electronic information sharing through developing a single unique identity number, developing a common assessment framework and introducing a lead professional. If these are achieved, it will go a long way to helping solve some of the current management problems for children with DCD and related developmental difficulties.

Prioritizing referrals

The increasing rate of referrals to an already under-resourced service means that services need to have clear management pathways to manage the caseloads. Often prioritization is based on the principle of the child with the parent who shouts loudest is the one that receives the support fastest and for longest. This results in some children with greater urgency not being prioritized and remaining at the bottom of a pile and the less urgent cases being seen first. A method of triage needs to be considered in order to assess children by level of need.

Screening first

At the present time, most referrals come from two routes; either from the GP or health visitor (either when the child has been identified in the surgery or prompted by a parent recognizing difficulties) or, alternatively, by educational services (when the child is not making adequate progress as compared with his peers and requires an assessment for diagnosis or for a potential statement of educational need). However, the GP often lacks time and training to understand the difficulties and the potential needs of the child (Dunford et al., 2004). This can be seen in how GPs view the management of ADHD. A study from Australia by Shaw et al. (2003) showed that GPs did not want to be the primary providers of care for patients. Participants in this study indicated a preference to refer the patient to medical specialists for diagnosis and treatment of ADHD and expressed low levels of interest in becoming highly involved in ADHD care. Concerns about over-diagnosis and misdiagnosis of the disorder, diagnostic complexity, time constraints, insufficient education and training about the disorder and concerns regarding misuse and diversion of stimulant medications were the reasons cited for their lack of willingness. Thapar and Thapar (2002) also reported that doctors working within Primary Care in the United Kingdom are willing to follow up children on medication for ADHD and carry out monitoring of physical status. However, many felt they lacked confidence in the management of ADHD and most had received little or no training in child psychiatry. There are also concerns that adverse media reports will have an undue influence on the attitudes of doctors within primary care to families with children suffering from ADHD. If this is considered in the context of the overlapping management of developmental disorders and, in particular, DCD, there is even less training existing in the area of DCD.

At present there is no 'gold standard', no one test or screening measure that can be used alone to confidently identify all the problems in the child and adult at different stages in the child's life. However, there are a small number of assessment instruments available: The Early Years Movement Skills Checklist (Chambers and Sugden, 2002) can be used to identify children between 3 and 5 years and Movement ABC (Henderson and Sugden, 1992) can be used with children up to 12 years of age for coordination difficulties. These tools look at the child as if he or she only has one potential label and do not take into consideration the overlap between different neurodevelopmental disorders. The other screening tools, such as Conner's Rating Scale (1997), assess symptoms consistent with ADHD but all are not able to consider where one factor may present as one symptom but may in fact be a part of another condition as well. Screening in isolation for motor difficulties only may fail to identify related difficulties in language or vision (for example see previous case histories) but may be of help in understanding the motor difficulties in greater depth.

Health visitors have used a number of developmental rating scales including Schedule of Growing Skills (Bellman, Lingam and Aukett, 1997), Griffiths Mental Development Scales (Griffiths, 1967) and Bayley Scales of Infant Development (Bayley, 1993). However, the use of these varies from one area to another. These scales look at variations from the developmental norm but do not consider the underlying aetiology.

The paediatrician's assessment, when a child is referred through this route, is important to exclude other conditions presenting with motor delay or difficulties which have an implication for diagnosis, treatment and ongoing management. However, with paediatricians reporting that their work load has increased in the past five years in this field of medicine, there is a need to consider other options for potential service delivery. An alternative community-based service could be GP/nurse led but supported by the paediatrician. Ward and Gupta (2000) have cited the use of General Practitioners with Special Interests (GPwSI) as a key to reducing hospital waiting lists and there are over 1000 GPs working successfully in this way in the UK at present, in specialties such as dermatology.

Where and when should screening take place and by whom?

At present, routine health examination of children is limited to certain times for conditions such as hearing and vision. In the past this has been led by school health services. However, the role of the school medical team has diminished in some areas in the past few years. Could and should screening take place in schools with the support of a school health team to look at those individuals who are causing concern and need greater assessment? This would allow for schools to be able to approach the school medical team if they were concerned about the development of a child and ask for an opinion and would allow for an easier transfer of information from education to health and even may allow for observation to take place in a more naturalistic setting.

Screening could then look across at all developmental areas and ensure that a one-stop screen takes place which may be both more cost and time effective. However, it is important to consider that there may be a further need to repeat screening at other times apart from school entry. Another time may be when starting in secondary school where, for example, a child may have been coping in one school and now starts to flounder once in a larger school with greater expectation on him or her, such as writing at speed, playing rugby rather than practising ball skills and a greater need for self-organization. The child may lack the foundation skills in order to do these tasks but may have coped until this time or been adequately supported. Use of screening tools at school entry and at different points in the school career needs to be uniform to ensure that all concerned are measuring the same thing and there is a process of referral with identification criteria for onward referral. If this is undertaken in school, a functional approach allowing for intervention, even while waiting for medical assessment, limits discrimination against those with and without a label.

The assessment process

Assessment is the process of gathering information about an individual in order to make decisions about his or her therapy needs or support. The assessment for the child with DCD and overlapping difficulties often needs a combination of standardized testing with good observational assessments. These usually include a combination of the following:

- assessments
- informal/natural assessments ideally within a home/school setting
- norm-referenced tests
- observation
- criterion-referenced tests
- play-based tests
- checklists and rating scales
- parent interviews
- child-centred interviews.

However, different professionals use different assessment tools to make the diagnosis and the label is often influenced by which professional undertakes the assessment.

Principles underpinning the assessment framework

Assessments ideally should:

- be child centred;
- be rooted in the development of the child;
- be ecological in approach;
- ensure equality of opportunity for input from both parent and the professionals;
- involve working with the child and the family;
- build on strengths as well as identifying difficulties;
- be inter-agency in the approach to assessment and the provision of services;
- be carried out in parallel with other action and provision of services;
- be grounded in evidence-based knowledge;
- consider the functional difficulties of the child.

The ideal assessment is a continuing process and not a single event and once need has been established then:

- the parent's views of the child's needs and services need to be established;
- the precise nature of the needs defined, e.g. both functionally and taking into consideration the underlying cause;
- a prioritization for action and resources is required;
- the best options need to be pursued;
- a plan of action with a care pathway needs to be established with goals and agreed measurable outcomes and a review date, if appropriate.

Care pathways have been used in many areas of surgical and medical practice. Magyary and Brandt (2002) have shown the use of care pathways and decision trees in the management of ADHD in children with some success but it does require planning and reviewing to ensure that *all* stakeholders are included in the development and delivery.

Assessment often continues throughout a period of intervention if immediate needs can easily be addressed. Intervention may also start at the beginning of the assessment. The undertaking of the assessment with a child and the family can often begin a process of understanding and change by key family members and the child himself.

The professional may, by undertaking this process of gathering information, be also instrumental in bringing about change by the questions asked, by listening to the family and the child and by validating the family's concerns and also by providing information and advice as the assessment goes along. This is often the case in managing children with overlapping difficulties as the assessment may offer the parents the first opportunity of off-loading their difficulties and may only require advice and guidance which can be given at the time of the assessment.

The value of being heard and opinions listened to as a concerned parent can be very valuable in supporting both the child and the family. While taking a history, the professional may offer guidance and support and at times provide both the assessment and a solution orientated session for the child and the family.

The process of assessment can also be therapeutic in itself. Action and services are often provided in parallel with the assessment, where necessary, and do not always await completion of the assessment. Directing parents to parent support groups can itself have merit at this time (Law et al., 2001).

There has been growing knowledge in other fields such as autism where the parents have in-depth knowledge of their children that it would take 'professionals' a much longer time to acquire. Hinojosa and colleagues (2002) have shown an increased interest in a family-centred approach in occupational therapy but therapists still need to expand their knowledge and expertise in working effectively with families and also to consider creative ways to address some of the psychosocial issues in this area. In 2001, the Department of Health launched the 'Expert Patient' programme, mainly targeting chronic diseases. However, for individuals with DCD and overlapping difficulties, many of the issues may be similar such as

> physical and psychological difficulties, socio-economic problems, reduced quality of life and sometimes social exclusion. (p. 13)

This highlights the need to see the child, adolescent and his or her family as expert in their condition and needs and requiring ongoing support often for many years but at differing times relating to uniquely different sets of social and environmental circumstances.

Communication and partnership working

Orelove and Sobsey (1996) have written about the need for transdisciplinary working and inter-agency partnerships in educating children with multiple disabilities. Government directives cite the need to forge greater parent partnerships and also to work with organizations outside the statutory services such as the voluntary and independent sectors. The DfES reported in the paper 'Excellence for all children: Meeting Special Educational Needs' (1997) that the Department expects all LEAs to provide a parent partnership service, including dispute resolution arrangements, ensuring parents of children with SEN have access to independent information and advice about SEN procedures, school-based provision, support available for their child and additional sources of help and information, such as voluntary organizations and childcare information services (DfES, 1997, pp. 24–30).

The SEN and Disability Act (2001) has moved this on further by making parent partnership services a statutory requirement since January 2002. It has also strengthened the rights of children with special educational needs to be supported in mainstream. The most recent Government Green Paper 'Every Child Matters' (2003) talks about 'supporting parents and carers at the heart of its approach to improving children's lives' (p. 13). However, Rathbone (2002), a national charity providing advice and support to parents of children with special educational needs, reported that the current education system is failing both the children and parents of those with special needs and that over half the parents of children with special educational needs believe the support their children are getting is inadequate. This is illustrated in the example below.

Case JT

'I have a son who is almost 10; he attends main stream school, with the help of a full time Support Worker. My son has Asperger's Syndrome, DCD and ADHD. He is as capable as any other 10 year old to take part in all activities offered in school. This weekend there is a school trip to xx. It is part of the school curriculum. My son had NOT been invited to this, yet all 30 of the class have paid for their trip. I have only found out this week, as a little boy from my son's class came to our fireworks display. He asked JT what he was taking with him on the trip. Last year the head teacher said to my husband and myself she would see how he settled back in school before making a decision on what would happen; my husband offered to give up his time to go along with him so he would not feel any different from the other children. The head said that it was not possible for this to happen as the whole idea of the weekend was to be away from parents. We took our son out of school last year, as the head teacher called me into the office and told me my son could not take his part in communion as it would be unfair on the other children's special day.'

■ *www.dyscovery.co.uk message centre (2003)*

Current practice within education

With the enforcement of the revised Code of Practice in England and Wales (2001), along with the Disability Discrimination Act (1995), identification and provision of appropriate support for children with DCD become an even greater issue. There is increasing risk for education and health authorities in receiving litigious claims retrospectively from parents on behalf of their children. This increases the onus on educational services to provide appropriate and differentiated support for children with DCD. In the past, the 'statement of educational need' has been seen as the goal for provision for parents. However, the statementing process has been reduced and support has been aimed at being delivered within the classroom as inclusive provision, although newly qualified teachers have received little or no training about DCD and overlapping difficulties and so often have limited skills to support the child. There remains a need for mainstream class teacher training in this area as inclusion becomes the norm, if the 'learning diverse' child is really going to be addressed. In order to change delivery, it may also be necessary to change attitudes as well. Research suggests that teachers' attitudes are a crucial factor in their behaviour towards inclusive diverse learners (Landrum et al., 1995). Negative attitudes towards diversity acquired early in teachers' careers are difficult to change, so the role of initial teacher education, in promoting a positive approach, is crucial at both undergraduate and postgraduate level. The classroom assistant also needs training to understand how to facilitate the child with DCD and not 'do for' the child.

Dyspraxia friendly schools packs have been developed in a number of education authorities such as Durham, Bridgend and in the Highlands regions in Scotland. The Dyspraxia Foundation and the Dyscovery Trust in the UK have fact sheets to aid parents with functional difficulties. This is a positive change over the past five years but if GPs are to take on a gatekeeping role there is still little material within this setting to address the practical difficulties if labels have not been given.

Therapeutic approaches for children with DCD

These should ideally:

- use knowledge from research practice about the needs of the child and the family and consider the evidence for interventions critically, to inform the assessment and planning;
- listen and learn from the views of the users, i.e. children and parents;
- evaluate continuously whether the intervention is effective in responding to the needs of the child and family and whether the aims of the intervention are being met or have changed over time;
- consider re-evaluating the level of input and type if progress is not being made and consider adapting the environment and not the child, if necessary, to allow the child access to the curriculum.

Awareness of difficulties may occur at the pre-school stage and may be recognized by health visitors or general practitioners; assessment and support may then be delivered by the community paediatric services. This help is not always linked into educational goals but may be more therapy orientated. Advice to teachers is often not provided, regarding how teachers may support the child and his or her needs. Conversely, the school may identify the child with coordination difficulties but education may not have effective routes of working with local health services to help the child practically unless the difficulties are severe.

Sugden and Chambers (1998) have identified one potentially successful and effective model where both health and education could work together. Further models of good practice using transdisciplinary methods of working have been developed and delivered with Bridgend Education Authority, based on a Dyscovery Model of Practice (Kirby, Drew and Jones, 2002). This model considers a joint health and educational approach and intervention within the context of the educational setting. It is goal-orientated and has a cognitive approach. At the same time, it also empowers the parent by giving the parent the functional guidance required to support the child appropriately at home while working in partnership with school, allowing continuity of care. The model has a two track approach; undertaking comprehensive training of educational personnel at all levels from the SENCO to the classroom assistant, as well as providing support and training for parents, at the same time as providing a joint health and educational package.

Which treatment approach is right?

Mandich and colleagues (2001a), in a review paper, considered the evidence for different treatment regimes and concluded that there was no one treatment that was more effective than another. Clinical practice, in reality, may often be guided not by the evidence base but by the particular interest or experience of the therapist in the area. Research suggests, however, that, given the heterogeneity of DCD with other disorders such as ADHD, no one single approach works for all children and a cognitive needs led approach is probably one of the most effective ways of working, especially for the older child. Intervention needs to be a team approach rather than styled by individuals and must be consistent for the child both at home and in all areas of schooling.

There are a number of treatment options currently being used which have been discussed in other chapters in this book in greater detail. The following are some of the methods that have been more widely reviewed in the literature:

- physiotherapy including sensory integration therapy, individually tailored movement programmes
- kinaesthetic treatment
- Sugden and Chambers educational approach (cognitive motor approach)
- cognitive approaches, e.g. CO-OP.

Sugden and Chambers (2003a) and CO-OP (Polatajko et al. 2001a; 2001b) both take a functional approach considering the child at the centre of the therapy, rather than working purely with the underlying deficits. Both approaches have a positive impact on the child's self-esteem. Some isolated movement programmes, while working on self-esteem, may only teach the child splinter skills that cannot always be incorporated into other activities and may not address some of the fundamental difficulties such as social interaction and independent living skills.

Case TW

'My 5 year old has been assessed as having dyspraxia by the paediatrician, but now will have to wait for two years before seeing the paediatric occupational therapist. The school has said that they are 'just learning' about this in the younger child, which although is great that they have admitted this it really does not give me confidence in what he will achieve or receive help for! From what I can gather he struggles through school, but returning home we get the 'fall-out'. He only has one friend who most of the time is with another stronger child who will not let my son play. This is having a really bad affect on my child's confidence and he is regularly upset that no-one invites him to parties, plays mostly on his own and even on a school trip yesterday was *the* child that was sat on the coach on his own. He can play really well with children much younger than himself, but being in the reception year this is not an option. The school wants to send him to be assessed by the speech therapist for his understanding of speech, which I have no objections to, but I am very concerned about his mental state due to these rejections. I have spoken to my son's paediatrician who has said that in the school aged child a referral to the educational psychologist has to be done by the school and not the NHS. What should I now do?

■ *www.dyscovery.co.uk message centre (2003)*

Long-term needs of the child with DCD – growing up

Skinner and Piek (2001) have shown the effect on worsening self-esteem in adolescence. Further, research by Kirby and Drew (1999) suggests that the DCD is not solely restricted to childhood. If the accurate assessments of needs are not undertaken and appropriate support not given, evidence suggests that this has ramifications and implications in the longer term for these individuals (Cousins and Smyth, Chapter 6 in this book; Losse et al., 1991). The child with overlapping difficulties is even more likely to require longer term support throughout their growing years and into adulthood. If the adult with a mixed profile of difficulties is considered, research by Biederman et al. (1993) has indicated that 50–80 per cent of children diagnosed with ADHD continue to experience symptoms into adulthood. In addition, much research suggests that adults with ADHD exhibit relatively higher rates of depression and anxiety. There is a need for further research to determine which adults with motor coordination difficulties will continue to have difficulties into adult life.

If continuity of care is important longer term, a key worker system is one option. Viner (1999) has discussed the need for a *key worker system* to be established that is central to the individual and stands alone to support the different areas of needs whether social, health or educational over time and especially at times of transition. Many children moving from child to adult fall through service gaps and may not be able to access child and adolescent mental health services or paediatric services any longer but health professionals in adult mental health services have little or no experience in this field.

Continuity of care means also effective health care integration and this requires effective communication, teamwork and the commitment to deliver this care. Integrated documentation is a key element for enhancing interprofessional collaboration and reducing the isolation of professionals and the individual in the middle of this system. This type of record-keeping has been successfully implemented in a range of other health care settings and could be used as a potential model (Atwal and Caldwell, 2002), especially in view of a move towards the use of electronic patient records.

The future

If shortages in specialist support are to be overcome, existing services must be utilized to greater effect. As well as traditional methods of delivery, there is also need to consider the use of information technology for both the purposes of assessing individuals as well as training professionals and, most importantly, ensuring information and practical advice gets out to all individuals and their parents who require it, regardless of where they are living. A paradigm shift needs to occur where it is acceptable to use pocket PCs or have access to laptops for a child with handwriting difficulties, where sport does not mean only a choice of rugby or football but a differentiated PE curriculum to meet the needs of the diverse learner. Full and appropriate support will only happen for the child with DCD when creative solutions are sought for the range of difficulties seen.

New technologies could provide:

- A computerized screening tool for a baseline measure of the range of neurodevelopmental difficulties, allowing for data to be collected in a more uniform way nationally and to help target services appropriately and recognize the individual, rather than the label.
- Webcam delivered services could be used especially for remote or rural settings or where providing full teams may be less cost-effective. For example, a project using tele-occupational therapy is currently being run by Liu and Miyazaki (2000) in Canada. This methodology could also be extended to using web cameras in classrooms and even in the child's home (with permission) to have a real understanding of the functional difficulties and for monitoring treatment programmes.

The next ten years will be exciting for the management of DCD and other overlapping disorders. There are still huge gaps in research into the management of the whole child with complex needs, with a continuation of often examining only one aspect in isolation of the other factors. Management is a challenge to both researchers and clinicians at all levels but it is essential not to lose sight of the child and the need for a pragmatic approach to helping the whole child and not just isolated parts.

LIBRARY, UNIVERSITY OF CHESTER

References

Adelson A, Fraiberg S (1974) Gross motor development in infants blind from birth. Child Development 45: 114–26.

Agostoni E, Coletti A, Orlando G et al. (1988) Apraxia in deep cerebral lesions. Journal of Neurology, Neurosurgery and Psychiatry 46: 804–8.

Allcock P (2001) The understated difficulties of slow handwriting. Handwriting Today 1: 56–60.

Alston J (1990) Aspects of handwriting in primary school children. Unpublished doctoral thesis, University of Manchester.

American Psychiatric Association (1987) DSM-III-R Diagnostic and Statistical Manual of Mental Disorders. Washington DC: APA.

American Psychiatric Association (1994) DSM-IV Diagnostic and Statistical Manual of Mental Disorders. Washington DC: APA.

American Psychiatric Association (2000) DSM-IV-TR Diagnostic and Statistical Manual of Mental Disorders. Washington DC: APA.

Amundson SJ (1995) Evaluation Tool of Children's Handwriting (ETCH). Homer, AK: O.T. Kids.

Anastasi A (1997) Psychological Testing. Upper Saddle River, NJ: Prentice Hall.

Andersen K, Strack L, Rosen I et al. (1984) The development of acoustic reaction time in children. Developmental Medicine and Child Neurology 26: 490–4.

Anderson E, Emmons P (1996) Unlocking the Mysteries of Sensory Integration. Arlington, TX: Future Horizons.

Arnheim D, Sinclair WA (1979) The Clumsy Child: A Program of Motor Therapy (2nd edn). St Louis: Mosby.

Arscott C (1997) Clumsiness in developmental co-ordination (DCD) and Asperger's Syndrome (AS). Unpublished MSc thesis, University of Amsterdam.

Ashby AA (1983) Developmental study of short term memory characteristics for kinesthetic movement information. Perceptual and Motor Skills 57: 649–50.

Athenes S, Guiard Y (1991) Is the inverted handwriting posture really so bad for left-handers? In J Wann, AM Wing, N Sovik (eds), Development of Graphic Skills: Research Perspectives and Educational Implications. London: Academic Press, pp. 137–48.

Atwal A, Caldwell K (2002) Do multidisciplinary integrated care pathways improve interprofessional collaboration? Scandinavian Journal of Caring Sciences 16: 360–7.

Ayres AJ (1971) Characteristics of types of sensory integrative dysfunction. American Journal of Occupational Therapy 7: 329–34.

Ayres AJ (1972a) Southern California Sensory Integration Test Manual. Los Angeles: Western Psychological Services.

Ayres AJ (1972b) Sensory Integration and Learning Disorders. Los Angeles: Western Psychological Services.

Ayres AJ (1979) Sensory Integration and the Child. Los Angeles: Western Psychological Services.

Ayres AJ (1989) Sensory Integration and Praxis Test Manual. Los Angeles: Western Psychological Services.

Bailey DB, Wolery M (1992) Teaching Infants and Preschoolers with Disabilities (2nd edn). New York: Macmillan.

Bandura A (1986) Social Foundations of Thought and Action: A Social Cognitive Theory. Englewood Cliffs, NJ: Prentice Hall.

Barnett A, Henderson SE (1992) Some observations on the figure drawings of clumsy children. British Journal of Educational Psychology 62: 341–55.

Barnett A, Henderson SE (1994) Button fastening as a prototype for manipulative action: some observations on clumsiness. In VA Rossum, JI Laszlo (eds), Motor Development: Aspects of Normal and Delayed Development. Amsterdam: University of Amsterdam Press.

Barnett A, Henderson S, Haataja L et al. (1999) Difficulties in applying the diagnostic criteria for DCD: examples from case studies. DCD IV International Conference, Groningen, The Netherlands.

Barnett AL, Henderson SE, Scheib B (2002) The development of a handwriting assessment for 11+ year olds: a pilot study. Unpublished conference proceedings, 5th biennial workshop on children with DCD, Banff, Canada.

Bax M, Whitmore K (1987) The medical examination of children on entry to school. The results and use of neurodevelopmental assessment. Developmental Medicine and Child Neurology 29: 40–55.

Bayley N (1993) Bayley Scales of Infant Development (2nd edn). San Antonio, TX: Therapy Skill Builders.

Beery KE (1967) Developmental Test of Visual-Motor Integration. Chicago: Follett.

Beery KE (1997) The Beery-Buktenica Test of Visual-Motor Integration with Supplemental Developmental Tests of Visual Perception and Motor Coordination. Parippany, NJ: Modern Curriculum Press.

Beery KE, Buktenica NA, Beery NA (2004) The Beery-Buktenica Developmental Test of Visual Motor Integration (5th edn). Los Angeles: Western Psychological Services.

Bellman M, Lingam S, Aukett A (1997) Schedule of Growing Skills II. Windsor: NFER Nelson.

Benbow M (2002) Hand skills and handwriting. In SA Cermak, D Larkin (eds), Developmental Coordination Disorder. Albany, NY: Delmar, pp. 248–79.

Benson DF (1991) The role of frontal dysfunction in Attention Deficit Hyperactivity Disorder. Journal of Child Neurology 6: S9–S12.

Berger W, Trippel M, Discher M et al. (1992) Influence of subjects' height on the stabilization of posture. Acta Otholaryngology 112: 22–30.

Berlyne DE (1960) Conflict, Arousal, and Curiosity. New York: McGraw-Hill.

Bernheimer LP, Keogh BK (1995) Weaving interventions into the fabric of every-day life: an approach to family assessment. Topics in Early Childhood Education 15: 415–33.

Berninger VW (2001) Process Assessment of the Learning (PAL). Test Battery for Reading and Writing. San Antonio, TX: The Psychological Corporation.

Berninger VW, Swanson HL (1994) Modifying Hayes and Flower's model of skilled writing to explain beginning and developing writing. Advances in Cognition and Educational Practice 2: 57–81.

Berninger VW, Fuller F, Whitaker D (1996) A process model of writing development across the life span. Educational Psychology Review 8: 193–218.

Berninger VW, Mizokawa D, Bragg R (1991) Theory based diagnosis and remediation of writing disabilities. Journal of School Psychology 29: 57–79.

Berninger VW, Yates C, Cartwright A et al. (1992) Lower-level developmental skills in beginning writing. Reading and Writing: An Interdisciplinary Journal 4: 257–80.

Berninger VW, Vaughan K, Abbott R et al. (1997) Treatment of handwriting fluency problems in beginning writing: Transfer from handwriting to composition. Journal of Educational Psychology 89: 652–66.

Bernstein N (1967) The Co-ordination and Regulation of Movement. Oxford: Pergamon Press.

Bernstein N (1984) Some emergent problems of the regulation of motor acts. In HTA Whiting (ed.), Human Motor Actions: Bernstein Reassessed. Amsterdam: North Holland.

Bertenthal B, Bai D (1989) Infants' sensitivity to optical flow for controlling posture. Developmental Psychology 25: 936–45.

Beunen GP, Malina RM, Van't Hof MA et al. (1988) Adolescent Growth and Motor Performance: A Longitudinal Study of Belgian Boys. Champaign, IL: Human Kinetics Books.

Biederman J, Faraone SV, Spencer T et al. (1993) Patterns of psychiatric comorbidity, cognition, and psychosocial functioning in adults with attention deficit hyperactivity disorder. American Journal of Psychiatry 150: 1792–8.

Biederman J, Newcorn J, Sprich S (1991) Comorbidity of attention deficit hyperactivity disorder with conduct, depressive, anxiety, and other disorders. American Journal of Psychiatry 148: 564–76.

Blote A, Hamstra-Bletz L (1991) A longitudinal study on the structure of handwriting. Perceptual and Motor Skills 72: 983–94.

Bly L (2000) Motor Skills Acquisition Checklist. London: Psychological Corporation.

Bornholt LJ (1996) The ASK-KIDS Inventory for Children. Test Manual and Test Booklets. Sydney, NSW: The University of Sydney.

Botting N, Powls A, Cooke RWI et al. (1998) Cognition and educational outcome of very-low-birthweight children in early adolescence. Developmental Medicine and Child Neurology 40: 652–60.

Bouffard M, Watkinson EJ, Thompson LP et al. (1996) A test of the activity deficit hypothesis with children with movement difficulties. Adapted Physical Activity Quarterly 13: 61–73.

Boyle T (2003) Assessment tools used to identify children with developmental coordination disorder. Unpublished honours thesis. Crawley, Western Australia: The University of Western Australia.

Brace DK (1927) Measuring Motor Ability. New York: AS Barnes.

Brake NA, Bornholt LJ (in press) The personal and social basis of children's self-concepts about physical movement. Perceptual and Motor Skills.

Brenner MW, Gillman S (1966) Visuomotor ability in schoolchildren: a survey. Developmental Medicine and Child Neurology 8: 686–703.

Briggs D (1970) The influence of handwriting on assessment. Educational Research 13: 50–5.

British Medical Journal (1962) Clumsy children. British Medical Journal 1665–6.

Bronfenbrenner U (1977) Towards an ecology of human development. American Psychologist 32: 513–31.

Bronfenbrenner U, Morris PA (1998) The ecology of developmental processes. In W Damon (ed.), The Handbook of Child Psychology (5th edn), Vol. 1. New York: Riley, pp. 993–1028.

Brown AL, Campione JC (1986) Training for transfer: guidelines for promoting flexible use of trained skills. In MG Wade (ed.), Motor Skill Acquisition of the Mentally Handicapped. Amsterdam: North Holland.

Bruininks RH (1978) Bruininks-Oseretski Test of Motor Proficiency. CirclePines, MN: American Guidance Service.

Burton AW (1990) Applying principles of coordination in adapted physical education. Adapted Physical Activity Quarterly 7: 126–42.

Burton AW, Rodgerson RW (2001) New perspectives on the assessment of movement skills and motor abilities. Adapted Physical Activity Quarterly 18: 347–65.

Butterworth G, Hicks L (1977) Visual proprioception and postural stability in infancy. A developmental study. Perception 6: 255–62.

Camp B, Blom G, Herbert F et al. (1976) Think aloud: a program for developing self-control in young aggressive boys. Unpublished manuscript, University of Colorado School of Medicine, Denver, CO, USA.

Campbell FA, Pungello EP, Miller-Johnson S et al. (2001) The development of cognitive and academic abilities: growth curves from an early childhood educational experiment. Developmental Psychology 37: 231–42.

Cantell M, Kooistra L, Ahonen TP et al. (2001) A school-based intervention program for 6 and 7 year old children with developmental coordination disorder. Presentation at the Sixth Biennial Motor Control & Human Skill Research Workshop, Fremantle, WA.

Cantell M, Smyth MM, Ahonen TP (1994) Clumsiness in adolescence: educational, motor and social outcomes of motor delay detected at 5 years. Adapted Physical Activity Quarterly 11: 115–29.

Cantell M, Smyth MM, Ahonen TP (2003) Two distinct pathways for developmental coordination disorder: persistence and resolution. Human Movement Science 22: 413–31.

Carello C, Turvey MT (2000) Rotational dynamics and dynamic touch. In M Heller (ed.), Touch, Representation and Blindness. Oxford: Oxford University Press, pp. 22–66.

Carpenter A (1942) The measurement of general motor capacity and general motor ability in the first three grades. Research Quarterly 13: 444–65.

Causgrove Dunn J (2000) Goal orientations, perceptions of the motivational climate and perceived competence of children with movement difficulties. Adapted Physical Activity Quarterly 17: 1–19.

Causgrove Dunn J, Watkinson EJ (1994) A study of the relationship between physical awkwardness and children's perceptions of physical competence. Adapted Physical Activity Quarterly 11: 275–83.

Causgrove Dunn J, Watkinson EJ (1996) Problems with identification of children who are physically awkward using the TOMI. Adapted Physical Activity Quarterly 13: 347–56.

Cermak SA, Henderson A (1989) The efficacy of sensory integration procedures, Part I. Sensory Integration Quarterly XVII: 5.

Cermak SA, Henderson A (1990) The efficacy of sensory integration procedures, Part II. Sensory Integration Quarterly XVIII: 1–5.

Cermak SA, Coster W, Drake C (1980) Representational and nonrepresentational gestures in boys with learning disabilities. American Journal of Occupational Therapy 34: 19–26.

Cermak SA, Gubbay SS, Larkin D (2002) What is developmental coordination disorder? In SA Cermak, D Larkin (eds), Developmental Coordination Disorder. Albany, NY: Delmar, pp. 2–22.

Cermak SA, Trimble H, Coryell J et al. (1990) Bilateral motor coordination in adolescents with and without learning disabilities. Physical and Occupational Therapy in Pediatrics 10: 5–18.

Cermak SA, Ward EA, Ward LM (1986) The relationship between articulation disorders and motor coordination in children. American Journal of Occupational Therapy 40: 546–50.

Chambers ME, Sugden DA (2002) The identification and assessment of young children with movement difficulties. International Journal of Early Years Education 10: 157–76.

Chaminade T, Meltzoff A, Decety J (2002) Does the end justify the means? A PET exploration of the mechanisms involved in human imitation. NeuroImage 15: 318–28.

Chiel HJ, Beer RD (1997) The brain has a body: adaptive behavior emerges from interactions of nervous system, body and environment. Trends in Neuroscience 20: 553–7.

Chow MM, Choy SW, Mui SK (2003) Assessing handwriting speed of children biliterate in English and Chinese. Perceptual and Motor Skills 96: 685–94.

Cisek P (1999) Beyond the computer metaphor: behaviour as interaction. In R Nunez, WJ Freeman (eds), Reclaiming Cognition: The Primacy of Action, Intention, and Emotion. Bowling Green, OH: Imprint Academic, pp. 125–42. (Reprinted from Journal of Consciousness Studies, 1999, 6: 125–42).

Clark A (1999) Visual awareness and visuomotor action. In R Nunez, WJ Freeman (eds), Reclaiming Cognition: The Primacy of Action, Intention, and Emotion. Bowling Green, OH: Imprint Academic, pp. 1–18. (Reprinted from Journal of Consciousness Studies, 1999, 6: 1–18).

Clark JE, Moore JE (1981) Young children's ability to use precued information to select and maintain a response. Perceptual and Motor Skills 52: 655–8.

Clark JE, Phillips SJ (1993) A longitudinal study of intralimb coordination in the first year of independent walking: a dynamical systems analysis. Child Development 64: 1143–57.

Cohen DJ, Volkmar FR (eds) (1997) Handbook of Autism and Pervasive Developmental Disorders. New York: Wiley.

Cohen L, Meer J, Tarkka I et al. (1991) Congenital mirror movements. Brain 114: 381–403.

Connelly V, Hurst G (2001) The influence of handwriting fluency on writing quality in later primary and early secondary education. Handwriting Review 2: 50–6.

Conner CK (1997) Conner's Rating Scale (revised edn) (CRS-R). USA: Multi-Health Systems.

Connolly KJ (1970) Skill development: problems and plans. In KJ Connolly (ed.), Mechanisms of Motor Skill. London: Academic Press, pp. 3–17.

Connolly KJ (ed.) (1998) The Psychobiology of the Hand. London: MacKeith Press.

Connor M (1995) Handwriting performance and GCSE concessions. Handwriting Review 9: 7–21.

Cools AR, Smits-Engelsman BCM (1998) Bewegen en beweeglijkheid van het brein. In BCM Smits-Engelsman, I Ham, P van Vaes et al. (eds), Jaarboek fysiotherapie. Bohn Stafleu Van Loghum: Houten, pp. 166–83.

Cousins M, Smyth MM (2003) Developmental coordination impairments in adulthood. Human Movement Science 22: 433–59.

Crawford SG, Wilson BN, Dewey D (2001) Identifying developmental coordination disorder: consistency between tests. Physical and Occupational Therapy in Pediatrics 20: 29–50.

Cronbach LJ (1957) The two disciplines of scientific psychology. American Psychologist: 671–83.

Daly CJ, Kelley GT, Krauss A (2003) Relationship between visual-motor integration and handwriting skills of children in kindergarten: a modified replication study. American Journal of Occupational Therapy 57: 495–62.

Daniel ME, Froude E (1998) Reliability of occupational therapist and teacher evaluations of handwriting quality of grade 5 and 6 primary school children. Australian Occupational Therapy Journal 45: 48–58.

Dare MT, Gordon N (1970) Clumsy children: A disorder of perception and motor organisation. Developmental Medicine and Child Neurology 12: 178–85.

Darrah J, Hodge M, Magill-Evans J et al. (2003) Stability of serial assessments of motor and communication abilities in typically developing infants – implications for screening. Early Human Development 72: 97–110.

Darrah J, Redfern L, Maguire TO et al. (1998) Intra-individual stability of rate of gross motor development in full-term infants. Early Human Development 52: 169–79.

Davis WE, Burton AW (1991) Ecological task-analysis: translating movement behaviour theory into practice. Adapted Physical Activity Quarterly 8: 154–77.

Deci EL, Ryan RM (1985) Intrinsic motivation and self-determination in human behavior. New York: Plenum.

Denckla MB (1974) Development of motor co-ordination in normal children. Developmental Medicine and Child Neurology 16: 729–41.

Denckla MB (1983) The neuropsychology of social-emotional learning disabilities (Editorial). Archives of Neurology 40: 461–2.

Denckla MB (1984) Developmental dyspraxia: the clumsy child. In MD Levine, P Satz (eds), Middle Childhood: Development and Dysfunction. Baltimore: University Park Press, pp. 245–60.

Dennis JL, Swinth Y (2001) Pencil grasp and children's handwriting legibility during different-length writing tasks. American Journal of Occupational Therapy 55: 175–83.

Dennison P, Dennison G (2001) Brain Gym. Ventura CA: Edu-Kinesthetics Inc.

Department for Education and Skills (1997) Excellence for All Children: Meeting Special Educational Needs. London: The Stationery Office.

Department for Education and Skills (2001) Special Educational Needs Code of Practice. Annesley: DfES.

Department for Education and Skills (2003) Every Child Matters (Green Paper). London: The Stationery Office.

Department for Work and Pensions (1995) Disability Discrimination Act. London: The Stationery Office.

Department of Health (2000) Meeting the Challenge: A Strategy for Allied Health Professionals. London: Department of Health.

Department of Health (2001) The Expert Patient: A New Approach to Chronic Disease Management for the 21st Century. London: Department of Health.

Department of Health (2002) Children's Trusts. London: Department of Health.

Dewey D (1991) Praxis and sequencing skills in children with sensorimotor dysfunction. Developmental Neuropsychology 7: 197–206.

Dewey D (1993) Error analysis of limb and orofacial praxis in children with developmental motor deficits. Brain and Cognition 23: 203–21.

Dewey D (1995) What is developmental dyspraxia? Brain and Cognition 29: 254–74.

Dewey D, Kaplan BJ (1992) Analysis of praxis task demands in the assessment of children with developmental motor deficits. Developmental Neuropsychology 8: 367–79.

Dewey D, Kaplan BJ (1994) Subtyping of developmental motor deficits. Developmental Neuropsychology 10: 265–84.

Dewey D, Wilson BN (2001) Developmental Coordination Disorder: what is it? Physical and Occupational Therapy in Pediatrics 20: 5–27.

Dewey D, Kaplan BJ, Crawford SG et al. (2002) Developmental coordination disorder: associated problems in attention, learning and psychosocial adjustment. Human Movement Science 21: 905–18.

Dewey D, Roy EA, Square-Storer PA et al. (1988) Limb and oral praxic abilities in children with verbal sequencing deficits. Developmental Medicine and Child Neurology 30: 743–51.

Disability Rights Commission (2001) Special Educational Needs and Disability Act. London: The Stationery Office.

Doudlah A (1976) Motor Development Checklist. Madison, WI: Central Wisconsin Center for the Developmentally Disabled.

Doyle AJR, Elliott JM, Connolly KJ (1986) Measurement of kinaesthetic sensitivity. Developmental Medicine and Child Neurology 28: 188–93.

Drillien C, Drummond M (1983) Development screening and the child with special needs. A population study of 5000 children. Clinics in Developmental Medicine, No. 86. London: S.I.M.P. with Heinemann Medical; Philadelphia: Lippincott.

Dunford C, Richards S (2003) 'Doubly Disadvantaged' Report of a survey on waiting lists and waiting times for occupational therapy services for children with developmental coordination disorder. London: College of Occupational Therapists.

Dunford C, Street E, O'Connell H et al. (2004) Are referrals to occupational therapy for developmental co-ordination disorder appropriate? Archives of Disease in Childhood 89: 143–7.

Dunford C, Street E, Sibert JR et al. (in preparation) Developmental coordination disorder and its impact on activities of daily living for children aged 5-11 years.

Dutton KP (1991) Writing under examination conditions: establishing a baseline. Handwriting Review 2: 80–101.

Dwyer C, McKenzie BE (1994) Impairment of visual memory in children who are clumsy. Adapted Physical Activity Quarterly 11: 179–89.

Edwards A (1946) Body sway and vision. Journal of Experimental Psychology: Learning, Memory, and Cognition 36: 526–35.

Elliot JM, Connolly KJ, Doyle AJR (1988) Development of kinaesthetic sensitivity and motor performance in children. Developmental Medicine and Child Neurology 30: 80–92.

Estil LB, Ingvaldsen RP, Whiting HTA (2002) Spatial and temporal constraints on performance in children with movement co-ordination problems. Experimental Brain Research 147: 153–61.

Ferrel-Chapus C, Hay L, Olivier I et al. (2002) Visuomanual coordination in childhood: adaptation to visual distortion. Experimental Brain Research 144: 506–17.

Fily A, Truffert P, Ego A et al. (2003) Neurological assessment at five years of age in infants born preterm. Acta Paediatrica 92: 1433–7.

Fitts PM (1964) Perceptual-motor skill learning. In AW Melton (ed.), Categories of Human Learning. New York: Academic Press, pp. 243–85.

Fitts PM, Posner MI (1967) Human Performance. Belmont, CA: Brooks/Cole.

Fitzpatrick D, Watkinson EJ (2003) The lived experience of physical awkwardness: adults' retrospective views. Adapted Physical Activity Quarterly 20: 279–97.

Flanagan JR, Wing AM (1993) Modulation of grip force with load force during point-to-point arm movement. Experimental Brain Research 95: 131–43.

Flavell JJ (1979) Metacognition and cognitive monitoring: a new area of cognitive-developmental inquiry. American Psychologist 34: 906–11.

Fletcher-Flinn C, Elmes H, Stragnell D (1997) Visual-perceptual and phonological factors in the acquisition of literacy among children with congenital developmental coordination disorder. Developmental Medicine and Child Neurology 39: 158–66.

Flouris AD, Faught BE, Hay J et al. (2003) Modelling risk factors for coronary heart disease in children with developmental coordination disorder. Annals of Epidemiology 13: 555–63.

Forget R, Lamarre Y (1995) Postural adjustments associated with different unloadings of the forearm: effects of proprioceptive and cutaneous afferent deprivation. Canadian Journal of Physiology and Pharmacology 73: 285–94.

Forssberg H, Nashner L (1982) Ontogenetic development of postural control in man: adaptation to altered support and visual conditions during stance. Journal of Neuroscience 2: 545–52.

Forssberg H, Eliasson AC, Kinoshita H et al. (1991) Development of human precision grip I. Basic coordination of force. Experimental Brain Research 85: 451–7.

Forssberg H, Eliasson AC, Kinoshita H et al. (1995) Development of human precision grip. IV. Tactile adaptation of isometric finger forces to the frictional condition. Experimental Brain Research 104: 323–30.

Forssberg H, Kinoshita H, Eliasson AC et al. (1992) Development of human precision grip II. Anticipatory control of isometric forces targeted for object's weight. Experimental Brain Research 90: 393–8.

Foudriat BA, Di Fabio RP, Anderson JH (1993) Sensory organisation of balance responses in children 3–6 years of age: a normative study with diagnostic implications. International Journal of Pediatric Otorhinolaryngology 27: 255–71.

Foulder-Hughes LA, Cooke RWI (2002) Do mainstream school children who were born preterm have motor problems? British Journal of Occupational Therapy 66: 9–16.

Foulder-Hughes LA, Cooke RWI (2003) Motor, cognitive, and behavioural disorders in children born very preterm. Developmental Medicine & Child Neurology 45: 97–103.

Francis-Williams J (1976) Early identification of children likely to have specific learning difficulties: report of a follow-up. Developmental Medicine and Child Neurology 18: 71–7.

Francis-Williams J, Davies PA (1974) Very low birthweight and later intelligence. Developmental Medicine and Child Neurology 16: 700–28.

Frith U (2001) Mind blindness and the brain in autism. Neuron 32: 969–79.

Gallahue DL, Ozmun JC (1989) Childhood perception and perceptual motor development. In DL Gallahue, JC Ozmun (eds), Understanding Motor Development. Madison, WI: Brown & Benchmark Publishers, pp. 319–41.

Gallahue DL, Ozmun JC (1995) Understanding Motor Development: Infants, Children, Adolescents, Adults. Madison, WI: W.C. Brown.

Garmoyle J (2003) Identifying slow writers; an examination of methods and norms in Key Stage 2. Unpublished Masters dissertation, Institute of Education, University of London.

Gentilucci M, Toni I, Chieffi S et al. (1994) The role of proprioception in the control of movements: a kinematic study in a peripherally deafferented patient and in normal subjects. Experimental Brain Research 99: 483–500.

Gernsbacher MA, Goldsmith HH (2000) Toward a dyspraxic subtype of Autism Spectrum Disorder: a research hypothesis. Editorial Review 1–14.

Gesell A (1946) The ontogenesis of infant behaviour. In L Carmichael (ed.), Manual of Child Psychology. New York: Wiley, pp. 295–331.

Geuze RH (2003) Static balance problems in children with Developmental Coordination Disorder. Human Movement Science 22: 527–48.

Geuze RH (in press) Characteristics of DCD: on problems and prognosis. In RH Geuze (ed.), Developmental Coordination Disorder A Review of Current Approaches. Collection Psychomotricité. Marseille: Solal Éditeurs.

Geuze RH, Börger JMA (1993) Children who are clumsy, five years later. Adapted Physical Activity Quarterly 10: 10–21.

Geuze RH, Börger H (1994) Response selection in clumsy children: Five years later. Journal of Human Movement Studies 27: 1-15.

Geuze RH, Kalverboer AF (1987) Inconsistency and adaptation in timing of clumsy children. Journal of Human Movement Studies 13: 421–32.

Geuze RH, Kalverboer AF (1994) Tapping a rhythm: a problem of timing for children who are clumsy and dyslexic? Adapted Physical Activity Quarterly 11: 203–13.

Geuze RH, van Dellen T (1990) Auditory precue processing during a movement sequence in clumsy children. Journal of Human Movement Studies 19: 11–24.

Geuze RH, Jongmans MJ, Schoemaker MM et al. (2001) Clinical and research diagnostic criteria for Developmental Coordination Disorder; a review and discussion. Human Movement Science 20: 7–47.

Gibson EJ, Pick AD (2000) An Ecological Approach to Perceptual Learning and Development. New York: Oxford University Press.

Gibson JJ (1966) The Senses Considered as Perceptual Systems. Boston: Houghton Mifflin Company.

Gibson JJ (1977) The theory of affordances. In R Shaw, J Bransford (eds), Perceiving, Acting and Knowing: Toward an Ecological Psychology. Hillsdale, NJ: Lawrence Erlbaum Associates, Inc. pp. 67–82.

Gibson JJ (1979) The Ecological Approach to Visual Perception. Boston: Houghton Mifflin Company.

Gillberg C (1983) Perceptual, motor and attentional deficits in Swedish primary school children: some child psychiatric aspects. Journal of Child Psychology and Psychiatry 24: 377–403.

Gilberg C (1998a) Asperger syndrome and high-functioning autism. British Journal of Psychiatry 172: 200–9.

Gillberg C (1998b) Hyperactivity, inattention and motor control problems: prevalence, comorbidity and background factors. Folia Phoniatrica et Logopaedica 50: 107–17.

Gillberg C, Rasmussen P (1982a) Perceptual, motor and attentional deficits in six-year-old children: screening procedure in pre-school. Acta Paedatrica Scandinavica 71: 121–9.

Gillberg C, Rasmussen P (1982b) Perceptual, motor and attentional deficits in seven-year-old children: background factors. Developmental Medicine and Child Neurology 24: 752–70.

Gillberg C, Carlström G, Rasmussen P (1983) Hyperkinetic disorders in seven-year-old children with perceptual, motor and attentional deficits. Journal of Child Psychology and Psychiatry 24: 233–46.

Gillberg C, Carlström G, Rasmussen P et al. (1983) Perceptual, motor and attentional deficits in seven-year-old children: neurological screening aspects. Acta Paedatrica Scandinavica 72: 119–24.

Gillberg C, Rasmussen P, Carlström G et al. (1982) Perceptual, motor and attentional deficits in six-year-old children: epidemiological aspects. Journal of Child Psychology and Psychiatry 23: 131–44.

Gillberg IC, Gillberg C (1983) Three years follow-up at age 10 of children with minor neurodevelopmental disorders. I: Behavioural problems. Developmental Medicine and Child Neurology 25: 438–49.

Gillberg IC, Gillberg C (1988) Generalised hyperkinesis: follow-up study from age 7 to 13 years. Journal of the American Academy of Child and Adolescent Psychiatry 27: 55–9.

Gillberg IC, Gillberg C (1989) Children with preschool minor neurodevelopmental disorders. IV: Behavioural and school achievement at age 13. Developmental Medicine and Child Neurology 31: 3–13.

Gillberg IC, Gillberg C, Groth J (1989) Children with preschool minor neurodevelopmental disorders. V: Neurodevelopmental profiles at age 13. Developmental Medicine and Child Neurology 31: 14–24.

Gillberg IC, Gillberg C, Rasmussen P (1983) Three-year follow-up at age 10 of children with minor neurodevelopmental disorders, II: school achievement problems. Developmental Medicine and Child Neurology 25: 566–73.

Glascoe FP (2001) Are overreferrals on developmental screening test really a problem? Archives of Pediatric and Adolescent Medicine 155: 54–9.

Goodale M, Jakobson LS, Servos P (1996) The visual pathways mediating perception and prehension. In AM Wing, P Haggard, JR Flanagan (eds), Hand and Brain. London: Academic Press, pp. 15–32.

Goodgold-Edwards SA (1984) Motor learning as it relates to the development of skilled motor behavior: a review of the literature. Physical and Occupational Therapy in Pediatrics 4: 5–18.

Goodman R (1997) The Strengths and Difficulties Questionnaire: a research note. Journal of Child Psychology and Psychiatry 38: 581–6.

Goodman R (2001) Psychometric properties of the Strengths and Difficulties Questionnaire. Journal of the American Academy of Child and Adolescent Psychiatry 40: 1137–1345.

Goodway JD, Branta C (2003) Influence of a motor skill intervention on fundamental motor skill development of disadvantaged preschoolers. Research Quarterly for Exercise and Sport 74: 36–46.

Goodway JD, Crowe H, Ward P (2003) Effects of motor skill instruction on fundamental motor skill development. Adapted Physical Activity Quarterly 20: 298–314.

Gordon N (1969) Helping the clumsy child in school. Special Education 58: 19–20.

Goswami U (2002) Rhymes, phonemes and learning to read: interpreting recent research. In M Cook (ed.), Perspectives on the Teaching and Learning of Phonics. Royston: United Kingdom Reading Association, pp. 41–60.

Goyen EA, Lui K, Woods R (1998) Visual-motor, visual perceptual and fine motor outcomes in very low birthweight children at 5 years. Developmental Medicine and Child Neurology 40: 76–81.

Graham S (1986) The reliability, validity and utility of three handwriting measurement procedures. Journal of Educational Research 79: 373–80.

Graham S, Weintraub N (1996) A review of handwriting research: progress and prospects from 1980 to 1994. Educational Psychology Review 8: 7–87.

Graham S, Berninger V, Abbott R et al. (1997) Role of mechanics in composing of elementary school students: a new methodological approach. Journal of Educational Psychology 89: 170–82.

Graham S, Berninger V, Weintraub N (1998) The relationship between handwriting style and speed and legibility. Journal of Educational Research 5: 290–6.

Graham S, Berninger V, Weintraub N et al. (1998) The development of handwriting fluency and legibility in grades 1 through 9. Journal of Educational Research 92: 42–52.

Graham S, Boyer-Schick K, Tippets E (1989) The validity of the handwriting scale from the Test of Written Language. Journal of Educational Research 82: 166–71.

Green D, Archer J (2000) Audit of a therapist training scheme of sensory integrative therapy. SENSOR NET 11: 7–14.

Green D, Arscott C, Barnett A et al. (in preparation) A preliminary report comparing the self-perception of social and motor competence of children with specific developmental disorder of motor function and those with Asperger's syndrome.

Green D, Baird G, Barnett AL et al. (2002) The severity and nature of motor impairment in Asperger's Syndrome: a comparison with specific developmental disorder of motor function. Journal of Child Psychology and Psychiatry 43: 1–14.

Green D, Baird G, Sugden D (submitted) A pilot study of emotional/behavioural problems in developmental coordination disorder. Archives of Disease in Childhood.

Green D, Bishop T, Sugden D (2004) The prevalence of handwriting problems amongst children identified with DCD. DCD Research. UK Conference, Lady Margaret Hall, Oxford.

Green D, Bishop T, Wilson B et al. (in press) Is questionnaire-based screening part of the solution to waiting lists for children with developmental coordination disorder? British Journal of Occupational Therapy.

Greydanus DE, Pratt HD, Sloane MA et al. (2003) Attention-deficit/hyperactivity disorder in children and adolescents: interventions for a complex costly clinical conundrum. Pediatric Clinics of North America 50: 1049–92.

Griffin NS, Keogh JF (1982) A model of movement confidence. In JAS Kelso, JE Clarke (eds), The Development of Movement Control and Coordination. New York: Wiley, pp. 213–36.

Griffiths R (1967) Griffiths Mental Development Scales for Testing Babies and Young Children from Birth to Eight Years of Age. Amersham, Bucks: Association of Research in Infant Development.

Gubbay SS (1975a) The Clumsy Child. London: Saunders & Co.

Gubbay SS (1975b) Clumsy children in normal schools. The Medical Journal of Australia 1: 233–6.

Gubbay SS, Ellis E, Walton JN et al. (1965) Clumsy children. A study of apraxic and agnosic defects in 21 children. Brain 88: 295–312.

Guedon O, Gauthier G, Cole J et al. (1998) Adaptation in visuomanual tracking depends on intact proprioception. Journal of Motor Behavior 30: 234–48.

Haas W (ed.) (1976) Writing Without Letters. Manchester: Manchester University Press.

Hadders-Algra M (1999) Differentiation of developmental coordination disorder with the help of a standardized neurological assessment. DCD IV International Conference, Groningen, The Netherlands.

Hadders-Algra M (2000) The neuronal group selection theory: promising principles for understanding and treating developmental motor disorders. Developmental Medicine and Child Neurology 42: 707–15.

Hadders-Algra M (2002) Two distinct forms of minor neurological dysfunction: perspectives emerging from a review of data of the Groningen Perinatal Project. Developmental Medicine and Child Neurology 44: 561–71.

Hadders-Algra M (2003) Developmental coordination disorder: is clumsy motor behavior caused by a lesion of the brain at early age? Neural Plasticity 10: 39–50.

Hadders-Algra M, Groothuis AM (1999) Quality of general movements in infancy is related to neurological dysfunction, ADHD and aggressive behaviour. Developmental Medicine and Child Neurology 41: 381–91.

Hadders-Algra M, Lindahl E (1999) Pre- and perinatal precursors of specific learning disorders. In K Whitmore, H Hart, G Willems (eds), A Neurodevelopmental Approach to Specific Learning Disorders. Suffolk: MacKeith Press.

Hadders-Algra M, Huisjes HJ, Touwen BCL (1988a) Perinatal correlates of major and minor neurological dysfunction at school age: a multivariate analysis. Developmental Medicine and Child Neurology 30: 472–81.

Hadders-Algra M, Huisjes HJ, Touwen BCL (1988b) Perinatal risk factors and minor neurological dysfunction: significance for behaviour and school achievement at nine years. Developmental Medicine and Child Neurology 30: 482–91.

Hadders-Algra M, Touwen BCL, Huisjes HJ (1986) Neurologically deviant newborns: Neurological and behavioural developmental at the age of six years. Developmental Medicine and Child Neurology 28: 569–78.

Hadders-Algra M, Touwen BCL, Olinga AA et al. (1985) Minor neurological dysfunction and behavioural development: a report from the Groningen perinatal project. Early Human Development 11: 221–9.

Haley SM, Coster WJ, Ludlow LH (1991) Pediatric functional outcome measures. Physical Medicine and Rehabilitation Clinics of North America 2: 689–723.

Haley SM, Coster WJ, Ludlow LH et al. (1992) Pediatric Evaluation of Disability Inventory (PEDI). Boston: New England Medical Center Hospitals.

Hall A, McCleod A, Counsell C et al. (1995) School attainment, cognitive ability and motor function in a Scottish very low birthweight population at eight years: a controlled study. Developmental Medicine and Child Neurology 37: 1037–50.

Hall DMB (1988) Clumsy children. British Medical Journal 296: 375–6.

Hamill DD, Pearson NA, Voress JK (1993) Developmental Test of Visual Perception (2nd edn), Austin, TX: Pro-Ed.

Hamilton SS (2002) Evaluation of clumsiness in children. American Family Physician 66: 1435–40.

Hamstra-Bletz E, DeBie J, Den Brinker BPLM (1987) Beknopte beoordelingsmethode voor kinderhandschriften [The concise assessment method for children's handwriting]. Lisse: Swets and Zeitlinger.

Hands B, Larkin D (1997) Gender bias in measurement of movement. ACHPER Healthy Lifestyles Journal 44: 12–16.

Hands B, Larkin D (2001a) Developmental Coordination Disorder: a discrete disability. New Zealand Journal of Disability Studies 9: 93–105.

Hands B, Larkin D (2001b) Using the Rasch model to investigate the construct of motor ability in young children. Journal of Applied Measurement 2: 101–20.

Hands B, Larkin D (2002) Physical fitness and developmental coordination disorder. In SA Cermak, D Larkin (eds), Developmental Coordination Disorder. Albany, NY: Delmar, pp. 172–84.

Harris SJ, Livesey DJ (1992) Improving handwriting through kinesthetic sensitivity practice. Australian Occupational Therapy Journal 39: 23–7.

Harter S (1981) The development of competence and motivation in the mastery of cognitive and physical skills: is there still a place for joy? In GC Roberts, DM Landers (eds), Psychology of Motor Behaviour and Sport. Champaign, IL: Human Kinetics, pp. 3–29.

Harter S (1982) The perceived competence scale for children. Child Development 53: 87–97.

Harter S (1985) Manual for the Self-Perception Profile for Children: Revision of the Perceived Competence Scale for Children. Denver: University of Denver.

Harter S, Pike R (1984) The pictorial scale of perceived competence and social acceptance for young children. Child Development 55: 1969–82.

Harvey C, Henderson SE (1997) Children's handwriting in the first three years of school: consistency over time and its relationship to academic achievement. Handwriting Review 11: 8–25.

Hatzataki V, Zisi V, Kollias I et al. (2002) Perceptual-motor contributions to static and dynamic balance control in children. Journal of Motor Behavior 34: 161–70.

Hay L (1979) Spatial-temporal analysis of movements in children: motor programs versus feedback in the development of reaching. Journal of Motor Behavior 11: 189–200.

Hayes JR, Flower LS (1980) Identifying the organisation of the writing process. In LW Gregg, ER Steinberg (eds), Cognitive Processes in Writing. Hillsdale, NJ: Erlbaum, pp. 3–30.

Haywood KM, Getchell N (2001) Life Span Motor Development. Champaign, IL: Human Kinetics.

Heiberger DM, Heiniger-White MC (2000) S'cool Moves for Learning: A Program Designed to Enhance Learning through Body–Mind Integration. Integrated Learner Press, USA.

Hellgren L, Gillberg CI, Bagenholm A et al. (1994) Children with deficits in attention, motor control and perception (DAMP) almost grown up: psychiatric and personality disorders at age 16 years. Journal of Child Psychiatry and Psychology 35: 1255–71.

Hellgren L, Gillberg C, Gillberg IC et al. (1993) Children with deficits in attention, motor control and perception (DAMP) almost grown up. General health at age 16 years. Developmental Medicine and Child Neurology 35: 881–92.

Henderson L (1982) Orthographic and Word Recognition in Reading. London: Academic Press.

Henderson L, Rose P, Henderson SE (1992) Reaction time and movement time in children with a developmental coordination disorder. Journal of Child Psychology and Psychiatry 33: 895–905.

Henderson SE (1992) Clumsiness or developmental coordination disorder: a neglected handicap. Current Paediatrics 2: 158–62.

Henderson SE (1993) Motor development and minor handicap. In AF Kalverboer, B Hopkins, R Geuze (eds), Motor Development in Early and Later Childhood. Cambridge: Cambridge University Press, pp. 286–306.

Henderson SE (1994) Editorial. Adapted Physical Activity Quarterly 11: 111–14.

Henderson SE, Barnett AL (1998) The classification of specific motor coordination disorders in children: some problems to be solved. Human Movement Science 17: 449–69.

Henderson SE, Green D (2001) Handwriting problems in children with Asperger's syndrome. Handwriting Review 2: 65–79.

Henderson SE, Hall D (1982) Concomitants of clumsiness in young schoolchildren. Developmental Medicine and Child Neurology 24: 448–60.

Henderson SE, Henderson L (2002) Towards an understanding of developmental coordination disorders. The Second G Lawrence Rarick Memorial Lecture. Adapted Physical Activity Quarterly 19: 11–31.

Henderson SE, Sugden DA (1992) Movement Assessment Battery for Children. London: The Psychological Corporation.

Henderson SE, Barnett AL, Henderson L (1994) Visuospatial difficulties and clumsiness: on the interpretation of conjoined deficits. Journal of Child Psychology and Psychiatry 35: 961–9.

Henderson SE, Knight E, Losse A et al. (1991) The clumsy child in school – are we doing enough? British Journal of Physical Education 9 (Research Supplement): 2–9.

Henderson SE, Markee A, Scheib B et al. (1999) Tools of the Trade. London: The Handwriting Interest Group.

Henderson SE, May DS, Umney M (1989) An exploratory study of goal-setting behaviour, self-concept and locus of control in children with movement difficulties. European Journal of Special Needs Education 4: 1–15.

Henry FM (1961) Reaction time–movement time correlations. Perceptual and Motor Skills 12: 63–6.

Hill EL (1998) A dyspraxic deficit in specific language impairment and developmental coordination disorder? Evidence from hand and arm movements. Developmental Medicine and Child Neurology 40: 388–95.

Hill EL (2001) Non-specific nature of specific language impairment: a review of the literature with regard to concomitant motor impairments. International Journal of Language & Communication Disorders 36: 149–71.

Hill EL, Wing AM (1998) Developmental disorders and the use of grip force to compensate for inertial forces during voluntary movement. In KC Connolly (ed.), The Psychobiology of the Hand. London: MacKeith Press, pp.199–212.

Hill EL, Wing AM (1999) Coordination of grip force and load force in developmental coordination disorder: a case study. Neurocase 5: 537–44.

Hill EL, Bishop DVM, Nimmo-Smith I (1998) Representational gestures in developmental co-ordination disorder and specific language impairment: error-types and the reliability of ratings. Human Movement Science 17: 655–78.

Hinojosa J, Sproat CT, Mankhetwit S et al. (2002) Shifts in parent–therapist partnerships: twelve years of change. American Journal of Occupational Therapy 56: 556–63.

Hoare D (1991) Classification of movement dysfunctions in children: descriptive and statistical approaches. Unpublished doctoral thesis. University of Western Australia, Nedlands, W. Australia.

Hoare D (1994) Subtypes of developmental coordination disorder. Adapted Physical Activity Quarterly 11: 158–69.

Hoare D, Larkin D (1991) Kinaesthetic abilities of clumsy children. Developmental Medicine and Child Neurology 33: 671–8.

Holsti L, Grunau RVE, Whitfield MF (2002) Developmental coordination disorder in extremely low birthweight children at nine years. Developmental and Behavioral Pediatrics 23: 9–15.

Horn TS (1987) The influence of teacher-coach behavior on the psychological development of children. In D Gould, MR Weiss (eds), Advances in Pediatric Sport Science: Vol. 2. Behavioral issues. Champaign, IL: Human Kinetics, pp. 121–41.

Howlin P (2000) Assessment instruments for Asperger Syndrome. Child Psychology & Psychiatry Review 5: 120–9.

Hughes C (1996) Brief report: planning problems in autism at the level of motor control. Journal of Autism and Developmental Disorders 26: 101–9.

Hulme C, Biggerstaff A, Moran G et al. (1982) Visual, kinaesthetic and cross-modal judgements of length by normal and clumsy children. Developmental Medicine and Child Neurology 24: 461–71.

Hulme C, Smart A, Moran G (1982) Visual perceptual deficits in clumsy children. Neuropsychologica 20: 475–81.

Hulme C, Smart A, Moran G et al. (1983) Visual, kinaesthetic and crossmodal development: relationships to motor skill development. Perception 12: 477–83.

Hulme C, Smart A, Moran G et al. (1984) Visual, kinaesthetic and cross-modal judgements of length by clumsy children: a comparison with young normal children. Child: Care, Health and Development 10: 117–25.

Humphries T, Wright M, McDougall B et al. (1990) The efficacy of sensory integration therapy for children with learning disability. Physical and Occupational Therapy in Pediatrics 10: 1–17.

Hurt H, Brodsky NL, Betancourt L et al. (1995) Cocaine-exposed children: follow-up through 30 months. Developmental and Behavioral Pediatrics 16: 29–35.

Hutton JL, Pharoah P, Cooke RWI et al. (1997) Differential effects of preterm birth and small gestational age on cognitive and motor development. Archives of Disease in Childhood 76: 75–81.

Illingworth RS (1968) Delayed motor development. Pediatric Clinics of North America 15: 569–80.

Iloeje SE (1987) Developmental apraxia among Nigerian children in Enugu, Nigeria. Developmental Medicine and Child Neurology 29: 502–7.

Ivry RR, Keele SW (1989) Timing functions of the cerebellum. Journal of Cognitive Neuroscience 1: 136–52.

Johnston LM, Burns YR, Brauer SG et al. (2002) Differences in postural control and movement performance during goal directed reaching in children with developmental coordination disorder. Human Movement Science 21: 583–601.

Johnston O, Short H, Crawford J (1987) Poorly coordinated children: a survey of 95 cases. Child: Care, Health and Development 13: 361–76.

Jones V, Prior MR (1985) Motor imitation abilities and neurological signs in autistic children. Journal of Autism and Developmental Disorders 15: 37–46.

Jongmans MJ (1994) Perceptuo-motor competence in prematurely born children at school age: neurological and psychological aspects. Unpublished doctoral dissertation, Institute of Education, University of London.

Jongmans MJ, Demetre JD, Dubowitz L et al. (1996) How local is the impact of a specific learning difficulty on premature children's evaluation of their own competence? Journal of Child Psychology and Psychiatry 37: 565–8.

Jongmans MJ, Henderson S, de Vries L et al. (1993) Duration of periventricular densities in preterm infants and neurological outcome at 6 years of age. Archives of Disease in Childhood 69: 9–13.

Jongmans MJ, Linthorst-Bakker E, Westenberg Y et al. (in press) Use of a task-oriented self-instruction method to support children in primary school with poor handwriting quality and speed. Human Movement Science.

Jongmans MJ, Mercuri E, Dubowitz LMS et al. (1998) Perceptual-motor difficulties and their concomitants in six-year-old children born prematurely. Human Movement Science 17: 629–53.

Jongmans MJ, Oomen A, Hoop A (2002) Measuring executive function in children with DCD: influence of manual dexterity on performance on the Tower of London task. DCD-V Conference Proceedings, Banff, Canada.

Jongmans MJ, Smits-Engelsman BCM, Schoemaker M (2003) Consequences of comorbidity of developmental coordination disorders and learning disabilities for severity and pattern of perceptual-motor dysfunction. Journal of Learning Disabilities 36: 528–37.

Junaid K, Harris S, Fulmer A et al. (2000) Teachers' use of the MABC checklist to identify children with motor difficulties. Pediatric Physical Therapy 12: 158–63.

Kadesjö B, Gillberg C (1999a) Attention deficits and clumsiness in Swedish 7-year-old children. Developmental Medicine and Child Neurology 40: 796–804.

Kadesjö B, Gillberg C (1999b) Developmental coordination disorder in Swedish 7-year-old children. Journal of American Academy of Child and Adolescent Psychiatry 38: 820–8.

Kakebeeke TH, Jongmans MJ, Dubowitz LM et al. (1993) Some aspects of the reliability of Touwen's examination of the child with minor neurological dysfunction. Developmental Medicine and Child Neurology 35: 1097–1105.

Kaplan BJ, Crawford SG, Wilson BN et al. (1997) Comorbidity of developmental coordination disorder and different types of reading disability. Journal of the International Neuropsychological Society 3: 54.

Kaplan BJ, Dewey D, Crawford S et al. (2001) The term co-morbidity is of questionable value in reference to developmental disorders: data and theory. Journal of Learning Disabilities 34: 555–65.

Kaplan BJ, Polatajko HJ, Wilson BN et al. (1993) Re-examination of sensory integration therapy: a combination of two efficacy studies. Journal of Learning Disabilities 26: 342–7.

Kaplan BJ, Wilson BN, Dewey D et al. (1998) DCD may not be a discrete disorder. Human Movement Science 17: 471–90.

Kaplan E (1968) Gestural representation of implement usage: an organismic developmental study. Unpublished doctoral thesis, Clarke University.

Karlsdottir R, Stefansson T (2002) Problems in developing functional handwriting. Perceptual and Motor Skills 94: 623–62.

Karmiloff-Smith A (1998) Development itself is the key to understanding developmental disorders. Trends in Cognitive Sciences 2: 389–98.

Kavale KA, Forness SR (1995) The Nature of Learning Disabilities. New Jersey: Lawrence Erlbaum Associates.

Kavale KA, Mattson PD (1983) 'One jumped off the balance beam': meta-analysis of perceptual-motor training. Journal of Learning Disabilities 16: 165–73.

Kavale KA, Nye C (1985–86) Parameters of learning disabilities in achievement, linguistic, neuropsychological, and social/behavioural domains. Journal of Special Education 19: 443–58.

Keele SW, Ivry R (1990) Does the cerebellum provide a common computation for diverse tasks? A timing hypothesis. In A Diamond (ed.), The Development and Neural Basis of Higher Cognitive Functions. New York: NYAS Press.

Kelso JAS (1988) Dynamic patterns. In JAS Kelso, AJ Mandell, MF Shlesinger (eds), Dynamic Patterns in Complex Systems. Singapore: World Scientific.

Kelso JAS, Tuller B (1984) A dynamical basis for action systems. In MS Gazzaniga (ed.), Handbook of Cognitive Neuroscience. New York: Plenum, pp. 321–56.

Keogh BJ (1982) The study of motor learning disabilities. In J Das, R Mulcahy, AE Wall (eds), Theory and Research in Learning Disabilities. New York: Plenum Press, pp. 237–51.

Keogh JF, Sugden DA (1985) Movement Skill Development. New York: Macmillan.

Keogh JF, Sugden DA, Reynard CL et al. (1979) Identification of clumsy children: comparisons and comments. Journal of Human Movement Studies 5: 32–51.

Kimura D, Archibald Y (1974) Motor functions of the left hemisphere. Brain 97: 337–50.

Kirby A, Drew SA (1999) Is DCD a diagnosis that we should be using for adults? DCD IV International Conference, Groningen, The Netherlands.

Kirby A, Davies R, Bryant A (in preparation) Health and educational professional awareness of specific learning difficulties – is there a need for training?

Kirby A, Drew SA, Jones N (2002) Integrated intervention for children with DCD: from theory into practice. DCD V International Conference, Banff, Alberta, Canada.

Klin A, Volkmar FR, Sparrow SS et al. (1995) Validity and neuropsychological characterization of Asperger's syndrome: convergence with non-verbal learning disabilities syndrome. Journal of Child Psychology and Psychiatry 36: 1127–39.

Knuckey NW, Gubbay SS (1983) Clumsy children: a prognostic study. Australian Paediatric Journal 19: 9–13.

Knudson DV, Morrison CS (1997) Qualitative Analysis of Human Movement. Champaign, IL: Human Kinetics.

Kooistra L, Snijders T, Schellekens JMH et al. (1997) Timing variability in early treated congenital hypothyroidism. Acta Psychologica 96: 61–73.

Kools JA, Tweedie D (1975) Development of praxis in children. Perceptual and Motor Skills 40: 11–19.

Korkman M, Kemp SL, Kirk U (2001) Effects of age on neurocognitive measures of children ages 5 to 12: a cross-sectional study on 800 children from the United States. Developmental Neuropsychology 20: 331–54.

Kugler PN, Turvey MT (1987) Information, Natural Law and the Self Assembly of Natural Movements. Hillsdale, NJ: Erlbaum.

Kugler PN, Kelso JAS, Turvey MT (1980) On the concept of coordinative structures as dissipative structures: I. Theoretical lines of convergence. In GE Stelmach, J Requin (eds), Tutorials in Motor Behavior. Amsterdam: Elsevier Science.

Kugler PN, Kelso JAS, Turvey MT (1982) On the control and co-ordination of naturally developing systems. In JAS Kelso, JE Clark (eds), The Development of Movement Control and Co-ordination. New York: John Wiley & Sons Ltd, pp. 5–78.

Kulp MT, Sortor JM (2003) Clinical value of the Beery visual-motor integration supplemental tests of visual perception and motor coordination. Optomology and Visual Science 80: 312–15.

Lajoie Y, Paillard J, Teasdale N et al. (1992) Mirror drawing in a deafferented patient and normal subjects: visuoproprioceptive conflict. Neurology 42: 1104–6.

Landgren M, Pettersson R, Kjellman B et al. (1996) ADHD, DAMP and other neurodevelopmental/psychiatric disorders in 6-year-old children: epidemiology and co-morbidity. Developmental Medicine and Child Neurology 38: 891–906.

Landrum M, Imbeau M, Hunsaker SL et al. (1995) Preservice teacher preparation in meeting the needs of gifted and other academically diverse students. (Research Monograph 95134). Storrs, CT: The National Research Center on the Gifted and Talented, University of Connecticut.

Largo RH, Fischer JE, Caflisch JA (eds) (2002) Zurich Neuromotor Assessment. Zurich: AWE Verlag.

Largo RH, Fischer JE, Rousson V (2003) Neuromotor development from kindergarten age to adolescence: developmental course and variability. Swiss Medical Weekly 133: 193–9.

Larkin D, Cermak SA (2002) Issues in identification and assessment of developmental coordination disorder. In SA Cermak, D Larkin (eds), Developmental Coordination Disorder. Albany, NY: Delmar, pp. 86–102.

Larkin D, Hoare D (1991) Out of step: coordinating kids' movement. Human Movement Studies, UWA. Nedlands: Active Life Foundation.

Larkin D, Parker H (2002) Task specific intervention for children for children with developmental coordination disorder: a systems view. In S Cermak, D Larkin (eds), Developmental Coordination Disorder. Albany, NY: Delmar, pp. 234–47.

Larkin D, Revie G (1994) Stay in Step: A Gross Motor Screening Test for Children K-2. Sydney, Australia: published by authors.

Larkin, D, Rose B (1999) Use of the McCarron Assessment of Neuromuscular Development for DCD identification. Paper presented at the 4th Biennial Workshop on Children with a Developmental Coordination Disorder, Groningen, The Netherlands.

Larkin D, Hoare D, Phillips S et al. (1988) Children with impaired coordination: kinematic profiles of jumping and hopping movements. In D Jones, T Cuddihy (eds), Progress through Refinement and Innovation. Proceedings of the 6th International Symposium of Adapted Physical Activity. Brisbane: Brisbane CAE Press.

Larkin D, Hoare D, Smith K (1989) Understanding and Teaching Children with Movement Dysfunction. Nedlands, Western Australia: Department of Human Movement and Recreational Studies.

Larsen S, Hammill D (1989) Test of Legible Handwriting. Austin, TX: Pro-Ed.

Laszlo JI, Bairstow P (1983) Kinaesthesis: its measurement, training and relationship to motor control. Quarterly Journal of Experimental Psychology 35: 411–21.

Laszlo JI, Bairstow P (1985a) Perceptual-motor Behaviour: Development, Assessment and Therapy. London: Holt, Rinehart & Winston.

Laszlo JI, Bairstow PJ (1985b) Test of Kinaesthetic Sensitivity. London: Senkit PTY in association with Holt, Rinehart & Winston.

Laszlo JI, Sainsbury KM (1993) Perceptual-motor development and prevention of clumsiness. Psychological Research 55: 167–74.

Laszlo JI, Bairstow PJ, Bartrip J (1988) A new approach to treatment of perceptuo-motor dysfunction: previously called 'clumsiness'. Support for Learning 3: 35–40.

Laszlo JI, Bairstow PJ, Bartrip J et al. (1988) Clumsiness or perceptuo-motor dysfunction? In A Colley, J Beech (eds), Cognition and Action in Skilled Behaviour. Amsterdam: North Holland, pp. 293–316.

Latash ML, Nicholas JJ (1996) Motor control research in rehabilitation medicine. Disability & Rehabilitation 18: 293–9.

Law M, King S, Stewart D et al. (2001) The perceived effects of parent-led support groups for parents of children with disabilities. Physical and Occupational Therapy in Pediatrics 21: 29–48.

Law M, Polatajko H, Schaffer R et al. (1991) The impact of heterogeneity in a clinical trial: motor outcomes after sensory integration therapy. Occupational Therapy Journal of Research 11: 177–89.

Lee DN (1980) The optic flow field: the foundation of vision. Philos Trans R Soc Lond B Biol Sci 290: 169–79.

Lee DN, Aronson E (1974) Visual proprioceptive control of standing in human infants. Perception and Psychophysics 15: 529–32.

Lee DN, Young DS, McLaughlin CM (1984) A roadside simulation of road crossing for children. Ergonomics 27: 1271–81.

Leemrijse C, Meijer OG, Vermeer A et al. (2000) The efficacy of Le Bon Depart and sensory integration treatment for children with developmental coordination disorder: a randomized study with six single cases. Clinical Rehabilitation 14: 247–59.

Levene M, Dowling S, Graham M et al. (1992) Impaired motor function (clumsiness) in 5 year old children: correlation with neonatal ultrasound scans. Archives of Disease in Childhood 67: 687–90.

Lindstrom K, Bremberg S (1997) The contribution of developmental surveillance to early detection of cerebral palsy. Acta Paediatrica 86: 736–9.

Liu L, Miyazaki M (2000) Telerehabilitation at the University of Alberta. Journal of Telemedicine and Telecare 6: 47–9.

Lord R, Hulme C (1987a) Perceptual judgements of normal and clumsy children. Developmental Medicine and Child Neurology 29: 250–7.

Lord R, Hulme C (1987b) Kinaesthetic sensitivity of normal and clumsy children. Developmental Medicine and Child Neurology 29: 720–5.

Lord R, Hulme C (1988a) Patterns of rotary pursuit performance in clumsy and normal children. Journal of Child Psychology and Psychiatry 29: 691–701.

Lord R, Hulme C (1988b) Visual perception and drawing ability in clumsy and normal children. British Journal of Developmental Psychology 6: 1–9.

Losse A, Henderson SE, Elliman D et al. (1991) Clumsiness in children – do they grow out of it? A 10-year follow up study. Developmental Medicine and Child Neurology 33: 55–68.

Lundy-Ekman L, Ivry R, Keele S et al. (1991) Timing and force control deficits in clumsy children. Journal of Cognitive Neuroscience 3: 367–76.

Lunsing RJ, Hadders-Algra M, Huisjes HJ et al. (1992a) Minor neurological dysfunction from birth to 12 years. I: Increase during late school-age. Developmental Medicine and Child Neurology 34: 399–403.

Lunsing RJ, Hadders-Algra,M, Huisjes HJ et al. (1992b) Minor neurological dysfunction from birth to 12 years, II: Puberty is related to decreased dysfunction. Developmental Medicine and Child Neurology 34: 404–9.

Luoma L, Herrgard E, Martikainen A (1998) Neuropsychological analysis of the visuomotor problems in children born preterm at ≤ 32 weeks of gestation: a 5-year prospective follow-up. Developmental Medicine & Child Neurology 40: 21–30.

Lyytinen H, Ahonen T (1988) Developmental motor problems in children: a 6-year longitudinal study. Journal of Clinical and Experimental Neuropsychology 10: 57.

McCarron LT (1982) MAND – McCarron Assessment of Neuromuscular Development (revised edn). Dallas, TX: Common Market Press.

McCloy CH (1934) The measurement of general motor capacity and general motor ability. Research Quarterly 5: 46–61.

McConaughy SH, Achenbach TM (1994) Comorbidity of empirically based syndromes in matched general population and clinical samples. Journal of Child Psychology and Psychiatry 35: 1141–57.

McGovern R (1991) Developmental dyspraxia: or just plain clumsy? Early Years 12: 37–8.

McGraw MB (1945) The Neuromuscular Maturation of the Human Infant. New York: Columbia University Press.

MacKeith R, Bax M (eds) (1963) Minimal cerebral dysfunction: papers from the international study group held at Oxford, September 1962. London: National Spastics Society in association with William Heinemann.

Macnab J (2003) Healthy development in childhood: the role of child factors, family factor, and parenting practices in the prediction of cognitive competence and behavioural dysfunction at school age. Unpublished doctoral dissertation, University of Western Ontario, Western Ontario, Canada.

Macnab JJ, Miller LT, Polatajko HJ (2001) The search for subtypes of DCD: is cluster analysis the answer? Human Movement Science 20: 49–72.

Maeland AF (1992) Identification of children with motor coordination problems. Adapted Physical Activity Quarterly 9: 330–42.

Maeland AF (1994) Self esteem in children with motor coordination problems (clumsy children). Handwriting Review 8: 128–33.

Maeland AF, Karlsdottir R (1991) Development of reading, spelling and writing skills from third to sixth grade in normal and dysgraphic school children. In J Wann, AM Wing, N Sovik (eds), Development of Graphic Skills. London: Academic Press, pp. 179–84.

Magill RA (2001) Motor Learning: Concepts and Applications (6th edn). Madison, WI: McGraw-Hill.

Magyary D, Brandt P (2002) A decision tree and clinical paths for the assessment and management of children with ADHD. Issues of Mental Health Nursing 23: 553–66.

Mandal AC (1985) The Seated Man. Copenhagen: Dafnia.

Mandich A (1997) Cognitive strategies and motor performance in children with developmental coordination disorder. Unpublished master's thesis, University of Western Ontario, Western Ontario, Canada.

Mandich A, Polatajko H (2003) Developmental coordination disorder: mechanisms measurement management. Human Movement Science 22: 406–11.

Mandich A, Buckolz E, Polatajko H (2003) Children with developmental coordination disorder (DCD) and their ability to disengage ongoing attentional focus: more on inhibitory function. Brain and Cognition 51: 346–56.

Mandich A, Miller LT, Polatajko HJ et al. (2003) A cognitive perspective on handwriting: cognitive orientation to daily occupational performance (CO-OP). Handwriting Review 2: 41–7.

Mandich A, Polatajko HJ, Macnab JJ et al. (2001a) Treatment of children with developmental coordination disorder: what is the evidence? Physical and Occupational Therapy in Pediatrics 20: 51–68.

Mandich A, Polatajko HJ, Missiuna C et al. (2001b) Cognitive strategies and motor performance in children with developmental coordination disorder. Physical and Occupational Therapy in Pediatrics 20: 125–44.

Mandich A, Polatajko H, Rodger S (2003) Rites of passage: understanding participation of children with developmental coordination disorder. Human Movement Science 22: 583–95.

Manitoba Department of Education (1980) Manitoba Physical Fitness Performance Test Manual and Fitness Objectives. Ottawa, Ontario: CAPHER .

Manjiviona J, Prior M (1995) Comparison of Asperger Syndrome and high functioning autistic children on a test of motor impairment. Journal of Autism and Developmental Disorders 25: 23–41.

Marchiori GE, Wall AE, Bedingfield EW (1987) Kinematic analysis of skill acquisition in physical awkward boys. Adapted Physical Activity Quarterly 4: 305–15.

Marlow N, Roberts BL, Cooke RWI (1989) Motor skills in extremely low birth weight children at the age of 6 years. Archives of Disease in Childhood 64: 839–47.

Martin G, Pear J (1996) Behavior Modification: What It Is and How To Do It (5th edn). Upper Saddle River, NJ: Prentice Hall.

Martini R (1994) Verbal self-guidance as an approach to the treatment of children with developmental coordination disorder: a systematic replication study. Unpublished master's thesis, University of Western Ontario, London, Ontario, Canada.

Martini R, Polatajko HJ (1998) Verbal self-guidance as a treatment approach for children with developmental coordination disorder: a systematic replication study. The Occupational Therapy Journal of Research 18: 157–81.

Mathai J, Anderson P, Bourne A (2002) The Strengths and Difficulties Questionnaire (SDQ) as a screening measure prior to admission to a Child and Adolescent Mental Health Service (CAMHS). Australian e-Journal for the Advancement of Mental Health 1: 1–12.

Meichenbaum D (1977) Cognitive-behavior Modification: An Integrative Approach. New York: Plenum Press.

Meichenbaum D (1991) Cognitive-behavior Modification. Workshop presented at the Child and Parent Research Institute Symposium, London, Ontario, Canada.

Meltzer H, Garward R, Goodman R et al. (2000) Mental Health of Children and Adolescents in Great Britain. London: The Stationery Office.

Miller LT, Missiuna CA, Macnab JJ et al. (2001a) Clinical description of children with developmental coordination disorder. Canadian Journal of Occupational Therapy 68: 5–15.

Miller LT, Polatajko HJ, Missiuna C et al. (2001b) A pilot trial of a cognitive treatment for children with developmental coordination disorder. Human Movement Science 20: 183–210.

Missiuna C (1994) Motor skill acquisition in children with developmental coordination disorder. Adapted Physical Activity Quarterly 11: 214–35.

Missiuna C (1998) Development of 'All About Me', a scale that measures children's perceived motor competence. The Occupational Therapy Journal of Research 18: 85–108.

Missiuna C, Polatajko H (1995) Developmental dyspraxia by any other name: are they all just clumsy children? The American Journal of Occupational Therapy 49: 619–27.

Missiuna C, Mandich AD, Polatajko HJ et al. (2001) Cognitive Orientation to Daily Occupational Performance (CO-OP): Part 1-Theoretical foundations. Physical and Occupational Therapy in Pediatrics 20: 69–82.

Miyahara M (1994) Subtypes of students with learning disabilities based upon gross motor functions. Adapted Physical Activities Quarterly 11: 368–82.

Miyahara M, Möbs I (1995) Developmental dyspraxia and developmental coordination disorder. Neuropsychology Review 5: 245–68.

Miyahara M, Tsukii M, Hori M et al. (1997) Brief report: motor incoordination in children with Asperger Syndrome and learning disabilities. Journal of Autism and Developmental Disorders 27: 597–602.

Mon-Williams MA, Mackie RT, McCulloch DL et al. (1996) Visual evoked potentials in children with developmental coordination disorder. Ophthalmic and Physiological Optics 16: 178–83.

Mon-Williams MA, Pascal E, Wann JP (1994) Ophthalmic factors in developmental coordination disorder. Adapted Physical Activity Quarterly 11: 170–8.

Mon-Williams MA, Wann JP, Pascal E (1999) Visual-proprioceptive mapping in children with developmental coordination disorder. Developmental Medicine and Child Neurology 41: 247–54.

Morris A, Williams J, Atwater A et al. (1982) Age and sex differences in motor performances of 3 through 6 year old children. Research Quarterly for Exercise and Sport 53: 214–21.

Morris PR, Whiting HTA (1971) Motor impairment and compensatory education. London: G. Bell & Sons.

Morton J (2004) Understanding Developmental Disorders: A Causal Modelling Approach. Oxford: Blackwell.

Moxley-Haegert L, Ladd HW (1989) Follow-up of children identified with and treated for a motor delay of nonspecifiable etiology. Infant Mental Health Journal 10: 45–58.

Mulder T (1991) A process-oriented model of human motor behaviour: toward a theory-based rehabilitation approach. Physical Therapy 71: 157–64.

Müller K, Hömberg V (1992) Development of speed of repetitive movements in children is determined by structural changes in corticospinal efferents. Neuroscience Letters 144: 57–60.

Müller K, Ebner V, Hömberg V (1994) Maturation of fastest afferent and efferent central and peripheral pathways: no evidence for a constancy of central conduction delays. Neuroscience Letters 166: 9–12.

Mutch L, Leyland A, McGee A (1993) Patterns of neuropsychological function in a low-birth-weight population. Developmental Medicine and Child Neurology 35: 943–56.

Nelson JK, Thomas JR, Nelson KR et al. (1986) Gender differences in children's throwing performance: biology and environment. Research Quarterly for Exercise and Sport 57: 280–7.

Ness Research Team (2004) The national evaluation of Sure Start local programmes in England. Child and Adolescent Mental Health 9: 2–8.

Netelenbos JB, Koops W (1988) Ontwikkeling van de motoriek (Motor development). In W Koops, JJ van der Werff (eds), Overzicht van de empirische ontwikkelingspsychologie 2. De ontwikkeling van functies en cognitie. Groningen: Wolters-Noordhoff.

Newell KM (1986) Constraints on the development of coordination. In MG Wade, HTA Whiting (eds), Motor Development in Children: Aspects of Coordination and Control. Dordrecht: Martinus Nijhoff, pp. 341–61.

Newnham C, McKenzie BE (1994) Cross-modal transfer of sequential visual and haptic shape information by clumsy children. Perception 22: 1061–73.

Nicholls JG (1984) Achievement motivation: conceptions of ability, subjective experience, task choice, and performance. Psychological Review 91: 328–46.

Nichols PL, Chen TC (1981) Minimal Brain Dysfunction: A Prospective Study. Hillsdale, NJ: Erlbaum.

Nicolson RI, Fawcett AJ (1994) Comparison of deficits in cognitive and motor skills in children with dyslexia. Annals of Dyslexia 44: 147–64.

Nicolson RI, Fawcett AJ (1999) Developmental dyslexia: the role of the cerebellum. Dyslexia 5: 155–77.

Nicolson RI, Fawcett AJ, Berry EL et al. (1999) Association of abnormal cerebellar activation with motor learning difficulties in dyslexic adults. Lancet 353: 1662–7.

Niemeijer AS, Smits-Engelsman BCM, Reynders K et al. (in press) Verbal actions of physiotherapists to enhance motor learning in children with DCD. Human Movement Science.

O'Beirne C, Larkin D, Cable T (1994) Coordination problems and anaerobic performance in children. Adapted Physical Activity Quarterly 11:141–9.

Odenrick P, Sandstedt P (1984) Development of postural sway in the normal child. Human Neurobiology 3: 241–3.

O'Hare A, Khalid S (2002) The association of abnormal cerebellar function in children with developmental coordination disorder and reading difficulties. Dyslexia 8: 234–48.

O'Hare A, Gorzkowska J, Elton R (1999) The development of an instrument to measure manual praxis. Developmental Medicine and Child Neurology 41: 597–607.

Oliver M (1996) Understanding Disability from Theory to Practice. Basingstoke: Macmillan.

Orelove F, Sobsey D (1996) Educating Children with Multiple Disabilities: A Transdisciplinary Approach (3rd edn). Baltimore, MD: Paul Brookes.

Ornstein R (1998) The Right Mind. London: Harcourt Brace International.

Orton ST (1937) Reading, Writing and Speech Problems in Children. New York: Norton.

Ottenbacher K (1986) Evaluating Clinical Change: Strategies for Occupational and Physical Therapists. Baltimore, MD: Williams & Wilkins.

Ottenbacher KJ, Msall ME, Lyon N et al. (1999) Measuring developmental and functional status in children with disabilities. Developmental Medicine and Child Neurology 41: 186–94.

Overton W, Jackson J (1973) The representation of imagined objects in action sequences: a developmental study. Child Development 44: 309–14.

Owen SE, McKinlay IA (1997) Motor difficulties in children with developmental disorders of speech and language. Child: Care, Health and Development 23: 315–25.

Parker GM (1995) A study of the motor phenomena in chorea. Psychological Review 12: 370–85.

Parker HE, Larkin D, Wade M (1997) Are motor timing problems subgroup specific in children with developmental coordination disorder. Australian Educational and Developmental Psychologist 14: 35–42.

Parr JR, Ward A, Inman S (2003) Current practice in the management of Attention Deficit Disorder with Hyperactivity (ADHD). Child: Care, Health and Development 29: 215–18.

Parush S, Yehezkehel I, Tenenbaum A et al. (1998) Developmental correlates of school age children with a history of benign congenital hypotonia. Developmental Medicine and Child Neurology 40: 448–52.

Pasamanick B, Knobloch H (1966) Retrospective studies on epidemiology of reproductive casualty: old and new. Merrill Palmer Quarterly of Behavioral Development 12: 7–26.

Passenger T, Stuart M, Terrel C (2000) Phonological processing and early literacy. Journal of Research in Reading 23: 55–66.

Pereira HS, Landgren M, Gillberg C et al. (2001) Parametric control of fingertip forces during precision grip lifts in children with DCD (developmental coordination disorder) and DAMP (deficits in attention motor control and perception). Neuropsychologia 39: 478–88.

Peters J, Barnett A, Henderson SE (1999) Clumsy, Dyspraxia and Developmental Coordination Disorder: Same or Different? How do Health and Educational Professionals in U.K. Define the Terms? DCD IV International Conference, Groningen, The Netherlands.

Peters J, Henderson S, Dookun D (2004) Provision for children with developmental coordination disorder (DCD): audit of the service provider. Child: Care, Health and Development 30: 463–79.

Peters M, Pedersen K (1978) Incidence of left-handers with inverted writing position in a population of 5910 elementary school children. Neuropsychologia 16: 743–6.

Phelps J, Stempel L (1991) The identification of dyslexic handwriting through graphoanalysis. In J Wann, AM Wing, N Sovik (eds), Development of Graphic Skills. New York: Academic Press, pp. 191–204.

Phelps J, Stempel L, Speck G (1985) The Children's Handwriting scales: a new diagnostic tool. Journal of Educational Research 79: 46–50.

Phillips DM, Longlett SK, Mulrine C et al. (1999) School problems and the family physician. American Family Physician 59: 2816–24.

Piaget J-P (1952) The Origins of Intelligence in Children. New York: International Universities Press.

Piek JP (2003) The role of variability in early motor development. Infant Behavior and Development 25: 452–65.

Piek JP, Coleman-Carman R (1995) Kinaesthetic sensitivity and motor performance of children with developmental co-ordination disorder. Developmental Medicine and Child Neurology 37: 976–84.

Piek JP, Dworcan M, Barrett NC et al. (2000) Determinants of self-worth in children with and without developmental coordination disorder. International Journal of Disability, Development and Education 47: 259–72.

Piek JP, Pitcher RM, Hay DA (1999) Motor coordination and kinaesthesis in boys with attention deficit-hyperactivity disorder. Developmental Medicine and Child Neurology 41: 159–65.

Piper MC, Pinell LE, Darrah J et al. (1992) Construction and validation of the Alberta Infant Motor Scale (AIMS). Canadian Journal of Public Health 83: 46–50.

Pless M (2001) Developmental coordination disorder in pre-school children. Effects of motor skills intervention, parents' descriptions, and short-term follow-up of motor status. Unpublished doctoral thesis.

Pless M, Carlsson M (2000) Effects of motor skill intervention on Developmental Coordination Disorder: a meta-analysis. Adapted Physical Activity Quarterly 17: 381–401.

Pless M, Carlsson M, Sundelin C et al. (2000) Effects of group motor skill intervention on five-to six-year-old children with developmental coordination disorder. Pediatric Physical Therapy 12: 183–9.

Pless M, Carlsson M, Sundelin C et al. (2001) Pre-school children with developmental coordination disorder: self-perceived competence and group motor skill intervention. Acta Paediatrica 90: 532–8.

Pless M, Persson K, Sundelin C et al. (2001) Children with developmental coordination disorder: a qualitative study of parents' descriptions. Advances in Physiotherapy 3: 128–35.

Pochon JB, Levy R, Poline JB et al. (2001) The role of dorsolateral prefrontal cortex in the preparation of forthcoming actions: an fMRI study. Cerebral Cortex 11: 260–6.

Polatajko HJ (1999) Developmental coordination disorder (DCD): alias the clumsy child syndrome. In K Whitmore, H Hart, G Willems (eds), A Neurodevelopmental Approach to Specific Learning Disorders. London: MacKeith Press, pp. 119–33.

Polatajko HJ, Fox AM (1995) Final Report on the Conference. Children and Clumsiness: A Disability in Search of Definition. London, Ontario: International Consensus Meeting.

Polatajko HJ, Mandich A (2004) Enabling Occupation in Children: The Cognitive Orientation to daily Occupational Performance (CO-OP) Approach. Ottawa, ON: CAOT Publications ACE.

Polatajko HJ, Fox M, Missiuna C (1995) An international consensus on children with developmental coordination disorder. Canadian Journal of Occupational Therapy 62: 3–6.

Polatajko HJ, Kaplan BJ, Wilson BN (1992) Sensory integration treatment for children with learning disabilities: its status 20 years later. Occupational Therapy Journal of Research 12: 323–41.

Polatajko HJ, Law M, Miller J et al. (1991) The effect of a sensory integration program on academic achievement, motor performance and self-esteem in children identified as learning disabled: results of a clinical trial. Occupational Therapy Journal of Research 11: 155–76.

Polatajko HJ, Macnab J, Anstett B et al. (1995) A clinical trial of the process-oriented treatment approach for children with developmental co-ordination disorder. Developmental Medicine and Child Neurology 37: 310–19.

Polatajko HJ, Mandich AD, Martini R (2000) Dynamic performance analysis: a framework for understanding occupational performance. American Journal of Occupational Therapy 54: 65–72.

Polatajko HJ, Mandich AD, Miller L et al. (2001a) Cognitive orientation to daily occupational performance: Part II – The evidence. Physical and Occupational Therapy in Paediatrics 20: 83–106.

Polatajko HJ, Mandich A, Missiuna C et al. (2001b) Cognitive orientation to daily occupational performance (CO-OP): Part III – The protocol in brief. Physical and Occupational Therapy in Pediatrics 20: 107–24.

Porter CS, Corlett EN (1989) Performance differences of individuals classified by questionnaire as accident prone or non-accident prone. Ergonomics 32: 317–33.

Portwood M (1999) Developmental Dyspraxia: Identification and Intervention. London: David Fulton.

Powell RP, Bishop DVM (1992) Clumsiness and perceptual problems in children with specific language impairment. Developmental Medicine and Child Neurology 34: 755–65.

Prechtl HFR (1977) Minimal brain dysfunction syndrome and the plasticity of the nervous system. In AF Kalverboer, HM van Praag, J Mendelwicz (eds), Minimal Brain Dysfunction: Fact or Fiction? (Advances in Biological Psychiatry, vol. 1). Basle: Karger.

Prechtl HFR (1997) State of the art of a new functional assessment of the young nervous system: an early predictor of cerebral palsy. Early Human Development 50: 1–11.

Pressley M, Borkowski JG, Schneider W (1987) Cognitive strategies: good strategy users coordinate metacognition and knowledge. In R Vasta (ed.), Annals of Child Development (Vol. 4). London: JAI Press, pp. 89–129.

Pyke JE (1986) Australian School Fitness Test for Students Aged 7–15. Parkside, South Australia: ACHPER Publications.

Qualifications and Curriculum Authority (2003) Assessment and Reporting Arrangements. Key Stage 3. London: QCA.

Rasmussen P, Gillberg C (1983) Perceptual, motor and attentional deficits in seven-year-old children: pediatric aspects. Acta Paedatrica Scandinavica 72: 125–30.

Rasmussen P, Gillberg C (2000) Natural outcome of ADHD with developmental coordination disorder at age 22 years: a controlled, longitudinal, community-based study. Journal of the American Academy of Child & Adolescent Psychiatry 39: 1424–31.

Rasmussen P, Gillberg C, Waldenstrom E et al. (1983) Perceptual, motor and attentional deficits in seven year old children: neurological and neurodevelopmental aspects. Developmental Medicine and Child Neurology 25: 315–33.

Rathbone Charity (2002) Could Do Better: An Analysis of How Well Mainstream Schools Involve the Parents of Pupils with Special Educational Needs. Manchester: Rathbone Charity.

Raynor AJ (1998) Fractionated reflex and reaction time in children with developmental coordination disorder. Motor Control 2: 114–24.

Raynor AJ (2001) Strength, power, and coactivation in children with developmental coordination disorder. Developmental Medicine and Child Neurology 43: 676–84.

Reed ES (1982) An outline theory of action systems. Journal of Motor Behavior 14: 98–134.

Reisman JA (1999) Minnesota Handwriting Assessment. San Antonio, TX: The Psychological Corporation.

Revie G, Larkin D (1993a) Looking at movement: problems with teacher identification of poorly coordinated children. The ACHPER National Journal 40: 4–9.

Revie G, Larkin D (1993b) Task specific intervention with children reduces movement problems. Adapted Physical Activity Quarterly 10: 29–41.

Revie G, Larkin D (1995) Screening for movement intervention. The ACHPER Healthy Lifestyles Journal 42: 4–7.

Riach CL, Hayes KC (1987) Maturation of postural sway in young children. Developmental Medicine and Child Neurology 29: 650–8.

Rintala P, Pienimaki K, Ahonen T et al. (1998) The effects of a psychomotor training programme on motor skill development in children with developmental language disorders. Human Movement Science 17: 721–37.

Rispens J, van Yperen TA (1997) How specific are 'specific developmental disorders'? The relevance of the concept of specific developmental disorders for the classification of childhood developmental disorders. Journal of Child Psychology and Psychiatry 38: 351–63.

Roaf C (1998) Slow hand: a secondary school survey of handwriting speed and legibility. Support for Learning 13: 39–42.

Robertson SS (1985) Cyclic motor activity in the human fetus after midgestation. Developmental Psychobiology 18: 411–19.

Robinson RJ (1991) Causes and associations of severe and persistent specific speech and language disorders in children. Developmental Medicine and Child Neurology 33: 943–62.

Rodger S, Ziviani J, Watter P et al. (2003) Motor and functional skills of children with developmental coordination disorder: a pilot investigation of measurement issues. Human Movement Science 22: 461–78.

Roncevalles MNC, Jensen JL, Woollacott MH (2001) Development of lower extremity kinetics for balance control in infants and young children. Journal of Motor Behavior 33: 180–92.

Rösblad B, von Hofsten C (1994) Repetitive goal-directed arm movements in children with developmental coordination disorders: role of visual information. Adapted Physical Activity Quarterly 11: 190–202.

Rose B, Larkin D, Berger B (1997) Coordination and gender influences on the perceived competence of children. Adapted Physical Activity Quarterly 14: 210–21.

Rose B, Larkin D, Berger BG (1998) The importance of motor coordination for children's motivational orientation in sport. Adapted Physical Activity Quarterly 15: 316–27.

Rose E, Larkin D (2002) Perceived competence, discrepancy scores and global self-worth. Adapted Physical Activity Quarterly 19: 127–40.

Rose E, Larkin D, Cantell M et al. (2000) Development of a movement confidence scale: a measure of perceived competence, fear and positive affect. Unpublished manuscript.

Rosenbaum DA (1991) Human Motor Control. New York: Academic Press.

Rosenblum S, Parush S, Weiss PL (2003) Computerized temporal handwriting characteristics of proficient and non-proficient handwriters. American Journal of Occupational Therapy 57: 129–38.

Rosenblum S, Weiss PL, Parush S (2003) Product and process evaluation of handwriting difficulties. Educational Psychology Review 15: 41–81.

Rothberg AD, Goodman M, Jacklin LA et al. (1991) Six-year follow-up of early physiotherapy intervention in very low birth weight infants. Pediatrics 88: 547–52.

Rourke BP (1989) Nonverbal Learning Disabilities: The Syndrome and the Model. New York: Guilford Press.

Roussounis SH, Gaussen TH, Stratton P (1987) A 2-year follow up of children with motor coordination problems identified at school entry age. Child: Care, Health and Development 13: 377–91.

Roy EA (1983) Current perspectives on disruptions to limb praxis. Physical Therapy 63: 1998-2003.

Roy EA, Square PA (1985) Common considerations in the study of limb, verbal and oral apraxia. In EA Roy (ed.), Neuropsychological Studies of Apraxia and Related Disorders. North Holland: Elsevier Science Publishers, pp. 111–61.

Rubin N, Henderson SE (1982) Two sides of the same coin: variations in teaching methods and failure to learn to write. Special Education: Forward Trends. Research Supplement 9: 17–24.

Rutter M (1982) Syndromes attributed to 'Minimal Brain Dysfunction' in childhood. American Journal of Psychiatry 139: 21–33.

Sackett D, Straus S, Richardson W et al. (2000) Evidence-based Medicine: How to Practice and Teach Evidence Based Medicine. London: Churchill Livingstone.

Salokorpi T, Rautio T, Kajantie E et al. (2002) Is early occupational therapy in extremely preterm infants of benefit in the long run? Pediatric Rehabilitation 5: 91–8.

Samson G (1985) Writing Systems: A Linguistic Introduction. London: Hutchinson & Co. Ltd.

Samson JF, de Groot L, Cranendonk A et al. (2002) Neuromotor function and school performance in 7 year-old children born as high-risk preterm infants. Journal of Child Neurology 17: 325–32.

Sassoon R (1990) Handwriting. The Way to Teach It. Cheltenham: Stanley Thornes.

Sassoon R (1993) The Art and Science of Handwriting. Bristol: Intellect Books.

Schillings JJ, Meulenbrook JGJ, Thomassen AJWM (1996) Decomposing trajectory modification: pen tip versus joint kinematics. In MJ Simner, CG Thomassen, AJWM Leedham (eds), Handwriting and Drawing Research. Basic and Applied Issues. Amsterdam: IOS Press, pp. 71–85.

Schmidt RA (1975) A schema theory of discrete motor skill learning. Psychological Review 82: 225–60.

Schmidt RA (1988a) Motor Control and Learning: A Behavioral Emphasis. Champaign, IL: Human Kinetics.

Schmidt RA (1988b) Motor and action perspective on motor behavior. In OG Meijer, K Roth (eds), Complex Movement Behaviour: 'The' Motor–Action Controversy. Amsterdam: North-Holland.

Schmidt RA, Bjork RA (1992) New conceptualizations of practice: common principles in three paradigms suggest new concepts for training. Psychological Science 3: 207–17.

Schmidt RA, Lee TD (1999) Motor Control and Learning: A Behavioural Emphasis (3rd edn). Champaign, IL: Human Kinetics.

Schmidt RA, Wrisberg CA (2000) Motor Learning and Performance: A Problem-based Learning Approach (2nd edn). Champaign, IL: Human Kinetics.

Schneck CN (1991) Comparison of pencil-grip patterns in first graders with good and poor writing skills. American Journal of Occupational Therapy 45: 701–6.

Schoemaker MM (1992) Physiotherapy for clumsy children. An effect evaluation study. Unpublished doctoral thesis, University of Groningen, The Netherlands.

Schoemaker MM, Kalverboer AF (1994) Social and affective problems of children who are clumsy: how early do they begin? Adapted Physical Activity Quarterly 11: 130–40.

Schoemaker MM, Geuze RH, Kalverboer AF (1987) Evaluatie van behandeling van houterige kinderen (Evaluation of therapy of clumsy children). Nederlands Tijdschrift Fysiotherapie 97: 93–7.

Schoemaker MM, Hijlkema MGJ, Kalverboer AF (1994) Physiotherapy for clumsy children – an evaluation study. Developmental Medicine and Child Neurology 36: 143–55.

Schoemaker MM, Niemeijer AS, Reynders K et al. (2003) Evaluation of the effectiveness of neuromotor task training for children with developmental coordination disorder: a pilot study. Neural Plasticity 10: 155–65.

Schoemaker MM, Smits-Engelsman BCM, Jongmans M (2003) Psychometric properties of the movement assessment battery for children – checklist as a screening instrument for children with a developmental coordination disorder. British Journal of Educational Psychology 73: 425–41.

Schoemaker MM, Smits-Engelsman BCM, Kalverboer AF (1998) The classification of specific motor disorders: implications for intervention. In J Rispens, T van Yperen, W Yule (eds), Perspectives on the Classification of Specific Developmental Disorders. Dordrecht: Kluwer Academic, pp. 231–44.

Schoemaker MM, Wees M, van der Flapper B et al. (2001) Perceptual skills of children with Developmental Coordination Disorder. Human Movement Science 20: 111–33.

Schul R, Townsend J, Stiles J (2003) The development of attentional orienting during the school-age years. Developmental Science 6: 262–72.

Segal R, Mandich A, Polatajko H et al. (2002) Stigma and its management: a pilot study of parental perceptions of the experiences of children with developmental coordination disorder. American Journal of Occupational Therapy 56: 422–8.

Shapiro DR, Ulrich DA (2001) Social comparisons of children with and without learning disabilities when evaluating physical competence. Adapted Physical Activity Quarterly 18: 273–88.

Shaw K, Wagner I, Eastwood H et al. (2003) A qualitative study of Australian GPs' attitudes and practices in the diagnosis and management of attention-deficit/hyperactivity disorder (ADHD). Family Practice 20: 129–34.

Shelley EM, Riester A (1972) Syndrome of minimal brain damage in young adults. Diseases of the Nervous System: 335–8.

Shumway-Cook A, Woollacott MH (1985) The growth of stability: postural control from a developmental perspective. Journal of Motor Behavior 17: 131–47.

Shumway-Cook A, Woollacott MH (1995) Motor Control: Theory and Practical Application. London: Williams & Wilkins.

Sigmundsson H (1999) Inter-modal matching and bimanual co-ordination in children with hand–eye co-ordination problems. Nordisk Fysioterapi 3: 55–64.

Sigmundsson H, Hansen PC, Talcott JB (2003) Do 'clumsy' children have visual deficits? Behavioural Brain Research 139: 123–9.

Sigmundsson H, Ingvaldsen RP, Whiting HTA (1997) Inter- and intra-sensory modality matching in children with hand–eye co-ordination problems. Experimental Brain Research 114: 492–9.

Sigmundsson H, Pedersen AV, Whiting HTA et al. (1998) We can cure your child's clumsiness! A review of intervention methods. Scandinavian Journal of Rehabilitation Medicine 30: 101–6.

Sigurdsson E, van Os J, Fombonne E (2002) Are impaired childhood motor skills a risk factor for adolescent anxiety? Results from the 1958 UK birth cohorts and the National Child Development Study. American Journal of Psychiatry 159: 1044–6.

Silver AA, Hagin RA (1990) Disorders of Learning in Childhood. New York: John Wiley and Sons.

Simner ML (1991) Estimating a child's learning potential from form errors in a child's printing. In J Wann, AM Wing, N Sovik (eds), Development of Graphic Skills: Research Perspectives and Educational Implications. London: Academic Press, pp. 205–18.

Simner ML, Leedham CG, Thomassen AJWM (1996) Handwriting and Drawing Research. Basic and Applied Issues. Amsterdam: IOS Press.

Simoneau M, Paillard J, Bard C et al. (1999) Role of the feedforward command and reafferent information in the coordination of a passing prehension task. Experimental Brain Research 128: 236–42.

Sims K, Morton J (1998) Modelling the effects of kinaesthetic acuity measurement in children. Journal of Child Psychology and Psychiatry 39: 731–46.

Sims K, Henderson SE, Hulme C et al. (1996a) The remediation of clumsiness: I. An evaluation of Laszlo's kinaesthetic approach. Developmental Medicine and Child Neurology 38: 976–87.

Sims K, Henderson SE, Morton J et al. (1996b) The remediation of clumsiness: II. Is kinaesthesis the answer? Developmental Medicine and Child Neurology 38: 988–97.

Sinani C (PhD thesis in preparation) The Planning of Movements in Children with Developmental Coordination Disorder.

Skinner RA, Piek JP (2001) Psychosocial implications of poor motor coordination in children and adolescents. Human Movement Science 20: 73–94.

Skorji V, McKenzie B (1997) How do children who are clumsy remember modelled movements? Developmental Medicine and Child Neurology 39: 404–8.

Smith LB, Thelen E (2003) Development as a dynamic system. Trends in Cognitive Sciences 7: 343–8.

Smits-Engelsman BCM, Halfens JHG (2000) Bewegingsprogramma's bij mensen met centraal neurologische aandoeningen: welke benaderingswijzen? In BCM Smits-Engelsman, I Ham, P van Vaes et al. (eds), Jaarboek fysiotherapie. Houten: Bohn Stafleu Van Loghum, pp. 97–137.

Smits-Engelsman BCM, Teulings HL (1992) A cognitive model of motor behavior. Report for CEC project A-2002: Computer Aided Movement Analysis in a Rehabilitation Context II.

Smits-Engelsman BCM, Tuijl ALT (1998) Toepassing van Cognitieve Motorische Controle Theorieën in de Kinderfysiotherapie: het controleren van vrijheidsgraden en beperkingen. In BCM Smits-Engelsman, I Ham, P van Vaes et al. (eds), Jaarboek fysiotherapie. Houten: Bohn Stafleu Van Loghum, pp. 202–29.

Smits-Engelsman BCM, van Galen GP, Meulenbraek RGJ (1996) Handwriting and its temporal evolution: a process-oriented perspective. Journal of Forensic Document Examiners 9: 27–44.

Smits-Engelsman BCM, Niemeijer AS, van Galen GP (2001) Fine motor deficiencies in children diagnosed as DCD based on poor grapho-motor ability. Human Movement Science 20: 161–82.

Smits-Engelsman BCM, Reynders K, Schoemaker MM (2001) Kinderen met Developmental Coordination Disorder (DCD): symptomatologie, diagnostiek en Behandeling. In R van Empelen, R Nijhuis-van der Sande, A Hartman (eds), Kinderfysiotherapie. Maarssen: Elsevier Gezondheidszorg, pp. 505–23.

Smits-Engelsman BCM, Steenbergen B, van Galen GP (2001) Motorische handelen van het perspectief van een actiemodel. In R van Empelen, R Nijhuis-van der Sande, A Hartman (eds), Kinderfysiotherapie. Maarssen: Elsevier Gezondheidszorg pp. 45–56.

Smits-Engelsman BCM, van Galen GP, Schoemaker MM (1997) Theory-based diagnosis and subclassification in developmental coordination disorder. In JP Rispens, T van Yperen, W Yule (eds), Perspectives on the Classification of Specific Developmental Disorders. Dordrecht: Kluwer Academic.

Smits-Engelsman BCM, Westenberg Y, Duysens J (2003) Development of isometric force and force control in children. Cognitive Brain Research 17: 68–74.

Smyth MM, Anderson H (2000) Coping with clumsiness in the school playground: social and physical play in children with co-ordination impairments. British Journal of Developmental Psychology 18: 389–413.

Smyth MM, Anderson HI (2001) Football participation in the primary school playground: the role of coordination impairments. British Journal of Developmental Psychology 19: 369–79.

Smyth MM, Mason UC (1997) Planning and execution of action in children with and without developmental coordination disorder. Journal of Child Psychology and Psychiatry 38: 1023–37.

Smyth MM, Mason UC (1998) Use of proprioception in normal and clumsy children. Developmental Medicine and Child Neurology 40: 672–81.

Smyth TR (1994) Clumsiness in children: a defect of kinaesthetic perception? Child: Care, Health and Development 20: 27–36.

Smyth TR (1996) Clumsiness: kinaesthetic perception and translation. Child: Care, Health and Development 22: 1–9.

Smyth TR, Glencross DJ (1986) Information processing deficits in clumsy children. Australian Journal of Psychology 38: 13–22.

Sonnander K (2000) Early identification of children with developmental disabilities. Acta Paediatrica Supplement 89: 17–23.

Soorani-Lunsing RJ (1993) Neurobehavioural relationships and puberty: another transformation? Early Human Development 33: 59–67.

Soorani-Lunsing RJ, Hadders-Algra M, Olinga AA et al. (1993) Is minor neurological dysfunction at 12 years related to behaviour and cognition? Developmental Medicine and Child Neurology 35: 321–30.

Southard DL (1991) Coordinative structures and the development of relative timing in a pointing task. In J Fagard, PH Wolff (eds), The Development of Timing Control and Temporal Organization in Coordinated Action: Invariant Relative Timing, Rhythms and Coordination. Advances in Psychology 81. Oxford: North-Holland, pp. 281–304.

Sparrow SS, Balla DA, Cicchetti DV (1985) Vineland Adaptive Behavior Scales. Circle Pines: AGS.

Sporns O, Edelman GM (1993) Solving Bernstein's problem: a proposal for the development of coordinated movement by selection. Child Development 64: 960–81.

Stainthorp R, Henderson SE, Barnett AL et al. (2001) Handwriting policy and practice in primary schools. Unpublished conference proceedings, BPS Developmental and Education Sections Joint Annual Conference, Worcester, UK.

Stephenson E, McKay C, Chesson R (1991) The identification and treatment of motor/learning difficulties: parent's perceptions and the role of the therapist. Child: Care, Health and Development 17: 91–113.

Stoffregen TA (1985) Flow structure versus retinal location in the optical control of stance. Journal of Experimental Psychology, Human Perception and Performance 11: 554–65.

Stott DH, Moyes FA, Henderson SE (1972) The Test of Motor Impairment. Ontario: Brook Educational Publishing.

Stott DH, Moyes FA, Henderson SE (1984) The Henderson Revision of the Test of Motor Impairment. San Antonio, TX: The Psychological Corporation.

Sugden DA (1980) Movement speed in children. Journal of Motor Behavior 12: 125–32.

Sugden DA (1988) Skill generalisation and children with learning difficulties. In DA Sugden (ed.), Cognitive Approaches in Special Education. Lewes: Falmer Press, pp 82–99.

Sugden DA (1990) Role of proprioception in eye–hand coordination. In C Bard, M Fleury, L Hay (eds), Development of Eye–Hand Coordination Across the Life Span. Columbia: University of South Carolina Press, pp. 133–53.

Sugden DA (in press) Dynamic management of DCD. In RH Geuze (ed.), Developmental Coordination Disorder: A Review of Current Approaches. Collection Psychomotricité. Marseille: Solal Éditeurs.

Sugden DA, Chambers ME (1998) Intervention approaches and children with developmental coordination disorder. Pediatric Rehabilitation 2: 139–47.

Sugden DA, Chambers ME (2003a) Intervention in children with developmental coordination disorder: the role of parents and teachers. British Journal of Educational Psychology 73: 545–61.

Sugden DA, Chambers ME (2003b) Monitoring the Educational Performance of Children with Developmental Coordination Disorder. Grant Report to Action Medical Research.

Sugden DA, Henderson SE (1994) Help with movement. Special Children 75: Back to Basics 13.

Sugden DA, Keogh JF (1990) Problems in Movement Skill Development. Columbia: University of South Carolina Press.

Sugden DA, Sugden L (1991) The assessment of movement skill problems in 7- and 9-year-old children. British Journal of Educational Psychology 61: 329–45.

Sugden DA, Wann C (1987) The assessment of motor impairment in children with moderate learning difficulties. British Journal of Educational Psychology 57: 225–36.

Sugden DA, Wright HC (1995) Helping Your Child with Movement Difficulties. Leeds: Harmer Press.

Sugden DA, Wright HC (1996) Curricular entitlement and implementation for all children. In N Armstrong (ed.), New Directions in Physical Education: 3. Change and Innovation. London: Cassells, pp. 110–30.

Sugden DA, Wright HC (1998) Motor Coordination Disorders in Children. Thousand Oaks, CA: Sage Publications.

Sugden DA, Wright HC, Chambers ME et al. (2003) Developmental Coordination Disorder. A Booklet for Parents and Professionals. Leeds: University of Leeds.

Summers J, Larkin D (2002) Social relationships of children with developmental coordination disorder. Presentation at the World Federation of Occupational Therapy Conference, Sweden.

Symes, K. (1972) Clumsiness and the sociometric status of intellectually gifted boys. Bulletin of Physical Education 9: 35–40.

Szatmari P, Bremner R, Nagy JN (1989) Asperger's Syndrome: a review of clinical features. Canadian Journal of Psychiatry 34: 554–650.

Tan SK, Parker HE, Larkin D (2001) Concurrent validity of motor tests used to identify children with motor impairment. Adapted Physical Activity Quarterly 18: 168–82.

Taylor J (2001) Handwriting. A Teacher's Guide. Multisensory Approaches to Assessing and Improving Handwriting Skills. London: David Fulton.

Thapar A, Thapar A (2002) Is primary care ready to take on Attention Deficit Hyperactivity Disorder? BMC Family Practice 3: 7.

Thelen E (1995) Motor development: a new synthesis. American Psychologist 50: 79–95.

Thelen E, Cooke DW (1987) Relationship between newborn stepping and later walking: a new interpretation. Developmental Medicine and Child Neurology 29: 380–93.

Thelen E, Smith LB (1994) A dynamic systems approach to the development of cognition and action. Cambridge, MA: MIT Press.

Thomas JR, French KE (1985) Gender differences across age in motor performance: a meta-analysis. Psychological Bulletin 98: 260–82.

Torrioli MG, Frisone MF, Bonvini L et al. (2000) Perceptual-motor, visual and cognitive ability in very low birthweight preschool children without neonatal ultrasound abnormalities. Brain and Development 22: 163–8.

Touwen BCL (1979) The Examination of the Child with Minor Neurological Dysfunction (2nd edn). Clinics in Developmental Medicine, No. 71. London: S.I.M.P. with Heinemann Medical; Philadelphia: Lippincott.

Tseng MH (1998) Development of pencil grip position in pre-school children. Occupational Therapy Journal of Research 18: 207–24.

Tseng MH, Chow SMK (2000) Perceptual-motor function of school-age children with slow handwriting speed. American Journal of Occupational Therapy 54: 83–8.

Tseng MH, Murray EA (1994) Differences in perceptual-motor measures in children with good and poor handwriting. Occupational Therapy Journal of Research 14: 9–36.

Tucha O, Lange K (2001) Effects of methylphenidate on kinematic aspects of handwriting in hyperactive boys. Journal of Abnormal Child Psychology 29: 351–6.

Turvey MT (1990) Coordination. American Psychologist 45: 938–53.

Turvey MT, Carello C (1981) Cognition: the view from ecological realism. Cognition 10: 313–21.

Turvey MT, Fitzpatrick P (1993) Commentary: Development of perception-action systems and general principles of pattern formation. Child Development 64: 1175–90.

Turvey MT, Shaw RE (1999) Ecological foundations of cognition I. In R Nunez, WJ Freeman (eds), Reclaiming Cognition: The Primacy of Action, Intention, and Emotion. Bowling Green, OH: Imprint Academic, pp. 95–110. (Reprinted from Journal of Consciousness Studies 1999, 6: 95–110.)

Ulrich DA (1985) Test of Gross Motor Development. Austin, TX: Pro-Ed.

Ulrich DA (2000) TGMD-2 Test of Gross Motor Development (2nd edn) Examiners Manual. Austin, TX: Pro-ed.

Umble KE, Shay S, Sollecito W (2003) An interdisciplinary MPH via distance learning: meeting the educational needs of practitioners. Journal of Public Health Management and Practice 9: 123–35.

Usui N, Maekawa K, Hirasawa Y (1995) Development of the upright postural sway of children. Developmental Medicine and Child Neurology 37: 985–96.

Vaessen W, Kalverboer AF (1990) Clumsy children's performance on a double task I. In AF Kalverboer (ed.), Developmental Biopsychology: Experimental and Observational Studies in Children at Risk. Ann Arbor: University of Michigan Press, pp. 223–40.

van Dellen T, Geuze RH (1988) Motor response processing in clumsy children. Journal of Child Psychology and Psychiatry 29: 489–500.

van Dellen T, Geuze RH (1990) Experimental studies on motor control in clumsy children. In AF Kalverboer (ed.), Developmental Biopsychology: Experimental and Observational Studies in Children at Risk. Ann Arbor: University of Michigan Press, pp. 187–205.

van Dellen T, Vaessen W, Schoemaker MM (1990) Clumsiness: definition and selection of subjects. In AF Kalverboer (ed.), Developmental Biopsychology: Experimental and Observational Studies in Children at Risk. Ann Arbor: University of Michigan Press, pp. 135–52.

van der Meulen JHP, Denier van de Gon JJ, Gielen CCAM et al. (1991a) Visuomotor performance of normal and clumsy children I: Fast goal directed arm movements with and without visual feedback. Developmental Medicine and Child Neurology 33: 40–54.

van der Meulen JHP, Denier van de Gon JJ, Gielen CCAM et al. (1991b) Visuomotor performance of normal and clumsy children II: arm-tracking movements with and without visual feedback. Developmental Medicine and Child Neurology 33: 118–29.

van der Meulen JHP, Gooskens RHJ, Willemse J et al. (1990) Arm-tracking performance with and without visual feedback in children and adults: developmental changes. Journal of Motor Behavior 22: 386–405.

van Galen GP (1991) Handwriting: issues for a psychomotor theory. Human Movement Science 10: 165–91.

van Galen GP, Portier SJ, Smits-Engelsman BCM et al. (1993) Neuromotor noise and poor handwriting in children. Acta Psychologia 82: 161–78.

Viner R (1999) Transition from paediatric to adult care: bridging the gap or passing the buck? Archives of Disease in Childhood 81: 271–5.

Visser J (1998) Clumsy adolescents: a longitudinal study on the relationship between physical growth and sensorimotor skills of boys with and without DCD. Unpublished doctoral thesis, University of Groningen.

Visser J (2003) Developmental coordination disorder: a review of research on subtypes and comorbidities. Human Movement Science 22: 479–93.

Visser J, Geuze RH (2000) Kinaesthetic acuity in adolescent boys: a longitudinal study. Developmental Medicine and Child Neurology 42, 93–6.

Visser J, Geuze RH, Kalverboer AF (1998) The relationship between physical growth, the level of activity and the development of motor skills in adolescence: differences between children with DCD and controls. Human Movement Science 17: 573–608.

Volkmar FR, Szatmari P, Sparrow SS (1993) Sex differences in pervasive developmental delay. Journal of Autism and Developmental Delay 23: 579–91.

Volman MJ, Geuze R (1998) Relative phase stability of bimanual and visuomanual rhythmic coordination patterns in children with a Developmental Coordination Disorder. Human Movement Science 2: 541–72.

von Hofsten C, Rösblad B (1988) The integration of sensory information in the development of precise manual pointing. Neuropsychologia 26: 805–21.

Vreede CF (1988) The need for a better definition of ADL. International Journal of Rehabilitation Research 11: 29–35.

Wade MG (1973) Biorhythms and activity level of institutionalized mentally retarded persons diagnosed hyperactive. American Journal of Mental Deficiency 78: 262–7.

Wade MG (1990) Impact of optical flow on postural control in normal and mentally handicapped persons. In A Vermeer (ed.), Motor Development, Adapted Physical Activity and Mental Retardation. Amsterdam: Karger, pp. 21–9.

Wade MG, Ellis MJ (1971) Measurement of free-range activity in children as modified by social and environmental complexity. American Journal of Clinical Nutrition 24: 1457–60.

Wade MG, Ellis MJ, Bohrer RE (1973) Biorhythms in the activity of children during free play. J Exp Anal Behav 20: 155–62.

Waine L (2001) Writing speed: what constitutes 'slow'? An investigation to determine the average writing speed of Year 10 pupils. In R Rose, I Grosvenor (eds), Doing Research in Special Education: Ideas into Practice. London: David Fulton, pp. 75–87.

Wainwright A, Bryson SE (2002) The development of exogenous orienting: mechanisms of control. Journal of Experimental Psychology 82: 141–55.

Wall AE, McClements J, Bouffard M et al. (1985) A knowledge-based approach to motor development: implications for the physically awkward. Adapted Physical Activity Quarterly 2: 21–42.

Wallen M, Bonney M-A, Lennox L (1996) The Handwriting Speed Test. Adelaide: Helios.

Walter C (1998) An alternative view to dynamical systems concepts in motor control and learning. Research Quarterly for Exercise and Sport 69: 326–33.

Walter C, Swinnen SP (1994) The formation and dissolution of 'bad habits' during the acquisition of coordination skills. In SP Swinnen et al. (eds), Interlimb

Coordination: Neural, Dynamical, and Cognitive Constraints. San Diego: Academic Press.

Walton JN, Ellis E, Court SDM (1962) Clumsy children: developmental apraxia and agnosia. Brain 85: 603–12.

Wann JP (1987) Trends in the refinement and optimization of fine-motor trajectories: observations from an analysis of the handwriting of primary school children. Journal of Motor Behavior 19: 13–37.

Wann JP (1991) The integrity of visual-proprioceptive mapping in cerebral palsy. Neuropsychologia 29: 1095–1106.

Wann JP, Kardirkmanathan M (1991) Variability in children's handwriting: computer diagnosis of writing difficulties. In J Wann, AM Wing, N Sovik (eds), Development of Graphic Skills: Research Perspectives and Educational Implications. London: Academic Press, pp. 224–36.

Wann JP, Mon-Williams M, Rushton K (1998) Postural control and co-ordination disorders: the swinging room revisited. Human Movement Science 17: 491–513.

Ward J, Gupta R (2000) Skill-mix. Seams good to us. Health Service Journal 110: 30–1.

Warren WH Jr. (1984) Perceiving affordances: visual guidance of stair climbing. Journal of Experimental Psychology, Human Perception and Performance 10: 683–703.

Watkinson EJ, Dunn JC, Cavaliere N et al. (2001) Engagement in playground activities as a criterion for diagnosing developmental coordination disorder. Adapted Physical Activity Quarterly 18: 18–34.

Wechsler D (1974) Weschler Intelligence Scale for Children, 1st revision (WISC-R) San Antonio, TX: The Psychological Corporation.

Weil MJ, Cunningham Amundson SJ (1994) Relationship between visuomotor and handwriting skills of children in kindergarten. American Journal of Occupational Therapy 48: 982–8.

Weindling AM, Hallam P, Gregg J et al. (1996) A randomized controlled trial of early physiotherapy for high-risk infants. Acta Paediatrica 85: 1107–11.

Weintraub S, Mesulam MM (1983) Developmental learning disabilities of the right hemisphere: emotional, interpersonal and cognitive components. Archives of Neurology 40: 463–8.

Wender PH (1971) Minimal Brain Dysfunction in Children. New York: John Wiley.

Wessel JA (1976) I CAN Instructional Management System. Austin, TX: PRO-ED.

Whitmore K, Bax M (1999) What do we mean by SLD? A historical perspective. In K Whitmore, H Hart, G Willems (eds), A Neurodevelopmental Approach to Specific Learning Disorders. Suffolk: MacKeith Press, pp. 1–23.

Wickens CD (1974) Temporal limits of human information processing: a developmental study. Psychological Bulletin 81: 739–55.

Wilcox A (1994) Children with mild motor problems: exploring a client-centred, cognitive approach in OT intervention. Unpublished master's thesis, The University of Western Ontario, London, Ontario, Canada.

Wilcox A, Polatajko H (1993) Verbal self-guidance as a treatment technique for children with developmental coordination disorder. Canadian Journal of Occupational Therapy Conference Supplement, p. 20.

Wilcox A, Polatajko HJ (1994) The impact of verbal self-guidance on children with developmental coordination disorder. 11th International Congress of the World Federation of Occupational Therapists Congress Summaries 3: 1518–19.

Williams HG, Fisher JM, Tritschler KA (1983) Descriptive analysis of static postural control in 4, 6, and 8 year old normal and motorically awkward children. American Journal of Physical Medicine 62: 12–26.

Williams HG, Woollacott MH, Ivry R (1992) Timing and motor control in clumsy children. Journal of Motor Behavior 24: 165–72.

Wilson BN, Kaplan BJ (1994) Follow-up assessment of children receiving sensory integration treatment. The Occupational Therapy Journal of Research 14: 244–66.

Wilson BN, Dewey D, Campbell A (1998) The Developmental Coordination Disorder Questionnaire. Calgary Canada: published by the authors.

Wilson BN, Kaplan BJ, Crawford SG et al. (2000a) Reliability and validity of a parent questionnaire on childhood motor skills. American Journal of Occupational Therapy 54: 484–93.

Wilson BN, Kaplan BJ, Crawford SG et al. (2000b) Interrater reliability of the Bruininks-Oseretsky Test of Motor Proficiency – Long Form. Adapted Physical Activity Quarterly 17: 95–110.

Wilson PH, McKenzie B (1998) Information processing deficits associated with developmental coordination disorder: a meta-analysis of research findings. Journal of Child Psychology and Psychiatry 39: 829–40.

Wilson PH, Maruff P, McKenzie BE (1997) Covert orienting of visuospatial attention in children with developmental coordination disorder. Developmental Medicine and Child Neurology 39: 736–45.

Wilson BN, Pollack N, Kaplan BJ et al. (1994) Clinical Observation of Motor and Postural Skills. Tucson, AZ: Therapy Skill Builders.

Wilson PH, Thomas PR, Maruff P (2002) Motor imagery training ameliorates motor clumsiness in children. Journal of Child Neurology 17: 491–8.

Wing AM (1996) Anticipatory control of grip force in rapid arm movement. In AM Wing, P Haggard, R Flanagan (eds), Hand and Brain: Neurophysiology and Psychology of Hand Movements. San Diego: Academic Press, pp. 301–24.

Wing AM, Kristofferson AB (1973) The timing of interresponse intervals. Perception and Psychophysics 13: 455–60.

Wing AM, Keele SW, Margolin DI (1984) Motor disorder and the timing of repetitive movements. In J Gibbon, L Allan (eds), Timing and Time Perception. New York: New York Academy of Sciences, pp. 183–92.

Witkin HA, Wapner S (1950) Visual factors in the maintenance of upright posture. American Journal of Psychology 63: 31–50.

Wolpert DM, Miall RC, Kawato M (1998) Internal models in the cerebellum. Trends in Cognitive Sciences 2: 338–47.

Woolley SM, Rubin AM, Kantner RM et al. (1993) Differentiation of balance deficits through examination of selected components of static stabilometry. The Journal of Otolanryngology 22: 368–75.

World Health Organization (1980) International Classification of Impairments, Disabilities and Handicaps. A Manual of Classification Relating to the Consequences of Disease. Geneva: World Health Organization.

World Health Organization (1992a) International Statistical Classification of Diseases and Related Health Problems (10th edn) Vol. 1 ICD-10. Geneva: World Health Organization.

World Health Organization (1992b) Classification of Mental and Behavioural Disorders: Clinical Descriptions and Diagnostic Guidelines. Geneva: World Health Organization.

World Health Organization (1993) Classification of Mental and Behavioural Disorders – Diagnostic Criteria for Research. Geneva: World Health Organization.

World Health Organization (2001) International Classification of Functioning, Disability and Health (ICF). Geneva: World Health Organization.

Wright HC (1996) The identification, assessment and management of children with developmental coordination disorder. Unpublished doctoral thesis. University of Leeds.

Wright HC, Sugden DA (1996a) The nature of developmental coordination disorder: Inter- and intragroup differences. Adapted Physical Activity Quarterly 13: 357–71.

Wright HC, Sugden DA (1996b) A two-step procedure for the identification of children with developmental coordination disorder in Singapore. Developmental Medicine and Child Neurology 38: 1099–1105.

Wright HC, Sugden DA (1996c) The nature of developmental coordination disorder in children aged 6–9 years of age. Journal of Sports Sciences 14: 50–1.

Wright HC, Sugden DA (1998) A school based intervention programmes for children with developmental coordination disorder. European Journal of Physical Education, 3: 35–50.

Wright HC, Sugden DA, Ng R et al. (1994) Identification of children with movement problems in Singapore: usefulness of the Movement ABC Checklist. Adapted Physical Activity Quarterly 11: 150–7.

Wright-Strawderman C, Watson BL (1992) The prevalence of depressive symptoms in children with learning disabilities. Journal of Learning Disabilities 25: 258–64.

Yochman A, Parush S (1998) Differences in Hebrew handwriting skills between Israeli children in second and third grade. Physical and Occupational Therapy in Paediatrics 18: 53–65.

Zaichkowsky JD (1974) The development of perceptual motor sequencing ability. Journal of Motor Behavior 6: 255–61.

Ziviani J, Elkins J (1986) Effects of pencil grip on handwriting speed and legibility. Educational Review 38: 247–57.

Ziviani J, Watson-Will A (1998) Writing speed and legibility of 7–14-year-old school students using modern cursive script. Australian Occupational Therapy Journal 45: 59–64.

Zoia S, Pelamatti G, Cuttini M et al. (2002) Performance of gesture in children with and without DCD: effects of sensory input modalities. Developmental Medicine and Child Neurology 44: 699–705.

Index

Abecedarian Project (US) 163
academic achievement 16–17, 123–4
  ADL 19–22, 43–4
  assessment 148
  co-morbidity 99–103, 105–6, 107, 109,
    116, 250
  early identification 156, 163
  handwriting 170
  movement planning and organization
    52, 59
  nature of children 3–5, 7–9, 14, 16–17
  NTT 225–6
  progression 123–4, 126–9, 131, 134
accident-proneness 130
accuracy 11–12, 20, 35–7, 131
  co-morbidity 96, 101, 106
  NTT 218, 220–1, 222
action systems 49
activities of daily living (ADL) 16–17,
  39–46
  assessment 148
  co-morbidity 33, 45, 244
  CO-OP 228–9, 231
  early identification 156, 159, 160, 161
  eco-developmental approach 204,
    210–11
  handwriting 21, 25, 28, 30, 31, 37–8,
    40–6, 170
  movement planning and organization
    29, 31, 47, 52, 59, 62
  nature of children 3, 6–8, 16–17
  NTT 217, 219–21, 224
  progression 119, 128, 129, 131
acuity 12, 27–8, 38–9, 67, 68, 97
adaptability 92

adolescence 6, 17, 28, 121–3, 126,
  133–4
  balance and posture 31
  co-morbidity 95, 103, 109, 254, 259,
    263–4
  progression 119–20, 121–3, 126, 129,
    131, 133–4
aetiology 6, 14, 16, 21, 127, 136
  causal modelling framework 71
  co-morbidity 95–6, 107, 113, 116–17
  CO-OP 229
  DS 90, 89–90
  NTT 214
affective disorders 109
affordances 73–4, 92
age 1–2, 6–7, 17
  ADL 20–2, 27–36, 38, 39, 40–3, 45–6
  assessment 136, 139–47, 149, 151
  co-morbidity 96, 99–103, 105–6, 107,
    109–12
  co-morbidity and management 243,
    245, 253–4, 256, 260, 263
  CO-OP 232
  DS 88, 90
  early identification 155, 159–67
  eco-developmental approach 191, 196,
    206
  handwriting 169–71, 173, 178, 180–2,
    184
  movement planning and organization
    47, 50–1, 53, 55–7, 60, 62, 67
  NTT 224, 226
  progression 119–20, 121–33
agnosia 4
aiming tasks 56–7

Alberta Infant Motor Scale (AIMS) 165
alignment of letters 170, 180
All About Me Scale (AAMS) 153
American Psychiatric Association (APA) 3, 5–7, 15, 49
anticipation 11–12, 57, 60, 66
anxiety 103, 109, 129, 190, 254, 264
apraxia 4, 18, 42, 52–4
  co-morbidity 96, 98
art 123
ASK-KIDS inventory 153
Asperger's Syndrome (AS) 99–100, 104, 108, 111–12, 114, 243, 260
  handwriting 188
assessment 135–54, 156–61, 257–9
  co-morbidity 137, 245, 247–8, 251–9, 261–4
  DS 87
  early identification 155–67
  eco-developmental approach 194–6, 206–8, 210–11
  handwriting 148, 168–88
  nature of children 1–2, 4, 8–9, 15–16
  NTT 214–15, 224–5, 227
  Touwen's 127
attention 1, 14, 31–3, 98, 104–6
  ADL 20, 26, 31–3, 34–5, 37, 39
  co-morbidity 94, 98–101, 104–8, 110, 115, 243, 250, 251
  CO-OP 236, 241
  DS 72, 77
  eco-developmental approach 191
  handwriting 172
  NTT 215, 216
  progression 120, 127, 128, 131
attention deficit disorder (ADD) 2, 72, 117
attention deficit hyperactivity disorder (ADHD) 13
  ADL 33, 45
  co-morbidity 33, 94, 97–103, 104–6, 111, 114–15, 131–2
  co-morbidity and management 244, 246, 252–6, 258, 260, 262, 264
  DS 77
  early identification 165
  handwriting 172, 188
  NTT 225
  progression 127, 128, 131–2

atypical brain development 3, 14, 95, 118, 244
Australian Schools Fitness Test 148
autistic spectrum disorder (ASD) 108, 115, 117, 196
  co-morbidity and management 246, 259
AXIS I disorder 111
AXIS II disorder 100

balance 2, 30–1
  ADL 20, 26, 30–1, 38, 43, 45
  assessment 137, 140, 143, 145–6, 153
  co-morbidity 96–7, 246–51
  CO-OP 240–1
  DS 82, 87–8, 90
  dynamic 97, 131, 140, 246–50
  early identification 158
  progression 121–2, 128–9, 131, 133–4
  static 97, 131, 140, 143, 246–50
ball skills 1–2, 6, 10, 72, 173
  ADL 20, 23, 27, 29, 42–3
  assessment 137, 140, 142–6, 150, 153
  co-morbidity 96–7, 112, 246–50, 257
  early identification 159
  eco-developmental approach 191, 192, 202
  movement planning and organization 59, 66
  NTT 215, 216, 220, 226
  progression 121, 122–3, 131, 133–4
basal ganglia 34, 73, 77, 87
Bayley Scale of Infant Development 256
beads 1, 101, 121
Beery–Buktenka Developmental Test of Visual Motor Integration (VMI) 157–8
behaviour 14, 109–11, 123–4
  ADL 20, 24, 40, 43
  assessment 150
  co-morbidity 93–5, 98–106, 108–13, 115–16, 118
  co-morbidity and management 249–51, 253
  CO-OP 230, 232
  DS 72, 74–5, 78–9, 81–2, 84–5, 92
  early identification 160
  eco-developmental approach 198, 199
  handwriting 172
  movement planning and organization 71

nature of children 2–4, 6, 8–9, 13–16
NTT 219–20, 222, 225
progression 120, 123–4, 125–9, 134
Bender–Gestalt designs 129
benign congenital hypotonicity 116
Bernstein's problem 75
bicycles 30, 42–5, 139
    CO-OP 228, 231, 240
    early identification 159, 161
bipolar disorder 110
Birleson Depression Inventory 110
BMAT-R 144, 150
Bronfenbrenner model 197, 203
Bruininks–Oseretsky Test (BOT) 77
Bruininks–Oseretski Test of Motor
    Proficiency (BOTMP) 100
    assessment 138, 140, 149
    early identification 157, 159
brushing teeth 40
buttons and fastenings 6, 43, 56, 58,
    101, 200

Canadian Manitoba Fitness Test 148
catching 2, 10, 72, 121, 173, 250
    ADL 23, 27, 29
    assessment 137, 142, 145–6, 153
    early identification 159
    eco-developmental approach 191, 192,
    202
    movement planning and organization
    59, 66
    NTT 216, 220
central (endogenous) cues 33
central nervous system (CNS) 47, 48, 58,
    109
    DS 75, 79, 81
cerebellum 5, 34, 107, 115
    DS 73, 77, 87
    timing 59, 62–3
cerebral palsy 2, 7–8, 18, 49, 119, 165
    co-morbidity 95, 97, 116, 251
Child Behavior Checklist 33
Children's Trusts 254
choreiform dyskinesia 7, 103
Clinical Observation of Motor and
    Postural Skills
    (COMPS) 140
closed-loop control 36, 48
clumsiness 4–7, 9–10, 14, 128–30

ADL 21, 28–9, 31, 32, 37, 38, 42–3, 45
    assessment 143, 148, 149, 152
    co-morbidity 96, 99, 105, 108, 109, 114
    co-morbidity and management 243
    DS 77, 87, 91
    eco-developmental approach 195
    handwriting 172
    movement planning and organization
    52, 69
    progression 119–24, 126–30, 132–3
cognition and cognitive function 11–12,
    15, 55–70
    ADL 20, 26, 28, 34, 37
    co-morbidity 96, 113, 115, 117, 262–3
    CO-OP 228–41
    DS 74, 78, 81, 85, 92
    early identification 161, 162
    eco-developmental approach 190–1,
    193, 194, 198, 202, 204
    handwriting 170, 175, 176
    movement planning and organization
    47–71
    NTT 213, 217, 221
    progression 126, 132
Cognitive Orientation to Daily
    Occupational Performance (CO-OP)
    45, 193, 213, 228–41, 263
coincidence timing tasks 57
College of Occupational Therapists
    252–3
combing hair 53–4
co-morbidity (overlapping conditions)
    93–118, 242–65
    ADHD 33, 94, 97–103, 104–6, 111,
    114–15, 131–2
    ADHD and management 244, 246,
    252–6, 258, 260, 262, 264
    ADL 33, 45, 244
    assessment 137, 245, 247–8, 251–9,
    261–4
    DS 72, 77, 78, 92
    dyslexia 94–5, 98, 111–12, 115, 131–2,
    244, 247
    emotional problems 95, 99–106,
    109–11, 118, 247, 251
    management 242–65
    nature of children 3, 8, 14
    NTT 213–14, 222, 225
    PDD 94, 108–9, 111–12, 117

premature birth 112–14, 116, 118, 247
progression 120, 128, 131, 132, 134
reading and writing 94, 99–103, 107,
    111, 243, 246
social impairment 95, 98–105, 108–9,
    111–12, 114, 117–18
specific language impairment 94,
    98–108, 106, 111–12, 114–15, 117
computers 2, 44, 248, 249
    handwriting 168, 185, 188
concentration 2, 129, 131
    co-morbidity 105, 247, 249, 250, 251
conceptual system 49
Concise Assessment Method for
    Children's Handwriting (BHK) 180–1,
    226, 227
confidence 16, 152, 153, 253, 263
Congenital Mirrored Movements 116
Conner's Rating Scale 256
constraints 24–5
copying 9, 50, 91, 122, 140, 176
    ADL 27, 31, 43
    co-morbidity 93, 243
    handwriting 171, 176–7, 178, 182,
        183, 187
    movement planning and organization
        50, 52
crawling 6, 21, 40, 162
    co-morbidity 247, 249, 250
culture 24, 38, 40, 135, 204

dancing 25
decision-making 11–12
deficits in attention, motor control and
    perception (DAMP) 3, 33, 127
    co-morbidity 99–101, 104, 105–6, 109,
        110, 243
degrees of freedom 23–4, 36, 74–5, 137,
    198
depression 103, 109, 110–11, 264
depth perception 29
developmental coach 204–5, 210, 211
Developmental Coordination Disorder
    Questionnaire (DCDQ) 136, 145, 149,
    159
developmental pathways 132–3, 134,
    142, 166
Developmental Test of Visual Perception
    (DTVP) 29, 90

Developmental Test of Visuo-Motor
    Integration (VMI) 123
diagnosis 6–8
    assessment 136, 148
    co-morbidity 94, 96–8, 100, 104–5,
        108, 113, 116–18
    co-morbidity and management 243–4,
        246–7, 249–50, 253, 255–7, 264
    CO-OP 232
    DAMP 33
    DS 72–4, 77, 83, 86, 92
    early identification 158, 161, 164, 167
    handwriting 170, 172, 186
    movement planning and organization
        49, 56
    nature of children 2–3, 6–8, 12, 14–15
    NTT 213–14, 224, 227
    progression 120–1, 125–31
distance perception 63, 64
domain specific strategies (DSS) 235–6,
    237, 238
doubling classes 21–2, 44
drawing 9, 51, 132
    ADL 27, 29, 42–3
    assessment 148, 150, 152
    handwriting 186, 187
    mirror 27
    movement planning and organization
        51, 52, 56, 58, 65
dressing 1, 6, 40, 42–3, 44, 155
    assessment 148, 150
    movement planning and organization
        47, 52
driving a car 131–2
dropping things 1, 6–7, 21
DSM-III 94, 109
DSM-IV (Diagnostic Statistical Manual –
    Fourth Revision) 6–8, 21–2
    ADL 21–2, 39–41, 46
    assessment 148
    co-morbidity 94, 100, 108–9, 117, 244,
        246
    Criterion A 6–7, 21–2, 39–41, 46
    Criterion B 7, 16, 21–2, 40–1, 46
    Criterion C 7, 17, 108, 117, 158
    Criterion D 7, 17, 117
    early identification 158
    handwriting 170, 187
    movement planning and organisation 49

nature of children 2–3, 5–8, 14–18
NTT 213, 227
progression 120, 125, 127, 128
dynamic performance analysis (DPA)
234–5, 237
dynamic systems (DS) 8, 48, 72–92, 162
CO-OP 229, 241
eco-developmental approach 197–9,
203–4
dyscalculia 95
Dyscovery Centre 246–51, 252
Dyscovery Model of Practice 262
Dyscovery Trust 261
dysdiadochokinesis 121
dysgraphaesthesia 121
dysgraphia 95, 118, 187, 226
dyskinaesthesia 28
dyskinesia 158
dyslexia 2, 13, 111–12
co-morbidity 94–5, 98, 111–12, 115,
131–2, 244, 247
handwriting 172, 188
dyspraxia 42, 52–5, 120, 137, 203
co-morbidity 95, 115, 243–6, 261, 263
developmental 52, 55
nature of children 5–7, 18
Dyspraxia Foundation 6, 120, 261

Early Years Movement Skills Checklist
167, 256
eating 72, 130, 148, 155, 187
ADL 40, 42–5
movement planning and organization
47, 52, 62
eco-developmental approach 189–211
ecological approach 81–3, 161, 238, 258
DS 78–83, 85–6, 88, 91–2
Edinburgh Handedness Inventory 20
educational psychologists 4, 186
co-morbidity 245–7, 263
electromyographs 81
emotional difficulties 92, 109–11, 133–4
co-morbidity 95, 99–106, 109–11, 118,
247, 251
employment 119, 123, 131, 134
environment 16
ADL 19, 23–5, 29, 32, 39–40
assessment 137, 144, 154, 259
co-morbidity 97, 259, 261

CO-OP 230, 235, 237
DS 74–5, 78–9, 81–5, 86, 89, 92
early identification 162–3, 166
eco-developmental approach 193, 196,
198–9, 203–4, 211
movement planning and organization
47–8, 66, 71
NTT 215, 218–19
epilepsy 246
Erhlos Dahnlo syndrome 116
errors 12, 35, 57, 130, 193, 240
DS 80, 83, 90
NTT 218, 222
Evaluation Tool of Children's
Handwriting (ETCH) 173, 180
examinations 169, 188
Expert Patient programme 259
expert scaffolding 202

feedback 11–12, 36–7, 91, 201, 207,
222–3
ADL 26, 29, 35, 36–7, 38, 39
movement planning and organization
48, 66
NTT 217, 218, 222–3, 224
fine motor skills 7, 13, 44, 70, 192
assessment 139, 140, 142, 149, 153
co-morbidity 96–7, 102–3, 106, 116,
243, 246–7, 250–1
early identification 158–60, 166
handwriting 175, 184, 186–7
NTT 216, 224–5, 226–7
progression 122, 127, 128, 131, 132
Fine Motor Performance Test 224–5
fitness assessment 147–8, 154
fluency 20, 35–6, 169–70, 178, 183,
185–6
following instructions 247, 248, 250
force 60–2, 76–80
free writing 50, 176–7, 182
Frostig's milestone test battery 29
Functional Independence Measure for
Children (WeeFIM) 40

gender 117, 126, 141–2
ADL 22
assessment 141–2, 143, 145, 153
co-morbidity 96, 103, 109–10, 116,
117, 247–9

DS 90
  handwriting 178, 180, 182
  movement planning and organization
    60
  NTT 226
  progression 126, 127, 131, 133
General Motor Performance Test 224–5
general practitioners (GPs) 18, 189, 210
  co-morbidity 243, 252, 255–6, 261–2
  NTT 213, 226
General Practitioners with Special
  Interests (GPwSI) 256
generalization 230–1, 233, 235, 237
Gerstmann's syndrome 119
gestures 18, 42, 52, 53–5, 122
  co-morbidity 96, 106, 107, 112,
    114–15
  intransitive 53–4, 96
  transitive 53–4, 96
GOAL-PLAN-DO-CHECK strategy 235,
  237–8
graphic tablets 185–6
Griffiths Mental Development Scales 256
grip 60–2, 72, 122, 183–5, 202
  assessment 140, 145
  handwriting 183–5, 186
  motor effector system 34
Groningen Motor Observation (GMO)
  20, 22
Groningen Perinatal Project 125
gross motor skills 7, 13, 44, 70, 192
  assessment 136, 139–40, 142, 145–6,
    149–50, 153
  co-morbidity 96–7, 102, 243, 250–1
  early identification 158–60, 165–6
  NTT 225, 226–7
  progression 122, 131
Gubbay's Test 157
guided discovery 234, 236–7
gyms and gymnastics 1, 44, 47

handedness see laterality
handwriting 50, 107, 168–88
  ADL 21, 25, 28, 30, 31, 37–8, 40–6,
    170
  assessment 148, 168–88
  co-morbidity 106, 107, 243, 248–9,
    257, 264
  CO-OP 228, 231

early identification 155, 157, 159, 161
eco-developmental approach 192
movement planning and organization
  47, 50, 52, 168–70
nature of children 1–2, 6–7, 9, 11, 17
NTT 226–7
progression 123, 131
script styles 173–4, 179–81, 183,
  185–6
haptic perception 30, 75, 91–2
Harter's Perceived Competence Scale for
  Children 123–4
Harter's Self-Perception Profile for
  Children 109, 112, 152
health visitors 255, 256, 262
heterogeneity
  co-morbidity 97, 246, 262
  early identification 156, 167
  eco-developmental approach 189
  nature of children 3, 12, 15–16
  NTT 213–14, 224
holistic approach 87, 180, 251, 254
hopping 43, 47, 137, 145, 146
hyperkinesis 105, 129
hypothyroidism 62

ICD-10 (International Classification of
  Diseases and Related Health
  Problems) 40, 77, 94, 187
  nature of children 6–8, 14–15, 17–18
imitation 24, 122, 203
  co-morbidity 112, 115
  CO-OP 240, 241
  movement planning and organization
    53–5, 64
information processing (IP) 9–12, 114,
  197–8
  ADL 24, 28, 29, 34–5
  DS 73–6, 78–81, 86–7, 89
  movement planning and organization
    48, 63–6
  NTT 216, 217
intelligence 1–4, 6–8, 18, 21–2, 88, 139
  co-morbidity 93, 101, 117
  handwriting 186, 187
  progression 124, 129
International Classification of
  Functioning, Disability and Health
  (ICF) 159–60, 161, 230–1

jumping 1, 43, 47, 153
  from standing 140, 142, 145, 146

kicking 47
Kinaesthetic Acuity Test (KAT) 27–8, 67,
  68
Kinaesthetic Perception and Memory
  Test 32, 67
Kinaesthetic Sensitivity Test (KST) 67
kinaesthetics and kinaesthetic
  perception 27–8, 65–9, 122, 212
  ADL 26–30, 32, 35, 36–7, 38–9
  co-morbidity 97, 114, 263
  DS 89–90
  eco-developmental approach 191, 192
  movement planning and organization
    63–70
  nature of children 10–13
kinematic techniques 82
kinesiology 84
knitting 20, 21

latencies 56–7
laterality (handedness) 20, 129
  co-morbidity 96, 101
  handwriting 182, 184–5
learning difficulties 3, 13, 17, 28, 38
  assessment 135, 136, 137, 138
  co-morbidity 93–5, 97–8, 103, 105,
    107, 109, 112–14, 116–18
  co-morbidity and management 243,
    246
  movement planning and organization
    54
  NTT 225, 227
  progression 119–20, 125
  SIT 212
legibility 1–2, 37, 170, 175–86, 188, 248
lesions 4, 18, 113, 114
letter formation 2, 170, 178–83, 185–6
literacy 93, 107, 115, 175, 179, 187
  see also handwriting; reading
low birth weight 8, 125–6, 163
  co-morbidity 93, 95, 113, 116

manual dexterity and manipulation skills
  1–2
  ADL 20, 45
  assessment 140, 143, 145, 150, 153

co-morbidity 97, 114, 246–51
early identification 158
eco-developmental approach 194, 200
handwriting 186
NTT 226
progression 131, 134
mathematics 93–4, 131, 249
maturational theory 48
McCarron Assessment of Neuromuscular
  Development (MAND) 145–6, 157
  assessment 136, 138–40, 142, 143–4,
    145–6, 150, 152
Meichenbaum's global problem-solving
  strategy 232
memory 12, 31–3
  ADL 26, 31–3, 34, 39
  DS 91
  eco-developmental approach 191
  handwriting 176–7
  movement planning and organization
    57, 64–5, 67–8
  NTT 215
mental retardation 8, 18, 84
metacognition 235, 238, 240
milestones 6, 9, 44
  ADL 19, 21, 29, 40, 43–4
minimal brain damage or dysfunction
  (MBD) 127–8
  co-morbidity 93–4, 99, 101–2, 105–6,
    116, 118, 244
  progression 125, 127–8, 129
minor neurological dysfunction (MND)
  125–6
  co-morbidity 103, 117
  progression 125–6, 128
motivation 14, 16, 223–4
  ADL 20, 38
  co-morbidity 110–11, 252
  CO-OP 234, 238
  early identification 162
  eco-developmental approach 198–9,
    211
  handwriting 175
  NTT 214, 215, 218, 222–4
  progression 124, 132, 133
motor effector system 26, 33–4, 52, 65
motor imagery training 195
motor learning 24, 37–8, 114–15,
  199–208, 214–21

ADL 24, 26, 36, 37–8, 42
co-morbidity 93, 96, 98, 114–15
CO-OP 214–17, 229–33, 235, 237–8, 240–1
eco-developmental approach 190, 193, 199–208, 210
explicit 217, 223
implicit 217
NTT 213–25
phases 202, 217–18, 220, 222–3, 225, 238
motor-perceptual dysfunction (MPD) 127, 129
motor programming 11–12, 34–5, 56, 194, 245
assessment 135, 138–9
movement planning and organization 47–8, 56, 59, 68
NTT 215, 217, 224
motor skills and control 35–8, 41, 114–15, 121–3, 162–6, 168–70, 196–208, 214–17
ADL 19–46
adolescence 121–3, 126, 133–4
assessment 135–54
checklists and questionnaires 148–53
clumsiness 128–30
co-morbidity 93–118, 247, 250, 256
contextuality 220–1
CO-OP 229–38, 240–1
DS 72–6, 78, 80–1, 83–6, 89
early identification 155–67
eco-developmental approach 189–211
handwriting 168–70, 172, 175, 184–5
nature of children 1–18
NTT 212–27
planning and organization 47, 52, 56, 58–9, 64, 70
progression 119–34
tests 143–6
timing 56, 58–9
transfer 219–20, 222
young adults 129–30
Motor Standard 140
motor teaching theory 214–17, 221–5
Movement Assessment Battery for Children (ABC) 143–4, 153, 208–9, 246–50
ADL 30, 31, 36, 41, 45

assessment 136, 138–40, 142, 143–5, 149, 150, 153
Checklist 97
co-morbidity 97, 99–103, 106, 246–50, 256
DS 72, 88
early identification 157, 159
eco-developmental approach 193, 206–9, 210
handwriting 187
nature of children 1–2, 12–13, 15–17
NTT 226, 227
progression 126, 130, 133–4
Movement Confidence Model 153
movement preparation 34–5
ADL 26, 34–5, 36, 39
movement stability 165–6
movement variability 165–6
muscles
ADL 22–4, 27, 30–1, 33–4, 37, 39
co-morbidity 243
DS 75, 81
early identification 157, 160, 162, 165
eco-developmental approach 198
movement planning and organization 48–9, 66, 68
NTT 215, 219
music and musical instruments 20, 42–4, 47
myelination 24

neurological dysfunction 7, 17–18
assessment 138, 142, 145–6, 150
co-morbidity 93, 96, 103, 106, 109, 112–13, 116–18
co-morbidity and management 242–3, 256, 265
DS 73, 75, 76–80, 81, 86–7
early identification 158, 165
eco-developmental approach 200
NTT 213, 215
progression 120–1, 123, 125–9
timing 76–80
Neuromotor Task Training (NTT) 212–27
Neuronal Group Selection Theory (NGST) 219
nonverbal learning disabilities (NVLD) 114

obsessions 250
occupational therapy 4, 72
  assessment 151, 259
  co-morbidity 117, 245, 248, 251–4,
    259, 263
  CO-OP 230, 237
  early identification 157, 163
  eco-developmental approach 189, 191,
    205, 211
  SIT 212
open-loop control 35, 36–7, 47–8
oppositional defiant disorder (ODD)
  104–5
organization and organizational skills
  1–2, 8, 13, 47–71
  co-morbidity 248–9, 257
  DS 74–6, 78–9, 81, 86, 89, 91

parameterization 216
parents 148–50, 205–8
  ADL 20–2, 41, 43–5
  assessment 136, 145, 148–50, 154,
    257–9
  co-morbidity 94, 97, 105, 111, 113
  co-morbidity and management 243–5,
    247–51, 253–5, 257–62, 264
  CO-OP 229, 231, 233, 234, 237
  DS 72
  early identification 155–6, 158–64
  eco-developmental approach 189, 196,
    201–8, 210–11
  handwriting 170, 172, 186
  movement planning and organization
    52
  nature of children 1–2, 4, 6, 14, 17–18
  NTT 214, 225, 226
  partnership working 259–62
  progression 119–20, 122, 126, 132
Parkinson's disease 57
partnership working 259–62
Pediatric Evaluation of Development
  Inventory (PEDI) 40, 160–1
pegboards 101, 122, 142
perception
  co-morbidity 96–101, 104, 109–11,
    116
  DS 77, 79, 85, 89–92
  eco-developmental approach 192, 198,
    200

  handwriting 186
  NTT 216
  progression 127
  see also self–perception
perception–action system 77, 79, 85, 92
perceptual–motor function 5, 27–39,
  63–70
  ADL 19, 24–6, 27–39, 42, 46
  assessment 137
  co-morbidity 93, 97, 99–101, 104–6,
    108–10, 113
  CO-OP 229
  DS 78
  eco-developmental approach 191, 195
  handwriting 169, 172, 173, 175, 186,
    188
  movement planning and organization
    49, 57, 63–70
  NTT 213–14
  progression 127
periodicity 75, 83–6, 92
peripheral (exogenous) cues 33
persistence 13, 133
personality 128, 130, 225
pervasive developmental disorder (PDD)
  2, 7, 111–12, 225
  co-morbidity 94, 108–9, 111–12, 117
  early identification 158
phases of learning 202, 217–18, 220,
  222–3, 225, 238
physical education (PE) and exercise 40,
  42, 126, 136, 148
  see also sport
physical therapists 72, 151
  CO-OP 229, 233, 234–8, 240
  early identification 157, 161, 163, 164
  NTT 213, 215, 223–4, 226–7
  SIT 212
physiotherapy 4, 20
  co-morbidity and management 245–6,
    247, 251, 253–4, 263
  eco-developmental 189, 191, 211
Pictorial Scale of Perceived Competence
  and Social Acceptance (PCSA) 160–1
planning 47–71
  ADL 29, 31, 47, 52, 59, 62
  assessment 137
  co-morbidity 96, 97–8, 114–15
  CO-OP 235, 237

early identification 159
eco-developmental approach 191, 198, 203
handwriting 47, 50, 52, 168–70
microscopic 59–63
nature of children 8, 11, 13, 16
NTT 215, 216
play and playgrounds 1–2, 17, 84–5, 132–3, 169
ADL 19, 21, 40, 42–3
assessment 136, 139, 147, 148, 153, 257
early identification 155–6, 160
pointing 10, 25, 27–8, 68, 90
positron emission tomography (PET) 115
posture 30–1, 183–5
ADL 23, 27, 30–1, 38, 45
assessment 140
co-morbidity 103
CO-OP 236, 240
DS 82, 84, 85–6, 87–8
early identification 158, 160
handwriting 183–5
movement planning and organization 47, 68, 70
NTT 215
progression 133
practice 214, 217–20, 222–4, 226, 238, 240–1
Prechtl's optimality concept technique 125
pregnancy 84, 116
premature birth 8, 112–13
assessment 139–40
co-morbidity 112–14, 116, 118, 247
early identification 158, 163, 165
progression 125–6
Printing Performance School Readiness Test (PPRT) 180, 181
problem solving 80–1, 201
CO-OP 213, 230–2, 235–7
proprioception 10–11, 88, 90, 191
ADL 27, 29, 32, 36–7
movement planning and organization 48, 65–6, 68–9
psychiatry 128–9
co-morbidity 93–4, 105, 109, 118, 255
psychology 3–4, 15, 186, 196, 216
co-morbidity 98, 109, 243, 245–7, 253, 254, 259, 263

CO-OP 230
DS 75, 81, 85, 92
psycho-social problems 135, 151–2, 156, 164, 259
punctuation 176

reaction time 12, 34–5, 56–9, 68, 75–6
reading 1–2, 17, 107, 131
ADL 20, 44
co-morbidity 94, 99–103, 107, 111, 243, 246
eco-developmental approach 192
handwriting 172, 186, 187
reductionism 190
reflexes 19, 61, 96, 103
reflex-hierarchical model 229
remedial teaching 21–2
repetition 240
Resilience Theory 111
research 76–80, 88–92, 231–3
ADL 20, 21, 41
assessment 137–9, 141–2, 143–5, 147, 149–50, 152, 153–4
co-morbidity 94, 97, 98, 106, 108, 109–11, 112, 114
co-morbidity and management 242, 261, 262, 264, 265
CO-OP 228, 230, 231–3, 238, 240–1
DS 72–4, 76–80, 84, 86, 88–92
early identification 158, 160, 163, 165
eco-developmental approach 189–91, 194–6, 198–9, 201, 205–6, 210–11
handwriting 82, 184
movement planning and organization 56, 63, 65, 68, 70
nature of children 4–6, 9–10, 15–18
NTT 213–14, 216–17, 219–20, 221, 227
progression 120–1, 127, 130, 134
response selection 56–8
rhyming 187
rhythmicity 75–6, 83–4, 86–7
rotary pursuit tasks 11
running 1–2, 23, 43, 47, 83, 159
assessment 137, 145, 146, 150

Schedule of Growing Skills 256
schizoid disorder 110
Schmidt's Schema Theory of Motor Learning 194, 200, 221

schools 1–2, 4, 9, 13, 15, 18
  ADL 20–2, 40, 42–5
  assessment 140–1, 149–51, 153
  co-morbidity 93, 97, 100–1, 103,
    108–9, 112
  co-morbidity and management 242,
    244–5, 247–54, 256–7, 260–5
  early identification 155–6, 162, 163,
    165–7
  eco-developmental approach 189, 195,
    196–7, 206, 211
  handwriting 168–70, 172–3, 175–6,
    178, 184, 186–7
  movement planning and organization
    47
  NTT 213, 225, 226–7
  partnership working 260–2
  progression 122, 123, 129
  support staff 97, 260
  see also teachers
scissors and cutting 53–4, 72, 173, 187,
  231, 249
  ADL 20, 25, 44, 45
  early identification 155, 159, 162
screening 255–7
  co-morbidity 245, 255–7, 265
  early identification 156, 158, 159,
    162–4, 166
  handwriting 173, 176, 178, 180
self-concept 14, 16, 101
self-esteem 15, 124, 152, 192
  causal modelling framework 71
  co-morbidity 109, 117, 247–9, 251,
    253–4, 263
  CO-OP 228
  handwriting 170
self-organization 74–6, 78, 81, 89, 91
self-perception 109–10, 112, 223–4
  assessment 136, 145, 148, 151–2, 153
self-report 131, 151–3, 225
  assessment 136, 148, 151–3
self-worth 103, 109, 111, 124, 250–1,
  254
sensitivity 12, 92, 141
sensorimotor (sensory motor) system 22–6
  ADL 19, 20–1, 22–6
  assessment 137
  early identification 158
  eco-developmental approach 191–2

movement planning and organization
    49, 54
  progression 126
Sensory Integration Therapy (SIT)
    191–2, 194, 212, 219
  co-morbidity 245, 263
  Southern California 106, 127, 157
sequences and sequencing 47, 53–5,
    193, 203, 216
  co-morbidity 107, 115
  CO-OP 236
  DS 78–80, 91
  timing 58, 63
shape 90, 91, 157, 187
shoelaces 6, 43–5, 130
  CO-OP 228, 231
sitting 6, 21, 40, 186
skipping 43
social skills and sociability 108–9, 123–4
  ADL 19, 20, 40
  assessment 135, 137, 139, 148, 151–2
  co-morbidity 95, 98–105, 108–9,
    111–12, 114, 117–18
  co-morbidity and management 250–1,
    259, 263
  CO-OP 228
  DS 92
  early identification 156, 160–1, 164
  handwriting 169–70, 172
  nature of children 1, 15
  NTT 213
  progression 119, 123–4, 131, 133
socio-economics 116, 124, 162–3, 259
soft neurological signs 96–7, 121, 129
somato-sensory perception 30, 52
Southern California Sensory Integration
  Tests (SCSIT) 106, 127, 157
spacing of letters 170, 180–1, 183
spatial perception 90, 122, 186
  ADL 29, 32–3, 39
  movement planning and organization
    63–5, 70
  see also visuospatial perception
special educational needs (SEN) 189,
  210, 252
  partnership working 259–62
  statements 243, 255, 261
Specific Developmental Disorder of
  Motor Dysfunction 7

Specific Developmental Disorder of
   Motor Function (SDDMF) 94, 99, 111
specificity and motor abilities hypothesis
   219
speech 40, 42–3, 129
   co-morbidity 93, 114, 243, 248
   handwriting 169, 172, 186
speech and (specific) language impairment (SLI) 106–12
   co-morbidity 94, 98–103, 106, 111–12,
      114–15, 117
   co-morbidity and management
      247–51, 253, 256
   handwriting 172, 186
   movement planning and organization
      54
   progression 125–6
speech and language therapy 161–2,
   246–8, 251, 253, 263
speed 20, 35–6, 48, 181–3
   co-morbidity 96, 101, 257
   early identification 159
   handwriting 11, 168–71, 173, 175–8,
      181–4, 188
   NTT 218, 220, 222, 227
spelling 94, 99, 107, 176–7
sport 4, 7, 9, 224
   ADL 19, 21, 42–4
   assessment 147, 148–50, 152–3
   co-morbidity 109–10, 111
   co-morbidity and management 244,
      248–50, 257, 264–5
   early identification 159
   eco-developmental approach 199
   progression 119, 124, 133
   see also physical education (PE) and
      exercise
STAIC 102
stairs 162
standing 142, 186
   and jumping 140, 142, 145, 146
Stay in Step 142, 145
strabismus 29
Strengths and Difficulties Questionnaire
   104–5
substance abuse 100, 128
suicide 100, 110
Sure Start 163
swaying 85–6, 87–8

swimming 40, 42, 44, 247, 250
systems analysis approach 25–6

Tactile Performance Test 90
tactile perception 10, 55, 90, 191, 212
   movement planning and organization
      48, 65, 69
tapping 56, 58–9, 61–2, 76, 86
teachers 149–51, 205–8
   ADL 20–2, 41, 45
   assessment 136, 147, 148, 149–51,
      154
   co-morbidity 97, 105, 111, 112–13
   co-morbidity and management 243–5,
      247, 251, 252, 261–2
   DS 72
   early identification 155, 167
   eco-developmental approach 189,
      193–4, 196, 201–2, 205–8, 210–11
   handwriting 169–70, 172, 173–4, 175,
      181, 186
   movement planning and organization
      56
   nature of children 1–2, 4, 17
   NTT 225, 226
   partnership working 261–2
   progression 119–20, 126
   see also schools
television and videos 2, 44, 250
Test of Gross Motor Development
   (TGMD) 72, 136, 139
Test of Gross Motor Development 2
   (TGMD–2) 146–7, 227
   assessment 142, 143, 146–7
Test of Legible Handwriting 181
Test of Motor Impairment (TOMI) 56,
   58, 91
   ADL 20, 21–2, 29, 31
   assessment 138, 142, 143–4
   co-morbidity 99, 101–2, 106
   progression 121–2, 123
Test of Motor Proficiency (TMP) 100,
   138, 140, 149
   early identification 157, 159
throwing 2, 47, 123, 159, 250
   assessment 142, 146
   NTT 216, 220–1
timing 58–9, 76–80, 107, 122, 216
   ADL 20, 23, 34

assessment 137, 144
DS 76–80, 86–7
movement planning and organization
56–7, 58–9, 61–3, 66
Touwen's neurological assessments 103,
127
tracing 65
tracking 11, 33, 36–7
transfer of learning 219–20
CO-OP 230, 231, 233, 235, 237
typical treatment approach (TTA) 233
typing 20–1, 43

Ulrich's object control category 144

verbal instructions 53–5, 221–2, 247
vebalization 236, 238
vestibular perception 29, 30, 65, 70,
191, 212
Vineland Adaptive Behavior Scales
(VABS) 41, 160
vision and visual perception 10–13, 17,
29–30, 63–5, 87–8
ADL 23, 26–7, 29–30, 32–7, 38–9
assessment 137
co-morbidity 97, 114–15, 118, 243,
247–8, 256
DS 79, 87–8, 90–2
early identification 157–8
eco-developmental approach 191
handwriting 168
movement planning and organization
48, 55, 63–5, 67–70
progression 122
screening 256
SIT 212

Visual Motor Integration (VMI) 123, 140,
157–8, 187
Visual Motor Integration Supplemental
Developmental Test of Motor
Coordination (MC) 157–8
Visual Motor Integration Supplemental
Developmental Test of Visual
Perception (VP) 157–8
visuospatial perception 16, 18, 157, 200,
214
co-morbidity 96, 114, 118
DS 89–91
movement planning and organization
63–5, 70

WAIS 129
walking 6, 21, 29, 30, 40, 44
assessment 140, 153
co-morbidity 247–50
delay and handwriting 186
DS 72, 81–3
early identification 162, 165
eco-developmental approach 198–9
movement planning and organization
48, 52
washing 40
Wechsler Intelligence Scale for Children
15, 127
Wing–Kristofferson model 58–9
World Health Organization 6–7, 77, 230

Zaner–Bloser Evaluation Scales 181
Zurich Neuromotor Assessment (ZNA)
142